BLOOD CELL – AN OVERVIEW OF STUDIES IN HEMATOLOGY

Edited by **Terry E. Moschandreou**

Blood Cell – An Overview of Studies in Hematology
http://dx.doi.org/10.5772/2979
Edited by Terry E. Moschandreou

Contributors

Gökhan Cüce, Tahsin Murad Aktan, Mahmoud Rafea, Serhiy Souchelnytskyi, Filip Cristiana, Zamosteanu Nina, Albu Elena, Ambreen Shaikh, Deepa Bhartiya, Moneer Faraj, Nihaya Salem, Junko Takahashi, Akiko Takatsu, Masaki Misawa, Hitoshi Iwahashi, Osamu Hayashi, Karen A. Selz, Terry E. Moschandreou, Youngchan Kim, Kyoohyun Kim, YongKeun Park, Hisham Mohamed, A.B. Shrivastav, K.P. Singh, S. Druyan, Kikuji Yamashita, Clement E. Zeh, Collins O. Odhiambo, Lisa A. Mills, Nuri Mamak, İsmail Aytekin

Published by InTech

Janeza Trdine 9, 51000 Rijeka, Croatia

Publishing Process Manager Sandra Bakic
Technical Editor InTech Prepress, Novi Sad
Cover InTech Design team

Additional hard copies can be obtained from orders@intechopen.com

Blood Cell – An Overview of Studies in Hematology, Edited by Terry E. Moschandreou
p. cm.
ISBN 978-953-51-0753-8

For EU product safety concerns:
IN TECH d.o.o., Prolaz Marije Krucifikse Kozulić 3, 51000 Rijeka, Croatia,
info@intechopen.com or visit our website at intechopen.com.

Meet the editor

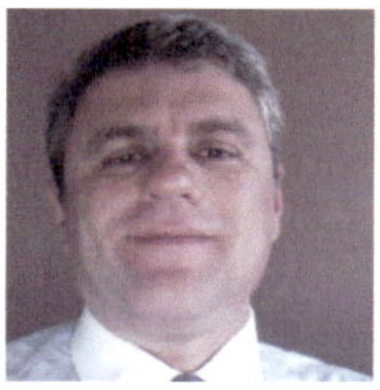

Dr Terry E. Moschandreou is a professor in applied mathematics and is currently working at the University of Western Ontario as a research associate in the department of medical biophysics. He also teaches at transport technology at Fanshawe College in London, Ontario Canada. He received his PhD in applied mathematics from the University of Western Ontario in 1996. The greater part of his professional life was spent at the University of Western Ontario and Fanshawe College in London, Ontario. For shorter times he worked at the National Technical University of Athens, Greece. Dr. Moschandreou is the author of several research articles in blood flow and oxygen transport in the microcirculation and general fluid dynamics. Also he has contributed in the field of finite element modelling of the upper airways in sleep apnea and surgical brain deformation modelling.

Contents

Preface

The editor has incorporated scientific contributions from a diverse group of leading researchers in the field of hematology and related blood cell research. This book aims to provide an overview of current knowledge pertaining to our understanding of hematology. The main subject areas will include blood cell morphology and function, the pathophysiology and genetics of hematological disorders and malignancies, blood testing and typing, and the processes governing hematopoiesis. Blood cell physiology, biochemistry and blood flow are covered in this book.

This text is designed for hematologists, pathologists and laboratory staff in training and in practice. Topics include platelets, whole blood RNA analysis, C-reactive protein, pluripotent stem cells, proliferation and differentiation of hematopoietic cells, homocysteine in red blood cells metabolism: pharmacological approaches, measurement techniques for red blood cells deformability, spontaneous alternation behaviour in human neutrophils, microfluidics technology for cell separation, effects of far infrared radiation on living body, laboratory reference intervals in Africa, RBC-ATP biochemistry and modelling, dynamics of RBC and antigens, transfusion principles, haematological and biochemical studies in tigers and ascites syndrome in broiler chickens.

The work presented in this book will be of benefit to medical students and to researchers of hematology and blood flow in the microcirculation. This book is written primarily for those who have some knowledge of chemistry, biochemistry and general hematology. The authors of each section bring a strong clinical emphasis to the book.

I am greatly indebted to many individuals who helped in the preparation of this book. Those whom I wish especially to thank for their help with this edition include Drs. Dan Goldman and Khoa Nguyen. I am also indebted to Dr. Jiandi Wan, who gave permission to use the referenced figure in the chapter contributed by the editor. I also would like to thank all those who took the time to email me offering helpful criticisms and suggestions. This includes Ms. Sandra Bakic, publishing process manager at InTech.

Dr. Terry E. Moschandreou
University of Western Ontario, Middlesex College,
London, Ontario,
Canada

Section 1

Main Concepts

Chapter 1

Platelets

Gökhan Cüce and Tahsin Murad Aktan

Additional information is available at the end of the chapter

http://dx.doi.org/10.5772/50969

1. Introduction

General information about platelets, origin of plateletes and granule contents of platelets were summarized.

2. Platelets

These cell fragments are morphologically small scale but functionally vital under life threatening conditions (1). They originate from megakaryocytes located mainly in the bone marrow, found in circulating blood and stored in spleen (2). Platelets don't contain a nuclei and during their inactive state they have a discoid morphology with a diameter of 2-4 micrometer (3, 4). But whenever they are active they can change their morphology very rapidly to an irregular branched spread form (5). Currently platelets are being used at wide spread clinic treatments from cosmetic needs to supporting insufficient heart (6, 7).

2.1. Development of Platelets

It is not exactly explained how platelets originate from megakaryocytes. There are several models to explain formation of platelets.

Megakaryocytes seem to locate as triple form. With their VEGF secretion capacity they hold vessel endothelial cells close to themselves (8). The most scientifically accepted three models are mentioned as,

1. Simply blebbing from the cell membrane of megakaryocytes (1).
2. In megakaryocytes there are special cell fields defined as "Demarcation Membrane System" where granules of platelets condense and fragments break away (9).
3. The most popular theory seems to be "Proplatelet Formation". Here megakaryocytes have long thin branch like extensions at the blood circulating site of blood vessels of

bone marrow and on these branches there are uprising small bodies where by the help of blood shear force platelets enter directly to circulating blood stream. It was suggested that the concept of platelet like bodies arise from pseudopods of Megakaryocytes, the forming platelets were named as "proplatelet" (10).

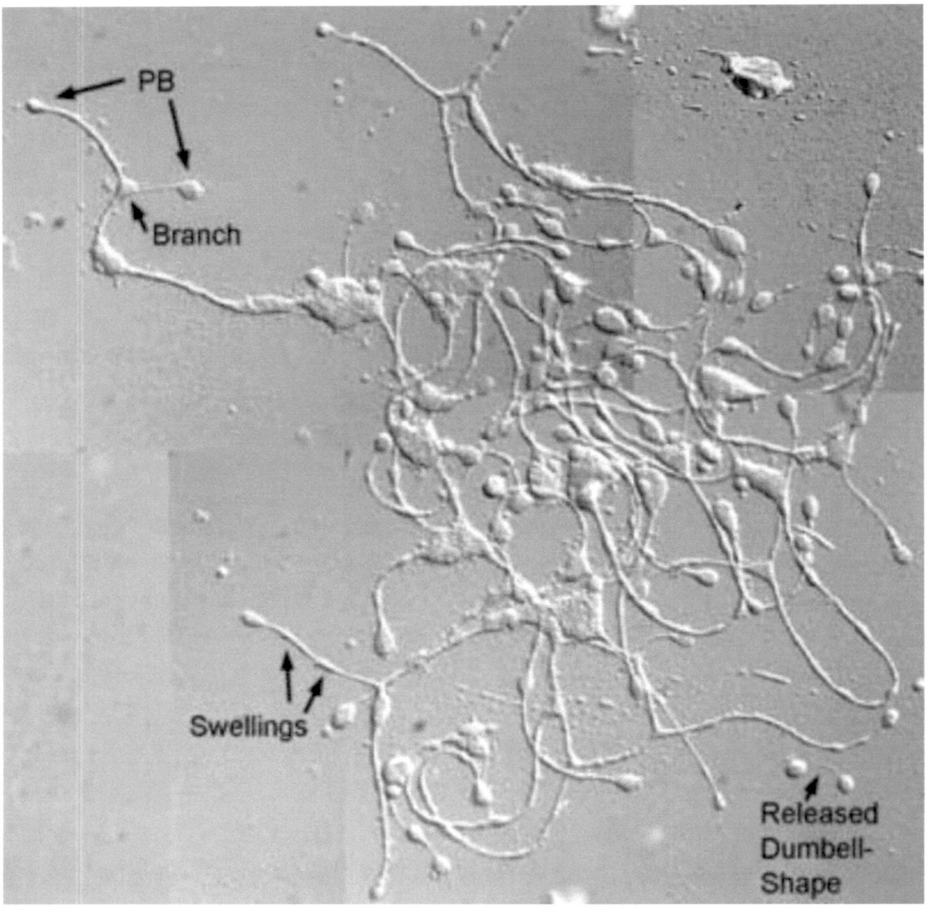

Figure 1. Megakaryocyte branches with Platelet Buds (PB) are seen. Proplatelets are released as Dumbell shaped bodies. This image is referenced from Hartwig and Italiano 2003 (Thanks for the kind permission of John Wiley and Sons to use this image) (11) .

Kinetics of platelets; they have a life span as 7-10 days and in 1 liter human blood it is estimated that there are 150-400X10^9 platelets so for a balanced number they are formed 15X10^9 -40X10^9 daily. Megakaryocytes located in the bone marrow sinusoids form a barrier to other bone marrow cells, it forms a physical barrier preventing direct contact to blood circulation. But there are canallicular openings in megakaryocyte membrane which permits cell migration to other cells to enter blood stream; this is named as "Emperipolesis" (8).

These small cell fragments have complex properties; 2 cytoplasmic regions can be seen in platelets

1. **Hyalomere:** The light blue homogeneous region of the peripheral cytoplasm is called Hyalomere. Hyalomere includes cytoplasmic filaments and circumferential microtubule bundle under the cell membrane. These elements of the cytoskeleton provide the movement and the protection of the platelets' shapes.
2. **Granulomere (Chromomere):** This is the central region and tight area. It is ranging in color from blue to purple-staining. Granulomere includes small Golgi complex, smooth endoplasmic reticulum, lysosome, scattered granules surrounded by a membrane and a variety of mitochondria (4).

Platelets have a simple appearance but carry very complex functional properties. By dividing this simple cell fragment to four regions helps for a better understanding of the functions of platelets.

1. Peripheral Zone:
   This region is composed from unit membrane with open canalicular system. Three parts are defined as;

a. Exterior outer layer:
   This is a glycocalix membrane with 10-20 nm thickness and thicker than the other blood cells, rich from glycoproteins that are mainly receptors for cell-cell and cell-vessel interactions(1, 8).

b. Platelet Unit Membrane:
   Platelet unit membrane has some similarities and appearance with other unit membranes of cells, it is composed from bilipid layer rich of phospholipids (12), it can distribute molecules according to phsico-chemical properties for passing the membrane. The membrane has anionic and cationic pumps. Platelet unit membrane is an important catalyst for liquid phase coagulation.

c. Submembrane Zone:
   Just located under the unit membrane a layer composed of microflament network. This network is anatomically and functionally related to membrane glycoproteins and cytoplasmic filament system.

2. Sol-Jel Zone:
   This is cytoplasm corresponding part of the cellular fragment, platelet. It is in soluble or gel phase according to changes of polymerization of the filaments; actin and microtubules(1).
   Just under the submembrane zone there are microtubules forming a peripheral ring which helps platelet to maintain its discoid shape in inactive form. When activated, the microtubules surround the organelles and with the contribution of other filaments (13), the organelles are tightly contracted. During silent form only 30-40 % of actin filaments are polymerized, when platelets are activated the polymerized amount increases(1).

3. Organel Zone:
   This is the zone where granule's, peroxisome's, lysosome's and mitochondria's are localized. There are enzymes, adenine nucleotids, calcium, serotonin and many other proteins in this region (1).

4. Membrane Zone
   There is a distinguishing feature of platelets that their plasma membrane contains wide spread invaginations that forms a network inside platelet. Finally with pore openings the inner network is directly in contact with outer zone. This system is named as "open canallicular system" (OCS) and with this system an extensive amount of surface area stays as potential in silent state. With this system also platelet gains a large area for molecular trafficking. A second canal system is composed from endoplasmic reticulum networks and named as "Dense Tubular System" (DTS). Here in DTS many enzymes and calcium ions that are important for activation are located. DTS is not directly connected to outer membrane (1, 14) but has close connections with OCS. These two systems actively exchange molecules (1).
   The granulles have diameters ranging between 200 to 500 nm and they are found as spherical or oval structures (15). There are 3 types of granules in platelets, Alfa Granules, Dense granules, lysosomes. Alpha granules are most prominent in terms of material content and majority. These granules include inflammatory molecules, cytokines, cell-activating molecules, proteins, Growth Factors, adhesion molecules, integrins and other proteins These granules are filled by megakaryocytes (3).

3. Alpha granules

It is widely accepted that these granules come from the budding of trans golgi apparatus organel of megakaryocytes (16, 17).

These are 200-400 nm diameter granules widespread in the cytoplasm (16) which gives the granular appearance in Romanoski stained smear preparations, each platelet contains around 50-80 of these granules. The content of granules is very diverse; a brief list is given in table 1 (14, 18, 19, 20, 21).

When platelets are activated these alpha granules fuse with each other, OCS and plasma membrane. The secretion of alpha granules is mediated by some proteins (such as SNARE) and membrane lipids (19).

The secretions effect platelet and cells in the environment (such as endothelial, leukocytes) for migration, adhesion and proliferation(14).

A rare syndrome named as Gray Thrombocyte Syndrome (GTS) is both involved with the quantity and quality of platelets which cases susceptibility for bleeding. In GTS the proteins synthesized by megakaryocytes are abnormal and don't enter platelets as they do in normal individuals and additionally the endocytotic mechanisms don't work properly. As a result the secretions spread to bone marrow and a fibrosis forms (miyelofibrozis)(22, 23).

Thrombospondin
P-selectin
platelet factor 4
beta thromboglobulinler
Factors V, XI, XIII fibrinogen
von Willebrand factor
fibronectin
vitronectin
high molecular weight complexes kininogen
chemokines
mitogenic growth factors (platelet-derived growth factor)
vascular endothelial growth factor
TGF-beta

Table 1. Some main components of alpha granules.

4. Dense granules

These are smaller granules with 150 nm diameter (24), because of the calcium and phosphate content there image seems dense under electron microscopic (EM) observation (21, 25). Each platelet contains 3-8 of these granules (14). The components of dense granules are briefly given in Table 2 (10, 14, 19, 20).

Ca
Mg
P
pyrophosphate Nucleotides ATP, GTP, ADP, GDP
Membrane proteins
CD63 (granulophysin)
LAMP 2
Serotonin
GPIb, GPIIb/IIIa
P-Selectin
Histamine
Epinephrine

Table 2. Some main components of dense granules.

In activated platelet these granules fuse with plasma membrane and expel their ingredients to their environment which causes other platelets to aggregate and a local vasoconstriction (especially by serotonin) in the involved vessels. Also the ADP content is a very important participant for homeostasis (14).

The importance of the components of dense granules for homeostasis is recognized when the diseases of the deficiency of dense granules was defined as Hermansky-Pudlak

Syndrome (26, 27, 28) and Chediak Higashi Syndrome. In both syndromes stoppage of bleeding is defective based on the impairment in dense granules (14).

5. Lysosomes

They have a diameter of 200-250 nm which places them to middle size granule (14). They can't be distinguished from alpha granules under EM observation because of the similarities in dense electron appearance. By the content of acid phosphates and arylsulphates cytochemical staining techniques can effectively distinguish lysosomes from alpha granules. In an activated platelet they expel their contents to environment as the other two granules by membrane fusing mechanisms. The difference for lysosomes to be involved in activation is that they need a more potent stimulus. The role of lysosomal components in homeostasis is not well understood as the other granules contribution. They are involved in thrombus formation and extracellular matrix remodeling (8).

It seems that lysosomes in platelets don't have any distinguished features, they share the common features with other cells lysosomes (29).

The components of dense granules are briefly given in Table 3 (8, 18, 30, 31, 32).

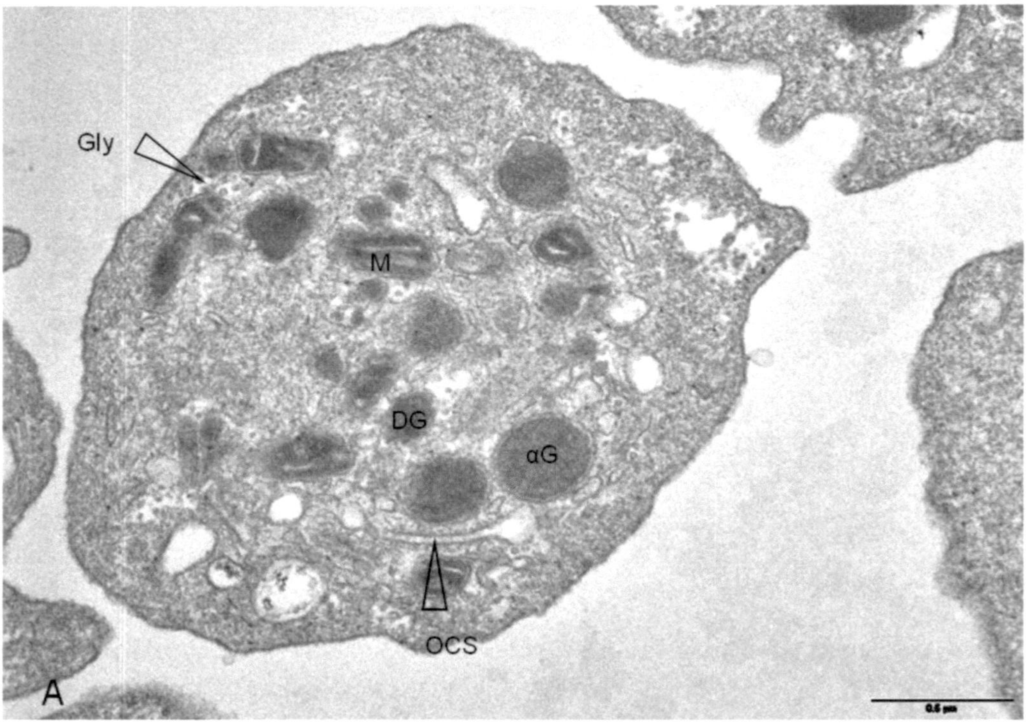

Figure 2. M: Mitochondria, αG: alfa-granules, DG: dense granules, Gly: glycogen particles and OCS: open canalicular system. The morphology can be seen in equatorial section of a human platelet. This image is referenced from Zufferey 2011 (Thanks for the kind permission of John Wiley and Sons to use this image)(33).

PF3
Acid phosphatase
Glucose-6 phosphatase
Arabinosidase
N-Acetyl-galactosominidase
ATP = adenosine triphosphate
TGF
CD63
Cathepsin
lysosomal membrane proteins (LAMP-1, LAMP-2)
acid hydrolases
cathepsins

Table 3. Some main components of platelet lysosomes

6. Autologous platelet rich plasma (PRP)

The application of growth factors in medical practice is one of the areas where basic clinical research has focused its attention but there are many problems associated with their local administration. For example, recombinant human growth factors are not cost effective, they have limited shelf life, and ineffectively delivered to target cells and in addition, to get efficient therapy, large doses are needed. The use of autologous platelets concentrates for tissue regeneration and wound healing has now become an alternative easy and cheap way to obtain high concentrations of these growth factors (34).

The autologous blood collected from a patient just before surgery can be prepared as platelet concentrates, platelet-rich plasma (PRP) and platelet gel for the treatment the patient specifically needs (35). These forms are prepared by gradient density centrifugation techniques to obtain high (x5) concentration of platelets (36). This autologous concentration includes a large amount of growth factors, especially PRP is an easy and inexpensive technique to accelerate the wound healing (37).

This quite new field is open for research, there are a lot of techniques still under development stage such as platelet gels can be obtained by adding thrombin to autologous platelet-rich plasma. The initiation of fibrin polymerization and the release of platelets factors and cytokines can be achieved by the specific activators such as thrombin, glass, freeze-thaw cycle to platelet-rich plasma depending on what is required during the surgery (35).

In spite of the distinct features of platelet-rich plasma (PRP) and its use by different fields of medicine, no adverse reactions were documented until now(38, 39, 40, 41).

Author details

Gökhan Cüce* and Tahsin Murad Aktan
Deparment of Histology and Embryology, Faculty of Meram Medicine University of Konya Necmettin Erbakan, Turkey

7. References

[1] Becker RC. Platelet Biology: The Role of Platelets in Hemostasis, Thrombosis and Inflammation. Platelets in Cardiovascular Disease. In:Bhatt DL. Imperial College Press. London, 2008:1-3.
[2] Mason KD, Carpinelli MR, Fletcher JI, Collinge JE, Hilton AA, Ellis S, Kelly PN, Ekert PG, Metcalf D, Roberts AW, Huang DC, Kile BT. Programmed anuclear cell death delimits platelet life span. Cell. 2007;128(6):1173-86.
[3] Rozman P, Bolta Z. Use of platelet growth factors in treating wounds and soft-tissue injuries. Acta Dermatovenerol Alp Panonica Adriat. 2007;16(4):156-65.
[4] Ovalle WK, Nahirney PC. Netter Essential Histology. Saunders; 2007;166.
[5] Klages B, Brandt U, Simon MI, Schultz G, Offermanns S. Activation of G12/G13 results in shape change and Rho/Rho- kinase-mediated myosin light chainphosphorylation in mouse platelets. J Cell Biol. 1999;144(4):745-54.
[6] Anitua E, Sánchez M, Nurden AT, Nurden P, Orive G, Andía I. New insights into and novel applications for platelet-rich fibrin therapies. Trends Biotechnol. 2006(5):227-34.
[7] Mishra A, Velotta J, Brinton TJ, Wang X, Chang S, Palmer O, Sheikh A, Chung J, Yang PC, Robbins R, Fischbein M. RevaTen platelet rich plasma improves cardiac function after myocardial injury. Cardiovasc Revasc Med. 2011;12(3):158-63.
[8] Drouin A, Cramer EM. Production of Platelets. Editor: Gresele P, Page CP, Fuster V, Vermylen J. Platelets in Thrombotic and Non-Thrombotic Disorders: Pathophysiology, Pharmacology and Therapeutics. Cambridge University Press; 2002;25.USA.
[9] Schulze H, Korpal M, Hurov J, Kim SW, Zhang J, Cantley LC, Graf T, Shivdasani RA. Characterization of the megakaryocyte demarcation membrane system and its role inthrombopoiesis. Blood. 2006;107(10):3868-75.
[10] Italiano JE Jr, Shivdasani RA. Megakaryocytes and beyond: the birth of platelets. J Thromb Haemost. 2003;1(6):1174-82.
[11] Hartwig J, Italiano J Jr. The birth of the platelet. J Thromb Haemost. 2003;1(7):1580-6.
[12] White JG. Platelet Structure. Editor:Michelson AD. Platelets. Elsevier: USA, Second Edition, 2007;45
[13] White JG. Views of the platelet cytoskeleton at rest and at work. Ann N Y Acad Sci. 1987;509:156-76.
[14] Rumbaut RE, Thiagarajan P. Platelet-Vessel Wall Interactions in Hemostasis and Thrombosis. Editör: Granger DN, Granger JP. Colloquium Series on Integrated Systems

* Corresponding Author

Physiology: From Molecule to Function to Disease. Morgan & Claypool Life Sciences; 2009-2011:5.

[15] Gassling VL, Açil Y, Springer IN, Hubert N, Wiltfang J. Platelet-rich plasma and platelet-rich fibrin in human cell culture. Oral Surg Oral Med Oral Pathol Oral Radiol Endod. 2009 ;108(1):48-55.

[16] King SM, Reed GL. Development of platelet secretory granules. Semin Cell Dev Biol. 2002(4):293-302.

[17] Blair P, Flaumenhaft R. Platelet alpha-granules: basic biology and clinical correlates. Blood Rev. 2009(4):177-89.

[18] McNicol A, Israels SJ. Platelet dense granules: structure, function and implications for haemostasis. Thromb Res. 1999;95(1):1-18.

[19] Reed GL. Platelet secretory mechanisms. Semin Thromb Hemost. 2004;30(4):441-50.

[20] Askari AT, Messerli AW, Lincoff M. Thrombosis and Antithrombotics in Vascular Disease. Management Strategies in Antithrombotic Therapy. Editör: Askari AT, Messerli AW.Wiley; USA. 2008:3.

[21] Ma AD, Key NS. Molecüler Basis of Hemostatic and thrombotic Diseases. Editör: Coleman WB, Tsongalis GJ, London. Molecular Pathology: The Molecular Basis of Human Disease. Academic Press; 1 edition, 2009:258.

[22] Di Paola J, Johnson J. Thrombocytopenias due to gray platelet syndrome or THC2 mutations. Semin Thromb Hemost. 2011(6):690-7.

[23] Nurden AT, Nurden P. The gray platelet syndrome: clinical spectrum of the disease. Blood Rev. 2007(1):21-36.

[24] Rendu F, Brohard-Bohn B. The platelet release reaction:granules' constituents, secretion secretion and functions. Platelets. 2001;12(5):261-73.

[25] Ruiz FA, Lea CR, Oldfield E, Docampo R. Human platelet dense granules contain polyphosphate and are similar to acidocalcisomes ofbacteria and unicellular eukaryotes. J Biol Chem. 2004;279(43):44250-7.

[26] King SM, McNamee RA, Houng AK, Patel R, Brands M, Reed GL. Platelet dense-granule secretion plays a critical role in thrombosis and subsequent vascularremodeling in atherosclerotic mice. Circulation. 2009;120(9):785-91.

[27] Nisal M, Pavord S, Oppenheimer CA, Francis S, Khare M. Hermansky-Pudlak syndrome: management of a rare bleeding disorder in a twin pregnancy. J Obstet Gynaecol. 2012 ;32(2):185-6.

[28] Saftig P, Klumperman J. Lysosome biogenesis and lysosomal membrane proteins: trafficking meets function. Nat Rev Mol Cell Biol. 2009;10(9):623-35.

[29] Skoglund C. Platelets in inflammation. Linköping University Medical Dissertations. 2010-Sweden;14.

[30] Gerrard JM, Phillips DR, Rao GH, Plow EF, Walz DA, Ross R, Harker LA, White JG. Biochemical studies of two patients with the gray platelet syndrome. Selective deficiency of platelet alpha granules. J Clin Invest. 1980;66(1):102-9.

[31] Nishibori M, Cham B, McNicol A, Shalev A, Jain N, Gerrard JM. The protein CD63 is in platelet dense granules, is deficient in a patient with Hermansky-Pudlaksyndrome, and appears identical to granulophysin. J Clin Invest. 1993;91(4):1775-82.

[32] Grau AJ, Reiners S, Lichy C, Buggle F, Ruf A. Platelet function under aspirin, clopidogrel, and both after ischemic stroke: a case-crossoverstudy. Stroke. 2003;34(4):849-54.

[33] Zufferey A, Fontana P, Reny JL, Nolli S, Sanchez JC. Platelet proteomics. Mass Spectrometry Reviews, 2011; 31, 331–351.

[34] Nikolidakis D, Jansen JA. The biology of platelet-rich plasma and its application in oral surgery: literature review. Tissue Eng Part B Rev. 2008 Sep;14(3):249-58.

[35] Soffer E, Ouhayoun JP, Anagnostou F. Fibrin sealants and platelet preparations in bone and periodontal healing. Oral Surg Oral Med Oral Pathol Oral Radiol Endod. 2003;95(5):521-8.

[36] Huang Q, Wang YD, Wu T, Jiang S, Hu YL, Pei GX. Preliminary separation of the growth factors in platelet-rich plasma: effects on the proliferation of human marrow-derived mesenchymal stem cells. Chin Med J (Engl). 2009;122(1):83-7.

[37] Napolitano M, Matera S, Bossio M, Crescibene A, Costabile E, Almolla J, Almolla H, Togo F, Giannuzzi C, Guido G. Autologous platelet gel for tissue regeneration in degenerative disorders of the knee. Blood Transfus. 2011;25:1-6.

[38] Edwards SG, Calandruccio JH. Autologous blood injection for refractory lateral epicondylitis. *J Hand Surg [Am]*. 2003;28(2):272-278.

[39] Mishra A, Pavelko T. Treatment of chronic elbow tendinosis with buffered platelet-rich plasma. *Am J Sports Med*. 2006;34(11):1774-1778.

[40] Kajikawa Y, Morihara T, Sakamoto H, et al. Platelet-rich plasma enhances the initial mobilization of circulation-derived cells for tendon healing. *Cell Physiol*. 2008;215(3):837-845.

[41] Sánchez M, Anitua E, Azofra J, Aguirre JJ, Andia I. Intra-articular injection of an autologous preparation rich in growth factors for the treatment of knee OA: a retrospective cohort study. *Clin Exp Rheumatol*. 2008;26(5):910-913.

Chapter 2

Rediscovering Red Blood Cells: Revealing Their Dynamic Antigens Store and Its Role in Health and Disease

Mahmoud Rafea and Serhiy Souchelnytskyi

Additional information is available at the end of the chapter

http://dx.doi.org/10.5772/48593

1. Introduction

The only identifiable function of Red Blood Cells (RBC) is the delivery of Oxygen. In mammals, RBC is a unique cell because:

- It does not have cellular organelles like any other cells in the body.
- It has a very especial protein: Hemoglobin which plays the role of carrying Oxygen to tissues and carries back carbon dioxide to lungs.
- It has a very especial cell membrane which carries a number of blood groups antigens' systems. Their functions include transporting other proteins and molecules into and out of the cell, maintaining cell structure, attaching to other cells and molecules, and participating in chemical reactions [1]. Those systems are genetically controlled with blood groups determining genes.

The work described in this chapter is based on the function carried out by the cell membrane antigens which are transporting other proteins and molecules into and out of the cell. The question is what are those proteins that are transported? In fact, this question identifies the knowledge gap about RBC role in health and disease. In the next section, some hypotheses will be inducted and deduced through analysis of available background knowledge. The experiments that can proof those hypotheses are described in section 3. This is followed by describing a theory about the role of RBC in health and disease based on the proved hypotheses and how we can benefit from this theory in diagnosing and treating of patients.

2. Knowledge analysis and hypotheses induction

Basically, when an antigen is introduced into a body, the immune system (IS) does either one of two reactions: immune tolerance (IT) or immune response (IR). IT-reaction is never absolute [2]. It is usually accompanied by a weak IR. In normal IR, one cannot identify if there is a degree of IT, because there is no defined laboratory method/test that can measure the degree of IT. Meanwhile, by logical implication, some degree of IT should exist with the normal IR. This entails that there is an equivalence relation between IT and IR.

Hypothesis I: There is no absolute immune tolerance, if and only if there is no absolute immune response

In central IT, immature self-reactive T lymphocytes recognize antigens in the thymus and undergo negative selection (deletion) [3]. Consequently, in normal IR against a particular antigen, measuring the concentration of this antigen in the thymus can be correlated to the degree of the accompanied IT. The transport mechanism of antigens to the thymus is a critical issue because of the remarkable capacity of IS which can recognize any antigen [4]. In [5], authors claim that Dendritic Cells (DCs) have several functions, not only, in innate and adaptive immunity, but also there is increasing evidence that DCs in situ induce antigen specific unresponsiveness or tolerance in central lymphoid organs and in the periphery. The evidence that DCs transport antigens to thymus in central tolerance is very weak while the evidence that DCs have role in peripheral tolerance is more acceptable based on the review article [6]. In conclusion RBC may be vehicles which transport self antigens to induce central IT.

The role of RBC in transporting antigens has not been investigated before. If RBC are capable of antigen transport to induce IT, this will unveil important knowledge. For instance, in hemolytic disease of fetus and newborn (HDFN), maternal anti D alloantibody and feto-maternal ABO incompatibility are the two major causes of HDFN, Meanwhile, with the implementation of Rhesus D immunoprophylaxis, hemolytic disease due to ABO incompatibility and other alloantibodies have now emerged as major causes of this condition. [7].

In pregnancy, most of delivered infants are normal when there is no anti D alloantibody which means that there is an efficient mechanism that can handle the other incompatibilities. The mechanisms explained in literature explain why ABO incompatibilities, only, do not occur [8], [9] and [10], but these mechanisms do not explain why those incompatibilities occur. The mechanism may be based on trapping those antibodies in placenta through RBC catering of ABO and other incompatible blood groups antigens. Consequently, the occurrence of HDFN may be due to depletion of those antigens' store from RBC. Also, if this RBC transport function is the mechanism a body tolerates his self antigens, this will explain how a pregnant woman is able to tolerate her fetus and placenta, assuming that they are part of self.

Hypothesis II: RBC hide antigens to transport them to target organs.

From these *hypotheses I & II*, if RBC play role in antigen transport, one can deduce that in any mammal, blood circulating antibodies against self and foreign, either antigens or tolergens, will react with hemolysate.

Hypothesis III: There is an injection function (one-to-one) between circulating antibodies and RBC's hemolysate antigens.

To proof that RBC have role in immune reactions (IR and IT), one need to proof that there is an inverse correlation between antibodies concentration in plasma and antigens concentration in RBC.

Hypothesis IV: In immune response, antibodies concentration in plasma against a particular antigen in hemolysate is higher than this antigen concentration in hemolysate. Meanwhile, in immune tolerance, antibodies concentration in plasma against a particular antigen in hemolysate is lower than this antigen concentration in hemolysate.

It should be remarked that Humans expressing a defective form of the transcription factor AIRE (autoimmune regulator) develop multi-organ autoimmune disease (autoimmune polyendocrinopathy syndrome type 1) [11]. Liston et all [12] prove that this autoimmune syndrome is caused by failure of a specialized mechanism for deleting forbidden T cell clones, establishing a central role for this tolerance mechanism.

3. Experiments

The methodology applied will demonstrate the existence of particular self tolerogens and particular foreign antigens in RBC (Hypothesis I & II) and show that innumerable antigens exist in RBC which react with innumerable antibodies that exist in plasma. This partially proves that RBC play a role in immune reaction. To proof Hypothesis IV, it will be demonstrated that the concentration of foreign antigens in RBC varies by time in relation to IR known behavior. The experiments done are the following:

1. RBC of pregnant females transport male spouse ABO blood group antigens
2. RBC of pregnant females transport male spouse HLA antigens
3. RBC transport self HLA antigens
4. RBC transport self Tissue Specific Antigens (TSAs).
5. RBC hemolysate antigens are precipitated by plasma obtained from the same individual and cross reacted with plasma from different individuals.
6. RBC transport bacterial antigens.
7. RBC antigens and plasma antibodies concentration vary with time.

3.1. Materials for experiments 1, 2, and 3

Couples that have children, pregnant females, and single females were selected from relatives and friends. The purpose of the experiments was explained to them. Not all the combinations could be found, after blood grouping. The combinations presented, in Table-1, were used to conduct the experiments. Blood samples were taken on heparin. Some of the blood samples were used to prepare RBC and plasma and the rest was used to prepare lymphocytes using the Ficoll hypaque technique [13].

RBC were washed several times using phosphate buffer saline (PBS). The male RBC were divided into two tubes. The first tube was divided into small aliquots that were frozen to rupture RBC. The second tube was used to prepare a 5% suspension. The female RBC were divided into small aliquots that were frozen to rupture RBC. Notice that we do not need female intact-RBC.

Female ABO group	Male ABO group
O	A
O	B
O	AB
A	O
A	B
B	A
O (SINGLE)	-

Table 1. The ABO blood groups of couples used in the experiments

3.2. RBC of pregnant females transport male spouse ABO antigens

To test RBC transport of male spouse ABO antigens, a technique based on competitive inhibition of RBC agglutination was followed. If the hemolysate contains ABO specific antigens, then those antigens will compete with RBC and prevent their agglutination. Figure 1 illustrates a schematic description of the experiment.

Method

The experiment was performed, for each couple, as follows:

- In positive control tubes which represent also reference tubes for comparison with test tubes, serial dilutions (up to 1/128) of female spouse plasma were made using normal saline. A drop of a male spouse's hemolysate was added before adding his RBC's suspension.
- In test tubes, serial dilutions of the female spouse's plasma were made using normal saline. A drop of the female spouse's hemolysate was added before adding a drop of her male spouse's RBC suspension.

Results

Whenever there is ABO incompatibility and the male spouse is not 'O', agglutination was inhibited by the female spouse hemolysate and was not inhibited by male spouse hemolysate. In most cases, agglutination was inhibited in the first tube. However, agglutination was never observed in subsequent tubes. The single virgin female RBC do not contain any ABO antigens.

3.3. RBC of pregnant females transport male spouse HLA antigens

This experiment was performed using commercial HLA Typing Trays for the identification and definition of HLA Class I Antigens using the microlymphocytotoxicity assay [14]. It is also based on competitive inhibition. Consequently, if typing wells that show positive reaction were inhibited in corresponding testing wells by adding hemolysate, this proves the existence of specific competing antigens. Figure 2 illustrate the experiment steps.

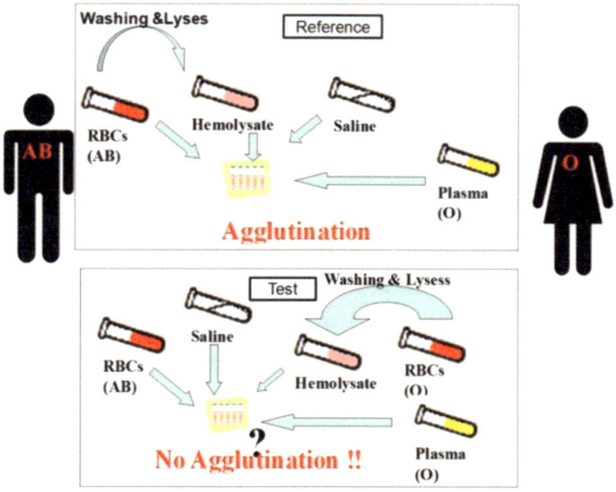

Figure 1. Schematic drawing of ABO antigen transport experiment, the upper part shows how the reference positive control is conducted, while the lower part shows how the test is conducted.

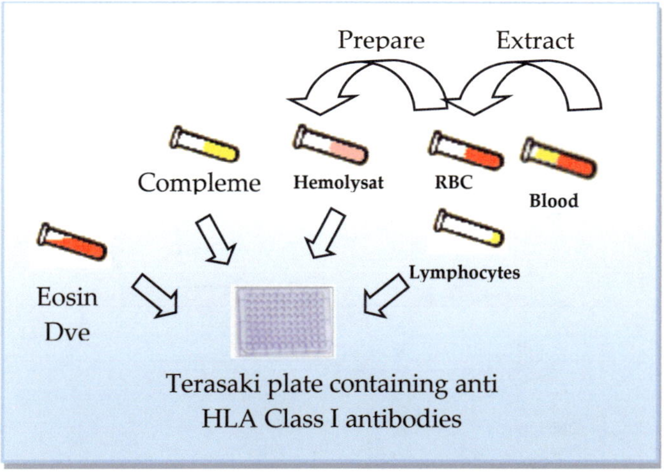

Figure 2. Re-typing of male spouse but using his female spouse hemolysate to compete with his lymphocytes

Method

First, each couple was HLA typed, and then the following was done:

- A hemolysate from a third person was added to control wells. The positive control should give positive reaction. In this way, we excluded inherent errors or non-specific reaction.
- Female spouse hemolysate (diluted 1/16) was added to typing wells

- Male spouse lymphocytes was added and followed by the complement and eosin dye as usual.
- Wells that gave positive reaction in typing were examined by contrast microscope.

Results

It was observed that female spouse hemolysate inhibited the typing reaction while the third person hemolysate did not. This indicates the existence of male spouse HLA antigens in female spouse hemolysate.

3.4. RBC transport self HLA antigens

This experiment is similar to the previous one. The only difference is the use of the male's own hemolysate instead of his female's spouse hemolysate. It was observed that a male hemolysate inhibited the typing reaction of his lymphocytes indicating the existence of self HLA antigens.

3.5. RBC transport Tissue Specific Antigens (TSAs)

If RBC transport antigens to central organs of the immune system to induce tolerance, then RBC will definitely transport TSAs. Otherwise this transport function has nothing to do with tolerance. Consequently, the objective of this experiment was to demonstrate that antibodies against TSAs can be prepared through injecting RBC of white mice into rabbits. Figure 3 illustrates the experiment.

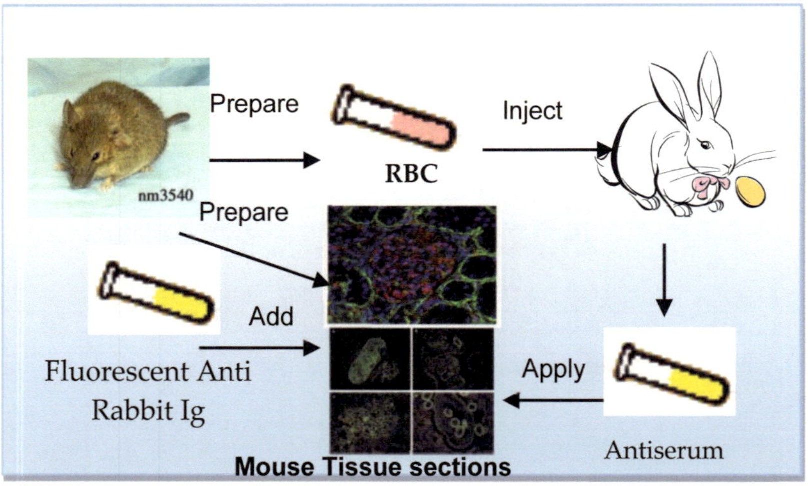

Figure 3. Preparing antibodies against white mice TSAs in rabbit

Materials

A number of white mice were slaughtered to collect their blood on sodium citrate and their organs (liver, kidney and spleen) were preserved on 10 % formalin. The separated RBC were washed many times with sodium citrate and then diluted with 3% formol-saline to kill any bacterial contamination. An ordinary rabbit was selected to prepare the antibodies.

Method:

- A rabbit was injected subcutaneously with one ml of white mice RBC for four times on weekly intervals.
- Blood was collected from ear-vein after 35 days from the first injection.
- The serum was examined for antibodies against mice RBC using direct agglutination slide test.
- The serum was examined for antibodies against TSAs of white mice (liver, kidney and spleen) using the sandwich technique in histo-pathology sections.

Results:

All sections showed florescence. Figure 4 illustrates some of the histopathology sections taken from a white mouse's organs.

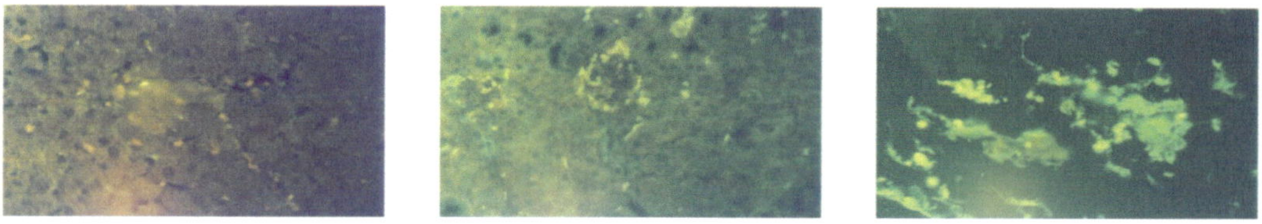

A B C

Figure 4. Histopathology sections from a white mouse's organs examined by florescent microscope showing florescence due to antigen-antibody reaction, A: kidney tissue, B: liver, and C: spleen.

3.6. RBC hemolysate antigens are precipitated by plasma

Ouchterlony immuno-precipitation test of normal serum against self and other normal hemolysate was conducted, Figure 5(a). We confirmed this finding by using Western Blot technique, and showed that serum from one individual recognized antigens in hemolysate from two normal persons, Figure 5(b). Further confirmation was obtained by using two-dimensional gel electrophoresis (2-DE) of co-immunoprecipitated hemolysate antigens using self-serum, Figure 5(c). Notice that the number of the immune-precipitated antigens is numerous and many spots were enriched by immune-precipitation because those antigens were not detected in 2-DE gel of hemolysate, Figure 5(d). Antigenicity of the separated proteins was confirmed by immune-blotting proteins separated by 2-DE with the same self-serum, Figure 5(e). This excluded co-precipitation of non-antigens, as they would not be detected in immune-blotting.

3.7. RBC transport bacterial antigens

As TB is a priority disease, trying to find Mycobacterium tuberculosis bacilli protein antigens (MTPAs) in TB-patient hemolysate was conducted through 2D electrophoresis, and then identifying gel spots with mass spectrometry. Fortunately, we discovered four MTPAs. This motivated us to do the experiments of the next section to identify more MTPAs in hemolysate of TB patients.

Identifying MTPAs in TB patients hemolysate

The goal is to find the set of antigens, in TB patients' hemolysate, which is related to Mycobacterium tuberculosis bacilli. The approach taken follows the following steps Figure 6:

1. The study resources are:
   - [A] Patients
   - [B] Mycobacterium tuberculosis (H37Rv)
2. For each patient:
   - Collect blood sample on anticoagulant (step 1)
   - Separate RBC and wash many times with saline (step 2)
3. Hemolysate [C] is prepared by rupturing RBC with low isotonic solution which is the binding buffer in affinity chromatography
4. Prepare hyper immune serum for M. *tuberculosis* (step 3)
5. Purify antibodies using Protein A Sepharose beads (step 4)
6. The purified antibodies are then used to separate antigens from hemolysate (step 5)
7. The disease related antigens are identified using in gel trypsin digestion and MALDI TOF mass spectrometry (step 6)

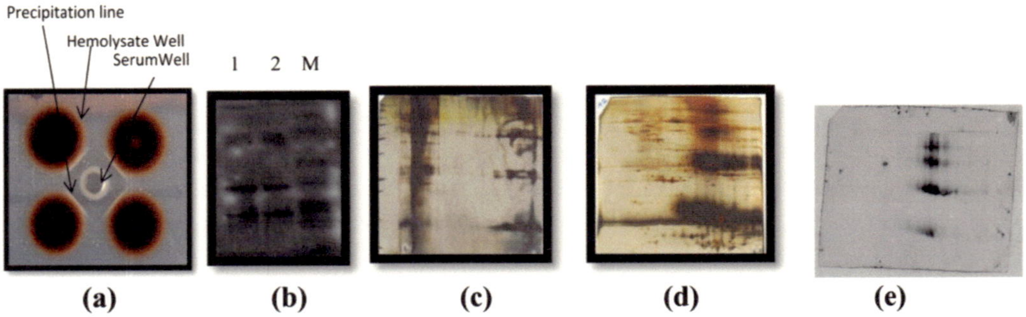

Figure 5. Detection of innumerable antigens in Red Blood Cells. (a) Ouchterlony test showing serum of normal against hemolysate of self and others (b) Western Blot using two normal hemolysate propped with serum of one of them (c) Silver stain of 2-DE of immune-precipitated hemolysate antigens (d) Silver stain of 2D electrophoresis of hemolysate (e) Western Blot of 2-DE of hemolysate propped with serum.

3.8. RBC antigens and plasma antibodies concentration vary with time

The objective of this experiment is to investigate the dynamics of foreign antigens in RBC. In effect, antibodies are taken at one instance of time, while RBC are taken at different instances.

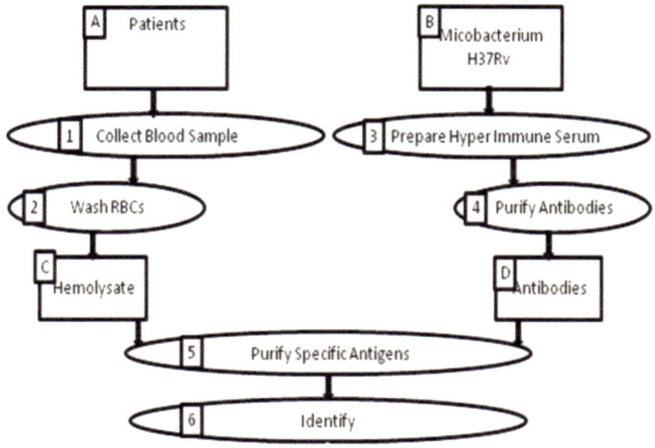

Figure 6. Flowchart depicting the resources and steps for identification of hemolysate antigens related to *Mycobacterium tuberculosis* (H37Rv)

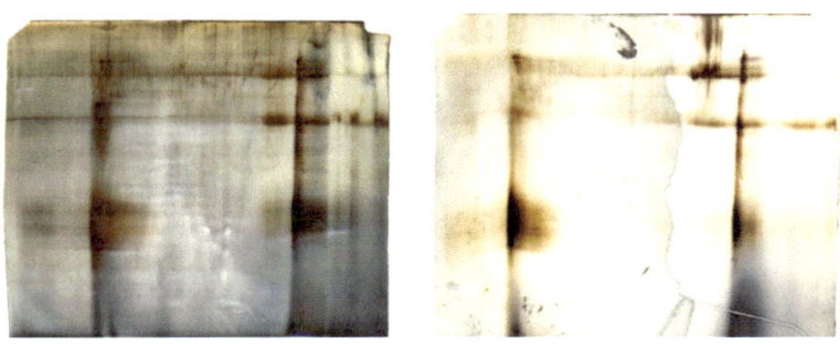

Figure 7. Precipitated Antigens separated using 2D electrophoresis Gel

Materials

- **Bacteria:** ***Escherichia coli*** O157:H7 strain[1] was inoculated onto SMAC agar (Oxoid). Colonies were tested by ***E. coli*** O157 latex kit (Oxoid DR 620) and confirmed biochemically. A single colony of ***E. coli*** bacterial growth from the plate was inoculated into Brain heart infusion broth (Oxoid) and incubated overnight at 37 °C and adjusted to a concentration of approximately 10^{10} CFU.
- **Animals:**
  1. A rabbit
  2. A baladi sheep between 8 to10 months.

The rabbit and sheep were tested serologically, to be negative, for ***Escherichia coli*** O157:H7.

Methods:

The first experiment method was done as follows, Figure 8:

1. Rabbits were vaccinated by Escherichia coli. Rabbits were injected subcutaneously with one ml on weekly basis for three weeks.
2. Blood was collected from the ear-vein after 21 days from the first injection.

[1] This strain is kindly provided by the serology department, Animal Health Research Institute (AHRI), Giza, Egypt.

3. Rabbits sera were separated and examined for antibodies against E. coli O157 using direct bacteria slide agglutination test.
4. A sheep was infected by oral administration of bacterial suspension.
5. Red blood cells were prepared from anti-coagulated sheep blood collected at 0 time (i.e., before inoculation), 1st week, 2nd week, and 3rd week. The collected blood was centrifuged at 4 °C for 25 minutes at 1170 g. Plasma and Buffy coat from each sample were removed. RBC were washed twice in normal saline solution by centrifugation at 4 °C for 5 minutes at 2000 g, and then re-suspended in Tris/Saline buffer pH 7.5 and subjected to lyses by freezing.
6. Nobel agar 1% in Tris/Saline was used as a supportive media for antigen-antibody precipitation, where the central well contained rabbit serum and peripheral wells contained sheep RBC hemolysate.

Results

The rabbit serum showed high titer (1/160) of antibodies against E. coli. Antigens of E. coli could be precipitated from sheep RBC of the 1st and 2nd week after infection, only, Figure 9.

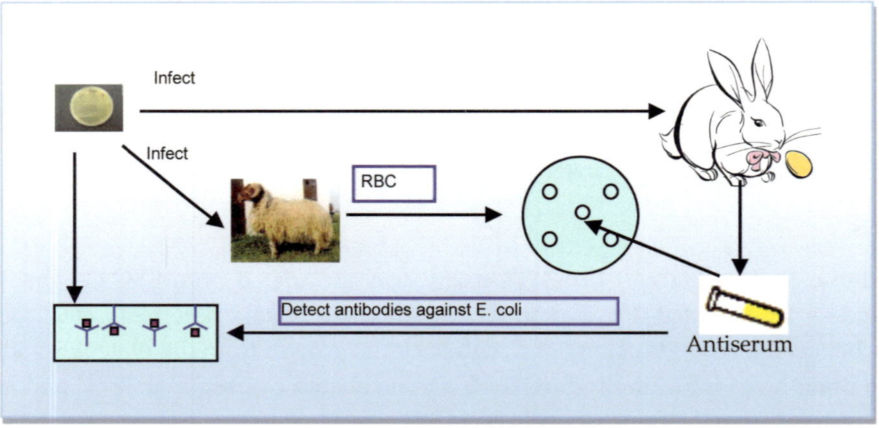

Figure 8. Preparing Antibodies against bacteria and preparing RBC carrying antigens of this bacteria. The purpose is to precipitate Bacteria antigens from RBC of infected animals using the prepared antibodies against those antigens.

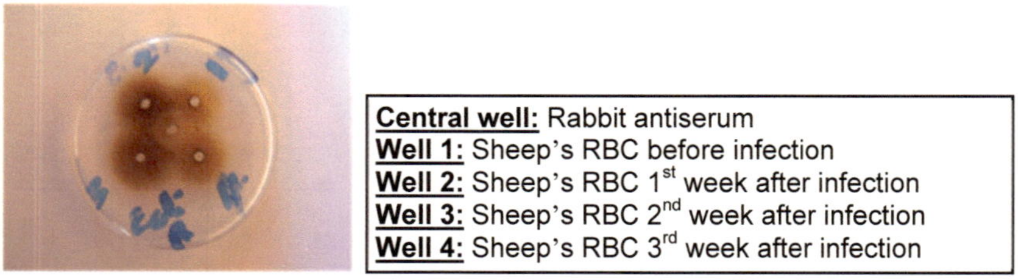

Figure 9. Illustrates the dynamics of RBC's antigens

4. The role of RBC antigens transport in health and disease

The RBC transport function maintains tolerance to self antigens. This function is exploited positively to protect a fetus from the immune system attack using the same mechanism of protecting the self. In effect, a fetus, which is an allograft, is considered part of self.

In humans and animals, not all microorganisms are capable of causing disease. Some of those microorganisms are equipped with the machinery that can overcome biological barriers and can cause disease in animals but not in humans and vice versa [15]. The role of RBC antigens transport in inducing tolerance to self-antigens is a feature that can be considered as a security-hole, as invaders can exploit this process to escape from the response of the immune system by disguising themselves as self. Tumors and parasites are negative examples.

Notice that this mechanism of tolerance induction does not contradict with all what we know about tolerance. Further, it explains the documented properties of tolerance. For instance, some of the properties that can be explained are:

- Artificially induced tolerance is of finite duration because antigen stores get depleted.
- Tolerance to self antigens is a process that continues throughout life but begins during fetal development because RBC are transporting self antigens all the time.

Notice that the discovered function of RBC fills a gap in the understanding of tolerance. Part of this gap can be expressed in the following questions:

1. Why soluble antigens administered intravenously favor tolerance while particulate antigens injected into the skin favor immunity.
2. Why ingested large doses of soluble proteins induce systemic T lymphocyte tolerance, whereas the components of vaccines such as the Sabin polio vaccine induce an effective local immune response.
3. Why tolerance is easier to induce in prenatal rather than postnatal life.

Answer of Question 1 and 2: RBC can easily absorb soluble antigens through pinocytosis while a particulate antigen needs receptor sites on RBC in order to be absorbed, which is the RBC membrane antigens function. Notice that the probability that the immune system will react to some processed antigens still exists. That is why the dose of antigens plays an important role. As far as there are enough stores of antigens in RBC, they are effectively tolerated.

Answer of Question 3: If antigens are introduced to a fetus while the immune system is still incapable of respond, there is a good chance for those antigens to be processed by the Antigen-Presenting-Cells (APC) and then absorbed by RBC. When mature lymphocytes production starts, later in life, antigen stores of RBC are used to induce tolerance. This may explain why tolerance is easier to induce in prenatal life.

Further, a pathogenesis mechanism of some autoimmune disease can be postulated. If RBC antigen-transport function is impaired for a particular self-antigen, for some reason, the tolerance to that antigen will eventually vanish. Consequently, an autoimmune response will be provoked to that antigen and autoimmune disease is established.

5. How this RBC antigens transport function can be exploited

This observed RBC antigens transport function creates an antigens' store. This store can be exploited in many directions. The proposed direction is to exploit functional proteomics approach [16] with the following three crucial aspects of the experimental design to produce products which are among diagnostic kits, vaccines or treatment components:

1. The strategy used for the selection, purification and preparation of the antigens to be analyzed by mass spectrometry
2. The type of mass spectrometer used and the type of data to be obtained from it
3. The method used for the interpretation of the mass spectrometry data and the search engine used for the identification of the proteins in the different types of sequence data banks available

The aim of this approach is to identify antigens which are relevant to a particular disorder.

5.1. Direct approach for products development

This approach is based on using a subset of antibodies which are specific against a subset of antigens of a particular disease to enable the use of those antibodies and those antigens in preparation of beneficial products.

Diagnostic kits can be prepared for all infectious microorganism and all tumors. In such disorders, simple kits can be prepared using the following steps:

1. Extract antigens from microorganism/tumor-cell-line cultures in coupling buffer
2. Prepare hyper immune serum using extracted antigens
3. Build an affinity column
4. Antibodies purification: Use affinity column containing antigens to separate their related antibodies from hyper immune serum
5. Adsorb purified antibodies to latex beads

A more advanced kits based on selection of antigen-determinant sites (epitopes) can be prepared. The problem of such kits, which uses a particular antigen, is in its validation which will be more sophisticated. One can expect that this particular antigen may not exist in RBC antigens' store of some population who are genetically different from the population used in preparation of the kit.

Active vaccines against all infectious microorganism and all tumors can be prepared by using the purified antibodies prepared for diagnostic kits in identifying related antigens existing in RBC antigens' store. The identified antigens can be prepared using the technology of recombinant proteins purification.

5.2. Bioinformatics approach for products development

The proposed mathematical model and a data mining algorithm will not only help in identifying proteins (antigens) that can be used in diagnosis and treatment of difficult disorders, but also will help in etiological diagnosis of idiopathic disorders and their treatment. This approach is based on building large databases of RBC antigens' store for patients and normal individuals. Consequently, a patient sample is collected on anticoagulant. RBC and plasma are separated. The plasma IgG is separated and then used as ligand in immunoaffinity chromatography to separate hemolysate antigens. The collected antigens are identified by mass spectrometry. The database record consists of the diagnosis and the set of identified antigens.

5.2.1. Mathematical model

It consists of four main parts; definitions of symbols, model of diseases caused by microorganisms, tumors, or foreign proteins; model of autoimmune diseases which result as a consequence of missed tissue proteins from RBC antigens' store; and model of diseases of unknown cause (Idiopathic).

Definitions

Let the assumption of this work be as the following:
p_i: protein amino acid sequence, where $i = 1 .. n$
d_j: health state, i.e., normal or disease name, where $j = 1 .. m$
$P = \{p_1, \ldots, p_n\}$, Set of all proteins of RBC antigens' store
$D = \{d_1, \ldots, d_m\}$, Set of all diseases
P_p: patient proteins where $P_p \subset P$ where p is the patient ID
O_p: (p_i, d_j), ordered pair of patient presented by protein sequence (i) and health state (j).

a. Model of Diseases caused by microorganisms, tumors, or foreign proteins

$$P_{dj} = \cap \{P_p\}_{dj}$$

Where P_{dj} is the set which contains all common proteins associated with d_j.

$$P_{normal} = \cup \{P_p\}_{normal}$$

Where P_{normal} is the set which contains proteins associated with normal.

P'_{normal} such that $\forall$ p in P_{normal} if the number of occurrence of $p \in P_{normal}$ is less than 5% of the total number of p in P_{normal} then remove p from P_{normal}.

$$P'_{dj} = P_{dj} - P'_{normal}$$

Where P'_{dj} is the set which contains proteins that can be used as biomarker or vaccines, Figure 10.

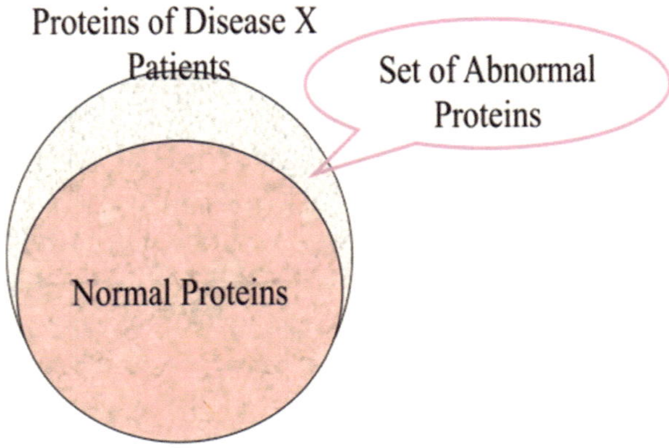

Figure 10. Venn diagram depicting set of abnormal protein of disease X (P'_{dj})

b. Model of Diseases caused as a result of missed tissue proteins

$$P^{u}_{dj} = \cup\{P_p\}_{dj}$$

The result is the set which contains all proteins associated with d_j

$$P''_{dj} = P_{normal} - P^{u}_{dj}$$

The result is the set which contains proteins that can be used to diagnose patients through detecting circulating auto-antibodies and to treat those patients through desensitizing them with the proteins that give positive reaction, Figure 11.

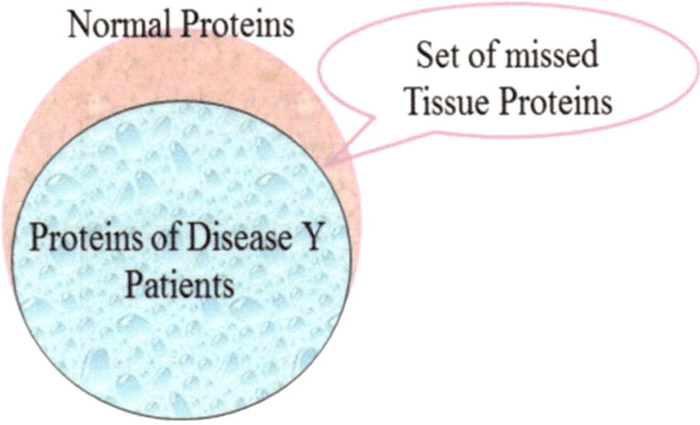

Figure 11. Venn diagram depicting set of missed normal proteins of disease Y (P''_{dj})

c. Model of Diseases of unknown cause (Idiopathic)

- There are many diseases that are identified as idiopathic.
- Those diseases can be caused due to existence of abnormal protein or absence of tissue proteins.

- Applying data mining methods (A and B) can help to identify new diseases and treat patients appropriately.

5.2.2. Scenario of the system in clinical environment

Patients' blood samples will be collected on anticoagulant. RBC and plasma are then separated in different tubes. Plasma is used as a ligand in immune-affinity chromatography to separate hemolysate antigens that can bind to plasma antibodies. The separated antigens are identified by MS and stored in the database indexed by the patient disorder.

In the same time, queries are done to verify the diagnosis and get a prognosis and a recommended treatment component. The following formulas describe the usage of this model in clinical practice.

Let Dp' is the set of all discovered P'_{dj}
Let Dp'' is the set of all discovered P''_{dj}

Then

$$\forall P'_{dj} \in Dp', \text{ if } P'_{dj} \subset P, \text{ then patient is diagnosed to have } d_j$$

Else

$$P''_{dj} \in Dp'', \text{ if } P''_{dj} \not\subset P, \text{ then patient is diagnosed to have } d_j$$

6. Conclusions

All the previous work in RBC proteomics neither has identified another function nor has mentioned the finding of: HLA, TSAs, or foreign proteins. The reasons are obvious. Firstly, it is not expected to find such proteins and consequently the method used for the interpretation of the mass spectrometry data, and the search engines used for the identification do not consider the right types of sequence data banks available. Secondly, the amount of most of the antigens which belong to the RBC antigens' store is little. This makes those antigens invisible and hence easily missed.

The work described is just a pilot study that throws some light on a new theory related to RBC. This theory is based on finding antigens' store consisting of self and non-self antigens. Although this theory can be related to immune tolerance by logical induction, the concrete evidence and mechanism need further research. Mainly, the logical induction is based on finding all kind of antigens in hemolysate, especially HLA antigens which are related to fetus. This existence of all kinds of antigens, definitely, plays some immunological role which may be immune tolerance.

The initial experiment, which shows the existence of ABO antigens in hemolysate of pregnant females, explains the mechanism of how HDFN occurs. Meanwhile, the experiment which shows that HLA antigens exist in their hemolysates proposes a new mechanism by which a pregnant woman is able to tolerate her fetus and placenta. Simply, it is the same mechanism a body tolerates his self antigens.

The experiments which use hemolysate against self-serum: Ouchterlony immune-precipitation test, Western Blot, and 2-DE of co-immunoprecipitated antigens demonstrated that RBC have an antigens' store. Mass spectrometry of spots obtained from 2-DE gel demonstrated the finding of all kind of antigens, self and non-self, in hemolysate. This indicates that blood circulating antibodies in any individual will react with his RBC's hemolysate antigens. In effect, there is no absolute immune response, too.

This directed our attention to use hyper immune serum against *Mycobacterium* antigens. This will help to get rid of other proteins and do better separation; and hence better identification. Consequently, we could identify 11 proteins from 60 gel spots belonging to H37Rv strain. The rest of spots are proteins related to bacterial commensals. Consequently, purification of specific antibodies from hyper immune serum is recommended to get further better separation.

In the experiment which investigates the dynamics of foreign antigens in RBC using sheep RBC which has been infected with *E. coli*, it was shown that the concentration of foreign antigens in RBC varies by time in relation to IR known behavior. This proves that RBC have role in immune reactions (IR and IT).

Whatever the reason of this existence of antigens in hemolysate this existence can help in designing diagnostic kits for different types of diseases. Further, it will help in discovering, not only, new immunological disorders which are, now, categorized under idiopathic disease, but also, identifying the obscure cause of many immunological disorders, including cancer. The identification of the cause of a disorder will help in its treatment and prevention.

Author details

Mahmoud Rafea and Serhiy Souchelnytskyi
Karolinska Biomics Centre, Department of Oncology-Pathology, Karolinska Institutet, Stockholm, Sweden

Acknowledgement

We would like to thank Dr. Saleh El-Ayouby, Dr. Essam Nasr, Professor Dr, Mervat El Anary, and Ms. Heba Zaki. Dr. El-Ayouby helped in preparation of antiserum and in conducting Ouchterlony immuno-precipitation test. Dr. Nasr has provided the H37Rv strain and helped in the preparation of the antigen extract. Professor El Ansary has provided lab facilities and reagents for HLA typing and has examined the typing trays. Ms. Zaki developed a computer program that implements the mathematical model to help in its verification.

7. References

[1] Daniels, G. (2007). Functions of red cell surface proteins. *Vox sanguinis , 93*, 331 - 340.

[2] Burek, C. L. (1998). Autoantibodies test for. In I. Roitt, & P. Delves (Ed.), *Encyclopedia of Immunology* (Second Edition ed., pp. 260-265). Baltimore, Maryland, USA: Elsevier Inc.

[3] Qin, S., Cobbold, S., Benjamin, R., & Waldmann, H. (1989). Induction of classical transplantation tolerance in the adult. *J. Exp. Med. , 169*, 799.

[4] Perelson, A. S., & Weisbuch, G. (1997). Immunology for physicists. *Rev. Mod. Phys. , 69* (4), 1219--1268.

[5] Steinman, R. M., Daniel, H., & Michel, N. C. (2003). TOLEROGENIC DENDRITIC CELLS. *Annu. Rev. Immunol , 21*, 685-711.

[6] Walker, L. S., & Abbas, A. K. (2002). THE ENEMY WITHIN: KEEPING SELF-REACTIVE T CELLS AT BAY IN THE PERIPHERY. *NATURE REVIEWS IMMUNOLOGY , 2*, 11-19.

[7] Basu, S., Kaur, R., and Kaur, G. (2011). Hemolytic disease of the fetus and newborn: Current trends and perspectives. Asian J Transfus Sci. 2011 January; 5(1): 3–7. doi: 10.4103/0973-6247.75963

[8] Mollison, P., Engelfriet, C., & Contreras, M. (1997). *Blood transfusion in clinical medicine* (10th ed.). Oxford: Blackwell Science.

[9] Hadley, A., & Soothill, P. (2002). *Blood diseases in pregnancy.* Cambridge University Press.

[10] Tawfik, H. (2005, March). *Management of Alloimmune Fetal Anemia*. Retrieved April 12, 2008, from ASJOG: http://www.asjog.org/journal/V2Issue1/262%20fetus&newborn-Fetal%20Anemia%20_dr.pdf

[11] Anderson, M. S., Venanzi, E. S., Klein, L., Chen, Z., Berzins, S. P., Tureley, S. J., et al. (2002). Projection of an immunological self shadow within the thumus by the aire protein. Science , 298 (5597), 1395-1401.

[12] Liston, A., Lesage, S., Wilson, J., Pletonen, L., & Doodnow, C. C. (2003). Aire regulates negative selection of organ-specific T cells. Nat. Immunol. , 4 (4), 350--4.

[13] Tamul, K., Schmitz, J. L., Kane, K., & Folds, J. D. (1995). Comparison of the Effects of Ficoll-Hypaque Separation and Whole Blood Lysis on Results of Immunophenotypic Analysis of Blood and Bone Marrow Samples from. CLINICAL AND DIAGNOSTIC LABORATORY IMMUNOLOGY , 337–342.

[14] Hopkins, K. (1990). The basic microlymphocytotoxicity assay. *The ASHI laboratory manual. 2nd edition* . ASHI Lenexa.

[15] Casadevall, A., & Pirofski, L. A. (2000). Host-Pathogen Interactions: Basic Concepts of Microbial Commensalism, Colonization, Infection, and Disease. *Infection and Immunity* , *12* (68), 6511-6518.

[16] Thomson, J. D., Schaeffer-Reiss, C., & Ueffing, M. (2008). Functional Proteomics Methods and Protocols. *Series: Methods in Mollecular Biology, 484* (XVIII), 115.

Chapter 3

Homocysteine in Red Blood Cells Metabolism – Pharmacological Approaches

Filip Cristiana, Zamosteanu Nina and Albu Elena

Additional information is available at the end of the chapter

http://dx.doi.org/10.5772/47795

1. Introduction

Red blood cells are responsible for oxygen transport from lung to tissues. Oxygen transport depends on reduced state of iron (Fe^{2+}) in hemoglobin. To accomplish their delivery function erythrocytes must accommodate to the environment conditions as they change along the vascular branches. Both element oxygen (O_2) and iron are able to quickly shift their oxidative state in response to different external/internal emerging stimuli. Moreover in erythrocyte nitric oxide (NO•) a vasodilalatory messenger is present. All these elements act in normal condition in well established mechanisms but they may generate alone or together high reactive species, named free radicals, that damage red blood cells as well as vascular endothelium. Free radicals may be generated from both oxygen and nitrogen and are known as reactive oxygen species (ROS) respectively nitrogen reactive species (RNS). However erythrocytes have intracellular enzyme/non enzyme defense system. When reactive species are quickly and intensely generated under external/internal stimuli the activity of antioxidant defense system is overwhelmed. Free radicals generation is triggered by normal, adaptive or pathological stimuli such as: superoxide detoxification, decreasing oxygen saturation in vascular branches, shear stress or atherosclerosis, ischemic attack and bacterial infections.

One of the most potent oxidant agents in living cells is homocysteine (Hcy) a metabolic compound from methionine metabolism. The already mention metabolism requires vitamin B_{12}, B_6 and folic acid involvement. Every deficiency in vitamins supplies or enzymes activity triggers the onset of different diseases and erythrocyte is first affected in megaloblastic or Biermer anemia. A secondary consequence of vitamins deficiency is hyperhomocysteinemia. HyperHcy represents a high risk in cardiovascular diseases and not only. Nowadays is generally accepted that Hcy disturbs the normal endothelial function, promoting thrombosis and inhibiting fibrinolysis through many mechanisms which can possibly integrate and are not mutually exclusive; oxidative processes, decreasing NO bioavailability and specific protein targeting.

The already specified free radicals are not all "bad". NO• can be regarded as a "good radical" but it is inactivated by many Hcy-dependent Mechanisms that finally impair its vasodilatatory function. Thus damaging Hcy effects expands to the environment where erythrocytes move and act. As a consequence directly and indirectly Hcy has a big impact on erythrocytes whose deformability in shear stress is crucial for circulatory function. Taken into account all these factors pharmacological approaches envisage lowering homocysteine levels by different ways such as: vitamins B supplementation, antioxidant drugs, hypotensive agent, antithrombotic drugs etc. Some of these patterns such is vitamins supplementation proved to have limited clinical benefits while others as nitrite/nitrate are still in debates. Because most pathological processes mentioned above involve oxidative pathway mechanism, pharmacological presentation will focus on drugs with antioxidant properties

As a conclusion the effect of elevated homocysteine appears multifactorial affecting both the vascular wall structure, function as well as erythrocytes metabolism.

2. Homocysteine and red blood cells

2.1. Red blood cells oxidative-reducing balance

Red blood cells are responsible for oxygen transport from lung to tissues. Their function depends on reduced state of iron (Fe^{2+}) in hemoglobin (Hb). Both element oxygen and iron are able to quickly shift their oxidative state in response to different emerging stimuli. Literature shows in [1] that hemoglobin may undergo oxidative reaction in the process of releasing oxygen. In this process iron is oxidized to Fe^{3+} and reactive oxygen species are generated. The bigger the reactive species release is the higher normal deformability and flexibility of erythrocytes is disturbed.

2.1.1. Reactive species generation

In erythrocyte are found together oxygen (O_2), nitrogen oxide (NO•) and iron (Fe^{2+}). All these elements act in normal condition in well established mechanisms but they may generate alone or together reactive species, named radicals, that damage red blood cells as well as vascular endothelium.

A radical is a chemical species that possesses a single unpaired electron in outer orbitals, and is able to independently exist, known also as free radical. Radicals are highly reactive in extracting an electron from any neighbor molecule in order to complete theirs own orbitals. There are two main groups of free radicals: ROS or reactive species of oxygen, RNS or reactive nitrogen species. ROS and RNS can act together damaging cells and causing nitrosactive stress. Therefore, these two species are often collectively referred to as ROS/RNS.

Transitional metals (Fe belongs to this group) particularly behave. They have a single unpaired electrons in theirs outer orbitals, but they don't behave as free radicals because within cells they are attached to proteins in most cases. However they are able to catalyze electron transfer in many processes and sometimes generate radicals.

2.1.2. Reactive oxygen species

Reactive species of oxygen refers to a group of highly reactive O_2 metabolites, including superoxide anion ($O_2^{\bullet -}$), hydrogen peroxide (H_2O_2), singlet oxygen ($^1O_2$), and hydroxyl radical ($OH\bullet$), that can be formed within cells. Reactive oxygen species are constantly formed as byproducts in normal enzymatic reaction in all human cells through normal aerobic processes as mitochondrial oxidative phosphorylation or as necessary products in neutrophils in order to kill invading pathogens. The above mentioned phenomena are consuming oxygen processes.

Erythrocytes must save oxygen for delivering it to the cells; as a consequence red blood cells lack mitochondrion the main oxygen consumer within cell. In this particular condition the source of ROS in erythrocyte may be the carried oxygen itself.

In order to understand oxygen behavior an inside in its structure is needed. The ground state of oxygen is triplet oxygen meaning that the molecule has two unpaired electrons occupying two different molecular orbitals.

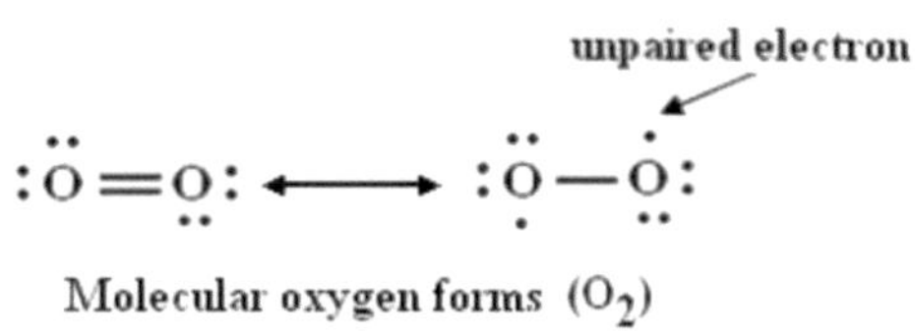

Figure 1. The structure of oxygen molecule

These electrons can't travel both in the same orbital because they have parallel spin (they spin in the same direction). As a consequence molecular oxygen is paramagnetic and from this feature it was concluded that the structure in the right may be assigned to O_2 (figure1). Although O_2 is very reactive from thermodynamic standpoint its single electrons cannot react rapidly with already paired electrons in the covalent bond of organic molecules (abundant in living cells). As a consequence it is harmless to these molecules. Instead molecular oxygen can rapidly react with single unpaired electrons from transitory metals (e.g. Fe, Cu, Mn). One mole of properly chelated cooper could catalyze consumption of all of the oxygen in an average room within one second in [2].

In fact oxygen O_2 is both kinetically stable thus not reactive and very reactive promoting fast reactions, depending the surrounding conditions.

Within cells where transitional metals are bounded to proteins (in metal containing proteins or enzymes) oxidative attack of O_2 tend to be slow, meaning that a first single electron is relatively difficult to add. As a consequence superoxid radical ($O_2^{\bullet -}$) will form very slow.

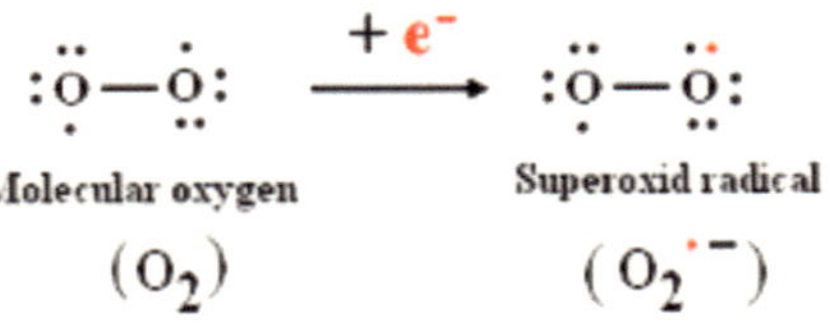

Figure 2. Superoxide radical generation

Once an electron acquired additional electrons are easier added, further reactions quickly occur in [3] and reactive species of oxygen are generated.

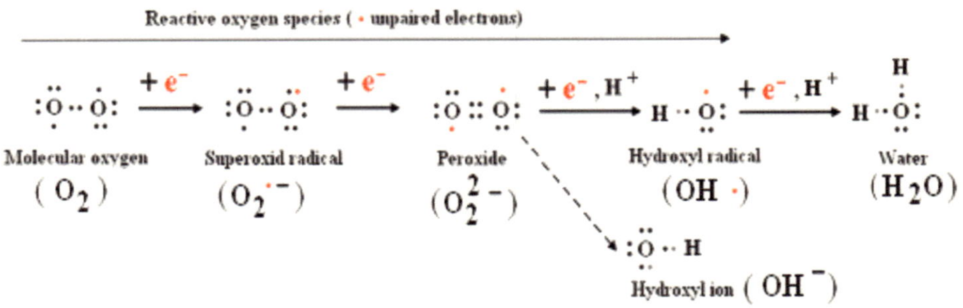

Figure 3. Reactive oxygen species generation

Superoxide ($O_2^{\bullet -}$) is formed when molecular oxygen (O_2) gains an additional electron, producing a molecule with only one unpaired electron (figure 2), generating a very reactive free radical. When accepts an electron, superoxide is reduced to hydrogen peroxide, which is not a radical. In the next one-electron reduction step hydrogen peroxide generates water and the hydroxyl radical ($OH\bullet$) which is probably the most reactive free radical. A final electron acceptance (figure 3) reduces hydroxyl radical to water in [4].

Superoxide radical ($O_2^{\bullet -}$) is a reactive radical, however it cannot diffuse to far having limited lipid solubility. Instead it might react in the presence of ferric iron with de hydrogen peroxide generating the most potent hydroxyl radical through a non-enzymatic reaction known as Haber-Weiss reaction.

The reaction takes place in two steps that involved ferric iron and superoxide as follows:

$$O_2^{\bullet -} + Fe^{3+} \rightarrow O_2 + Fe^{2+}$$

$$Fe^{2+} + H_2O_2 \rightarrow Fe^{3+} + OH^- + OH\bullet$$

The general non-enzymatic reaction occurring in living cells is:

$$O_2^{\bullet -} + H_2O_2 \rightarrow OH\bullet + OH^- + O_2$$

It appears that superoxide radical is also a source of hydroxyl radical in ferric iron presence.

Hydrogen peroxide (H_2O_2) is not a free radical but still classified as a ROS because it generates the most powerful hydroxyl radical ($OH\bullet$) in the presence of transitional metals (Fe^{2+}, Cu^+), the reaction above. Hydrogen peroxide (H_2O_2) is lipid soluble and as a consequence it can diffuse through lipid membranes. No matter where it meets proteins (including hemoglobin) that contain transition metals Fe^{2+}, Cu^{+}, H_2O_2 generates OH• at the specific site where these metals are located thus damaging protein structure.

Another reactive species (but not a radical) derived from molecular oxygen is singlet oxygen, designated as $^1O_2$. Singlet oxygen ($^1O_2$), a highly excited state created when molecular oxygen absorbs sufficient energy to shift an unpaired electron to a higher orbital, can be formed from superoxide radical in [5]:

$$2\,O_2^{\bullet\,-} + 2H^{+} \rightarrow H_2O_2 + {}^1O_2$$

Singlet oxygen is even more reactive than the hydroxyl radical, although it is not a radical.

As a conclusion the most reactive radical is hydroxyl (OH •) which indiscriminately extracts electrons from any other molecules around it whereas superoxide ($O_2^{\bullet-}$) and hydrogen peroxide (H_2O_2) are more selective in their reactions with biological molecules [6].

All the above reactions and processes take place in all human cells including erythrocytes. As for the other cells the main source for free radicals is mitochondrion, in the particular case of red blood cells the main source for radicals is the carried oxygen. Molecular oxygen is carried in order to be delivered to tissues and as a consequence it is found, for a short period of time, free, thus unbound. In this state it might be prone to generate the above described radicals.

Oxygen binds to hemoglobin at the ferrous iron. The ferrous state (Fe^{2+}) of iron is a condition for hemoglobin normal function. However a small percent of Fe^{2+} is slowly converted by O_2 to ferric form (Fe^{3+}) in resulting methemoglobin. An enzymatic system, methemoglobin reductase quickly restores Fe^{3+} to Fe^{2+} and reduces methemoglobin back to hemoglobin. Binding of oxygen to the iron in the hem is considered not to change the oxidation state of the metal. However oxygenated hem has some of the electronic characteristics of a Fe^{3+}–OO^{-} peroxide anion [3]. Misra and Fridovich demonstrate that the $Fe^{3+}O^{2-}$ complex is able to generate superoxide radical in [7] during the normal molecular oxygen transport to tissues through the hemoglobin auto-oxidation. Thus hemoglobin auto-oxidation causes superoxide formation within erytrocyte.

Other researchers show that hemoglobin may undergo oxidative reaction in the oxygen releasing process. Balagopalakrishna and coworkers demonstrate in [8] that at intermediate oxygen pressure, where hemoglobin partially releases molecular oxygen, the superoxide radical production increases. They show that superoxide radical is released in the hydrophobic hem pocket. The process in slow enough thus the formation of superoxide was followed for more than 15 min, and thus detected by low temperature electron paramagnetic resonance technique.

Being a radical superoxide reacts fast with other radicals or alternatively it is efficiently scavenged through the specific superoxide dismutase (SOD) activity.

When collides with other radicals $O_2^{\bullet-}$ gives birth to new reactive species as follows:

- $O_2^{\bullet-}$ reacts with itself generating molecular oxygen (O_2) and hydrogen peroxide (H_2O_2) a source for hydroxyl radical.

- $O_2^{\bullet-}$ reacts fast with NO• radical generating toxic peroxinitrite ($ONOO^-$), a reactive nitrogen specie (RNS). At physiological pH, $ONOO^-$ rapidly protonates to peroxynitrous acid, ONOOH. This powerful oxidizing and nitrating agent can directly damage proteins and lipids.

Thus, any system producing $O_2^{\bullet-}$ and NO• can cause biological damage, and erythrocytes make no exception in [6].

Hydrogen peroxide is not a radical because it doesn't have any unpaired electron. The limited reactivity of H_2O_2 allows it to cross membranes and to become widely dispersed. Even hydrogen peroxide is not a radical it can generates the short-lived but very active hydroxyl radicals via Harber-Weiss non-enzyme reaction in [9]. The hydroxyl radical (OH•), which is highly reactive, diffuses only a short distance before it reacts with whatever biomolecules it collides with. Recent study consider that the high and indiscriminate reactivity of the hydroxyl radical minimizes its ability to diffuse and makes it more damaging within cell or in the environment where it is generated in [10]. This consideration becomes more important when the oxidative events prevail within a specific cellular compartment. Hydroxyl radical are especially dangerous because it can initiate an autocatalytic radical chain reaction. Being so harmful cells carefully control hydroxyl radical by limiting the availability of both Fe^{2+} and H_2O_2 in [6].

The non-enzymatic decomposition of hydrogen peroxide described by Haber-Wiess and especially the mechanism through which hydroxyl radical (OH•) acts was highly debated.

Some researchers consider that hydroxyl radical is responsible for damaging cellular component on behalf of a radical mechanism. Others consider that ferryl ion ($Fe(IV)O^{2+}$), an oxidizing species where iron is in high oxidation state (Fe IV) in [11,12] is an active intermediate responsible for chain reaction propagation. Another group consider that conditions inside cell dictates whether metallo-oxo species or hydroxyl radical (OH•) is the main oxidant [in 13]. Some other like Prousek concluded in [14] that both oxidising species can be formed in living cells.

As a general conclusion in erythrocytes ROS are produced both accidentally and physiologically in different enzyme-catalyzed reactions (figure4).

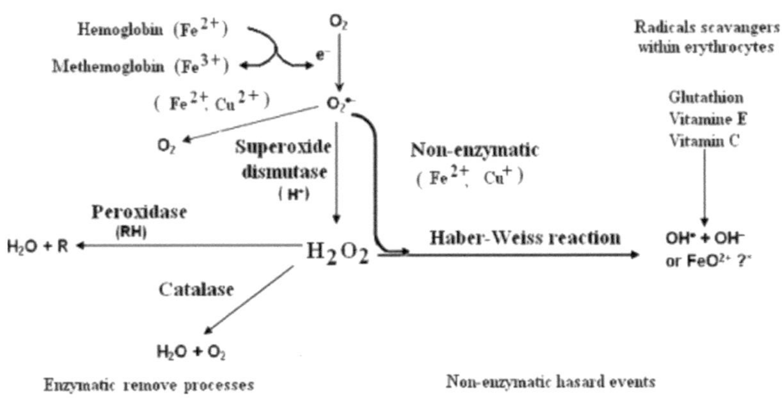

Figure 4. ROS generation in erythrocyte.

2.1.3. Damaging effects of ROS

ROS are considered "bad" radicals because can they indiscriminately interact with any biological molecule they meet causing DNA, lipids and protein damage. As a missing nucleus cell erythrocyte can undergoes the last two lesional processes but endothelium can undergoes all three mentioned injuries. Erythrocytes are particularly affected by oxidation of polyunsaturated fatty acids in membrane phospholipids which causes their peroxidation, degradation and fragmentation [15]. During lipid peroxidation other reactive species as peroxyl radicals are generated in a succession of chain reactions (fig.5). This reactive intermediates amplify the injury at the place were they are formed.

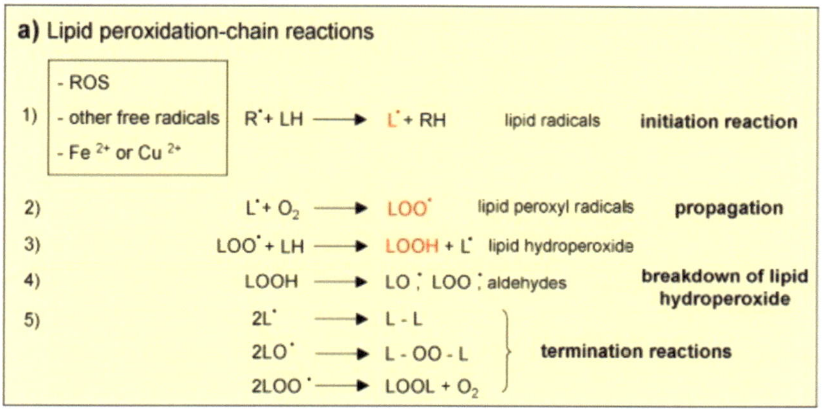

Figure 5. Lipid peroxidation and radical and non-radical intermediates formation [taken from 15]

Erythrocytes also undergo the amino acids and/or whole proteins oxidation. Protein oxidation leads to inactivation (if targeted proteins are enzymes), fragmentation, aggregation of fragments and/or increased susceptibility to proteolysis [**15**]. In addition if injured proteins belong to erythrocytes skeleton the deformability of erythrocytes is impaired [16]. ROS attack doesn't limit to erythrocytes it also affect endothelium cells, which in turn influence erythrocyte metabolism. In nucleus containing endothelium cell beside lipids and proteins oxidation ROS cause DNA injuries. Free radicals can interact with DNA leading to strand breaks or structural changes such as adduct formation (figure 6) [15].

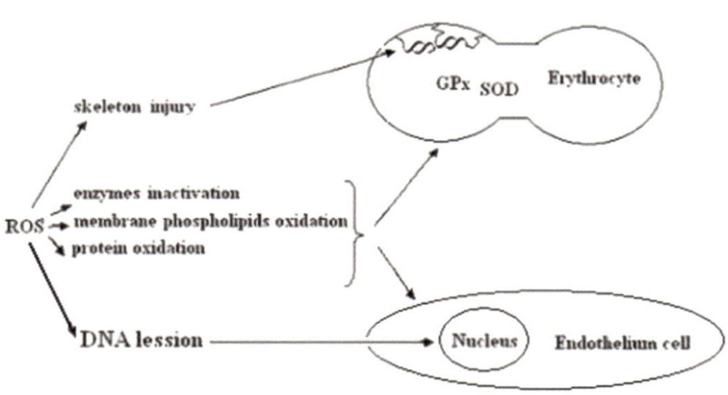

Figure 6. Over simplifying scheme of ROS damaging activity in erythrocytes and in endothelium cells

2.1.4. *ROS signaling*

Until recently reactive oxygen species were considered only oxidizing damaging factors. But it was demonstrated by in [**15, 17**] that ROS can be also "good" as they act as signaling molecules. In fact both authors show that ROS are neither "good" nor "bad", temporal length and intensity of free radicals generation make the difference between physiological, adaptive or pathological effect. Thus oxidizing molecules is not the end "of the road" for reactive species alternatively they trigger cellular responses which depending on the intensity of ROS attack, prepare the cell to survive or on contrary trigger cell death (figure 7).

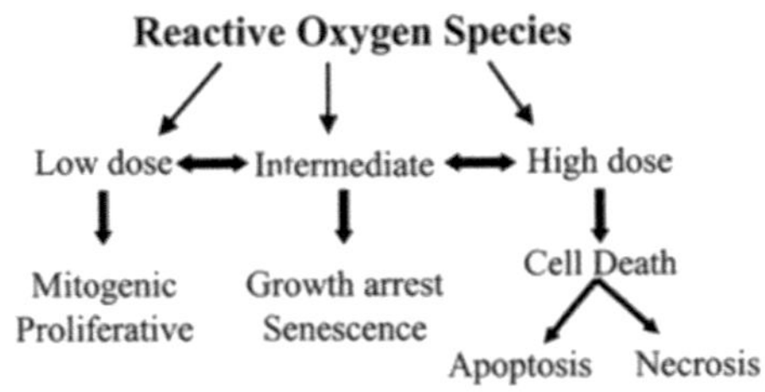

Figure 7. Cells response under ROS attack (taken from 17)

Being highly reactive ROS can intercept cell signaling pathways within successive steps in cascade events modulating the functions of many enzymes and transcription factors. Oxidative stress triggers cellular response by activating many signaling pathways. ROS can directly or indirectly modulate a) the function of different types of enzymes, b) the transcription factors activity and c) the activity of ion-channels.

a. Enzymes modulated by ROS include both kinases and phosphatases. The big class of kinase includes both tyrosine kinase as Src, Ras, JAK2, Pyk2, PI3K, and the mitogen-activated protein kinase (MAPK). The three best-characterized MAPK subfamilies are c-Jun N-terminal kinase (JNK), p38 MAPK and extracellular signal-regulated kinase (ERK) [18]. All these MAPK pathways are structurally similar, but functionally distinct. Importantly, ERK, JNK and p38 MAPK have all been shown to be activated by oxidative stress [19]. ERK and JNK are important in recruiting c-Fos and c-Jun to the nucleus where they activate the transcription factor AP—1 (activator protein -1), whereas activation of p38 and inhibitory kappa kinases (IKK) is important in the transcriptional activation of NF-κB. Both of these factors are important in regulating the diverse genes, which play key roles in the pathogenesis of inflammation, and in regulation of cell cycle, proliferation, and apoptosis. ROS may inhibit tyrosine phosphatase activity further contributing to tyrosine kinase activation.
b. ROS also influence gene and protein expression by activating transcription factors, such as the already mention NFkB and activator protein-1 (AP-1) and hypoxia-inducible factor-1 (HIF-1).
c. ROS stimulate ion channels, such as plasma membrane Ca2+ and K+ channels, leading to changes in cation concentration. The cytosolic Ca^{2+} level can be increased by ROS in various cell types, including epithelium cell, through the mobilization of intracellular Ca^{2+}stores and/or through the influx of extracellular Ca^{2+} [15]. The ROS-mediated increase

in Ca^{2+}concentration contributes to the oxidative stress-mediated activation of PKC and to the transcriptional induction of the AP-1 proteins c-Fos and c-Jun [20] (figure 8).

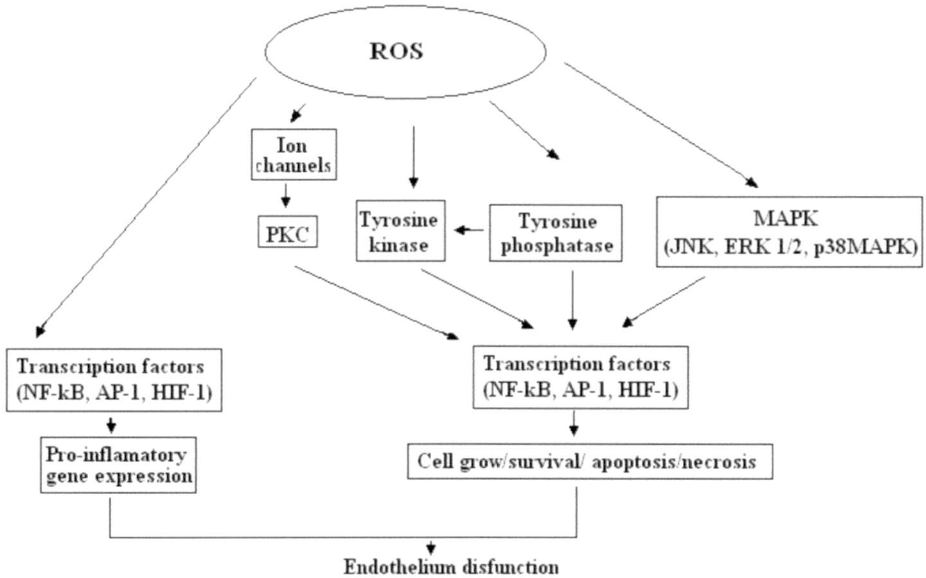

Figure 8. Major pathways activated by ROS generation (modified from **21)**.MAPK=mitogen-activated protein, JNK=c-Jun N-terminal kinases, ERK=extracellular signal-regulated kinases, NFκB=nuclear factor κB, AP-1=activator protein-1, HIF-1= hypoxia-inducible factor-1, PKC=protein kinase C

More details about the cellular response in ROS and other radical and non-radicals species attack in oxidative events can be found in [15,17,19]

2.1.5. Scavenging ROS

Erythrocytes have an impressing antioxidant enzyme and non-enzyme system that deals with an important amount of free radicals. Superoxide dismutase and glutathione peroxidase are the most efficient antioxidant enzyme in red blood cells.

Erythrocytes superoxide dismutase remove $O_2^{\bullet-}$ by catalyzing its dismutation, one $O_2^{\bullet-}$ being reduced to H_2O_2 and another oxidized to O_2 (figure 9).

$$2\,O_2^{\bullet-} + 2\,H^+ \xrightarrow{\text{Superoxide dismutase}} O_2 + H_2O_2$$

Figure 9. Superoxide dismutase activity

The dismutation of superoxide $O_2^{\bullet\,-}$by SOD is very efficient having the largest k_{cat}/K_M (an approximation of catalytic efficiency) of any known enzyme (~7 x 10^9 $M^{-1}s^{-1}$) [22]. SOD catalyst activity is limited only by the frequency of collision with superoxide. That means the reaction rate is limited only by the diffusion of superoxid radical. Diffusion limitation becomes canceled in radicals over production thus activating the process.

As seen in upper reaction (fig.9) superoxide dismutase must work with enzymes that remove H_2O_2.

Glutathione peroxidase (GPx) removes H_2O_2 by coupling its reduction to water (figure10) with oxidation of reduced glutathione (GSH), a thiol-containing tripeptide (glu-cys-gly). The product, oxidized glutathione (GS-SG), consists of two GSH linked by a disulphide bridge, and can be converted back to GSH by glutathione reductase enzymes in [6].

$$H_2O_2 + 2GSH \xrightarrow{\text{Glutathion peroxidase}} GSSG + 2H_2O$$

Figure 10. Glutathion peroxidase activity.

Beside enzyme antioxidant systems erythrocytes uses antioxidants agents (fig.4). These agents are preferentially oxidized by reactive species to preserve more important biomolecules and can be reversibly reduced back. For example, GSH and ascorbate can scavenge $O_2^{\bullet -}$, OH•, and also ONOOH. Tocopherols are good scavengers of peroxyl radicals and help to protect membranes against lipid peroxidation by interrupting the propagation-chain reaction (figure 5) in [6].

2.1.6. Reactive nitrogen species

Nitrogen compounds found in the body comes from exogenous sources as nitrites/nitrates or from endogen production of nitric oxide (NO•). The group of nitrogen derivatives includes:

- NO• nitric oxide a natural free radical also named nitrogen monoxide is involved in vasodilatation in mammals
- NO_2^- nitrogen dioxide or nitrite. In organism is found in its corresponding salts nitrites(from nitrous acid HNO_2)
- NO_3^- nitrate (from nitric acid HNO_3) also found in the body in corresponding salts

$$\underset{\text{Nitrate}}{NO_3^-} \rightleftharpoons \underset{\text{Nitrite}}{NO_2^-} \rightleftharpoons \underset{\text{Nitric oxid}}{NO\bullet}$$

Figure 11. Nitrogen derivatives

Nitrogen derivatives convert into each other forward and backward continuously under shifting conditions within cells (figure11).

Endogenous NO• is synthesized by nitric oxide synthases (NOS) in the endothelial and other cells, where is involved in vascular physiology.

Endothelial nitric oxide synthases (eNOS) synthesizes NO• (figure 12) from L-arginine with 1,5 consumption of 1.5 NADPH equivalents and two oxygen molecules per NO• formed in [23]. The reaction requires the presence of Ca^{2+}-Calmodulin and tetrahydrobiopterin (BH_4) as cofactors in[24].

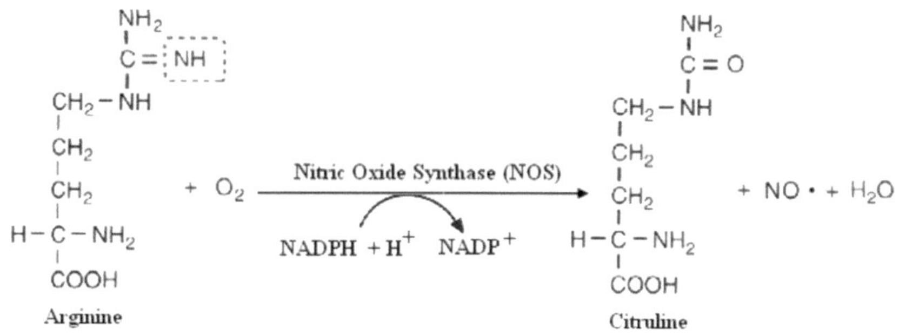

Figure 12. Nitric oxide generation

Generated NO• is a gaseous molecule with unpaired electrons and as a consequence a radical; it is lipophilic and diffuses rapidly through membranes. NO• is a messenger in many physiological processes: endothelial relaxation of the smooth muscle, inhibition of platelet aggregation, neurotransmission and cytoxicity in [25]. NO• pathology includes both low and high concentrations as follows: insufficient NO• production is involved in hypertension, the activation of platelet aggregation and atherogenesis while high NO• production generates septic shock, stroke, and carcinogenesis.

NO• released from endothelial cells diffuses through blood or to the underlining smooth muscle cells in the media where it triggers vasodilatation. In blood stream NO• will affect platelets, leucocytes and erythrocytes.

Recent studies show that:

a. e-NOS can produce NO • not only in normal oxygenation (figure 12) but also decreased oxygenation gradient across vascular branches. In addition eNOS can sometimes be a source of ROS generating $O_2^{\bullet-}$
b. endothelial cells are not the only ones able to generate NO•, blood erythrocytes are expressing functional NOS
c. Hemoglobin itself also "produces" NO• from nitrite in order to modulate vasodilatation.

a. It is only recently found that endothelial NOS may be a source of ROS generating $O_2^{\bullet-}$ depending the availability of its substrates within cell (figure 13) [23].

Endothelial nitric oxide synthetase activity is regulated by a combination of mechanisms that allow eNOS to modulate its activity under physio-pathological condition in [22]. eNOS contains 2 enzymatic domains, a flavin-containing reductase and a heme-containing oxygenase domain (Fe^{3+}) connected by a regulatory calmodulin-binding domain. Binding of the Ca^{2+}/calmodulin complex orients the other domains in such a position that NADPH-derived electrons generated on the reductase domain flow to the oxygenase domain in [26].

The oxygenase domain of eNOS contains an iron ion (Fe^{3+}) that binds oxygen on reduction Fe^{2+}, and this complex finally causes the conversion of L-arginine to NO• and L-citrulline. This sequence of events properly rules if the cofactor BH_4 "provides the connection" between the two domains. Deficiency of arginine or BH_4 causes the reductase uncoupling from oxygenase. At the oxygenase domain intermediate Fe^{2+}-O_2 complex dissociates to form superoxide and the original Fe^{3+} group of the eNOS)[27]. Thus eNOS releases $O_2^{\bullet -}$ instead of NO• (figure 9).

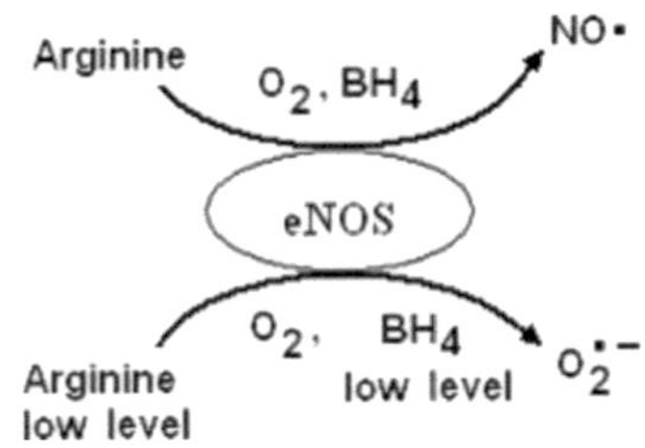

Figure 13. Endothelial NOS differently behaves generating either NO• or $O_2^{\bullet -}$ depending on the substrate availability.

Oxygen deficiency is known to halt the L-arginine cycle if the oxygen levels fall below a threshold level of ca $[O_2]$ ~ 10 μM [28]. However, eNOS is not wholly inactivated in hypoxia, instead, in the presence of nitrite (figure 14), it shifts again and produces NO• in [29].

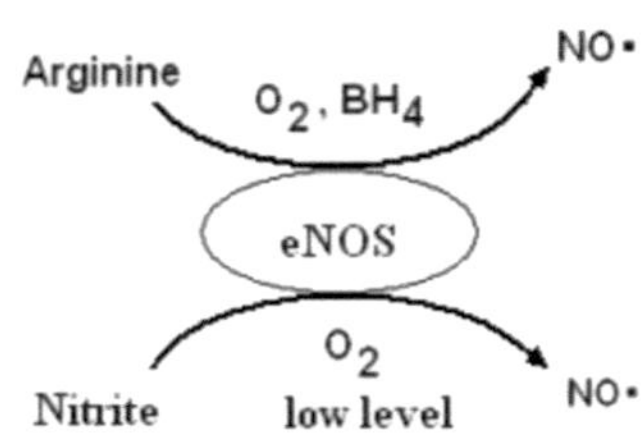

Figure 14. Endothelial NOS may generate NO• in both normal and low oxygenation

Stroes et al demonstrate in [30, 31] an intriguing activity for eNOS only, the simultaneous generation of both NO• and superoxide, even in the presence of BH_4 and L-arginine, under physiological conditions. The consequence is the production of peroxynitrite, a highly reactive molecule, by eNOS (figure 15).

Thus eNOS is a source of free radical producing "good" or "bad" radicals upon inside cell condition.

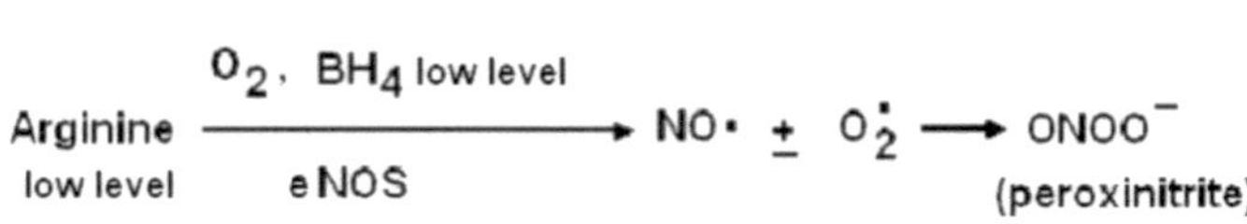

Figure 15. Peroxinitrite generation as a result of particularly eNOS activity

Peroxynitrite anion ($ONOO^-$) is a reactive species of increasingly recognized biological relevance that contributes to oxidative tissue damage. Recent research indicates in [32] that peroxynitrite is able to cross the erythrocyte membrane by two different mechanisms: in the anionic form through the anion exchange channel, and in the protonated form by passive diffusion. Entering the erythrocyte peroxynitrite causes nitration of intracellular hemoglobin, in a process that is enhanced in thiol-depleted erythrocytes.

To summarize NO• can be produced by eNOS from either L-arginine in good oxygenation physiological state or from nitrite in hypoxia. In vitamins deficiency (low BH4 levels) eNOS produces superoxide radical. Recent studies demonstrate that endothelium cells surprisingly produce ROS under hypoxia. The primary site of reactive oxygen species production was demonstrated to be complex III in electron transport in mitochondria. The paradoxically increase in ROS production under low oxygenation is still not fully understood but it is considered that reactive oxygen species released during hypoxia act as signalling agents that trigger induction of erythropoietin, endothelial growth factor and glycolytic enzymes. Systemically, these responses enhance the delivery of O_2 to cells and facilitate the production of glycolytic ATP instead of mitochondrion. Induction of these genes is mediated by "specialized" hypoxia inducible factor 1 (HIF-1) [33, 34]. As a conclusion in normal oxygenation NO is produced by eNOS. In hypoxia adaptive responses are onset; the release of NO from nitrite to sustain normal vascular function is one path. Alternatively when mitochondrion "senses" hypoxia it releases ROS as signaling molecules that activate diverse functional responses, including activation of gene expression that promote cell survival.

b. Kleinbongard demonstrates in [35] that red blood cells express functional eNOS which is located in both the internal side of the plasma membrane and the cytoplasm with a higher expression in the membrane. The enzyme has a similar activity and regulatory mechanism as the endothelial-derived NOS. Besides its vasodilatation activity NO• also regulates red blood cells deformability and inhibits platelet activation. In physiological condition where there is a normal supply of L-Arginine and subsequently a normal NO• production, nitric oxide sustains red blood cells deformability. On contrary decreased NO• levels reduces erythrocytes deformability preventing them to easily pass through microcirculation. The same effect was observed on platelet aggregation when decreased NO• levels promote thrombosis.

Ulker demonstrates in [36] that red blood cell-NOS is activated by mechanical factors and that export of NO from erythrocytes is enhanced by mechanical stress thus pointing erythrocyte contribution to the regulation of vascular tonus

c. NO• is a short life species as a consequence it quickly reacts with any encountered molecules or it is rapidly oxidized by hemoglobin in blood. In fact the general accepted theory is that Hb in the red blood cells is an extremely effective NO• scavenger in [37]. Oxigenated-Hb reacts with NO• which is rapidly converted into nitrate (figure 16). After reacting oxygenated hemoglobin is converted to methemoglobin (met-Hb). This reaction is considered to be limited only by the diffusion.

$$\underset{\text{oxyhemoglobin}}{\text{Hb-Fe (II)}O_2} + NO\bullet \longrightarrow \underset{\text{methemoglobin}}{\text{Hb (Fe III)}} + \underset{\text{nitrate}}{NO_3^-}$$

Figure 16. Oxyhemoglobin activity of scavenging the nitric oxide

Lundberg shows in [38] that NO• can be alternatively produced in hypoxic condition by deoxi-hemoglobin from nitrite. Inside erythrocyte Hb can interact with NO• in many ways depending on its oxygen saturation, as follows:

- in oxygenated form, oxi-Hb acts as a scavenger removing NO• as nitrate.
- in deoxygenated form deoxi-Hb acts in two different ways: first it binds NO• thus functioning as a transporter and second it reduces nitrite to generate NO• (figure17) Recently several authors suggest in [39-41] that this behavior represents a mechanism for NO• generation in regions of poor oxygenation where deoxy-Hb predominates

NO generation

Hb-Fe(II) deoxyhemoglobin	+	NO_2^- nitrite	→	Hb-Fe(III) methemoglobin	+	NO nitric oxide

NO binding/release

Hb-Fe(II) deoxyhemoglobin	+	NO	↔	Hb-Fe(II)NO nitrosyl-hemoglobin
Hb(β93-cys)	+	NO	↔	Hb(β93-cys-NO) S-nitrosohemoglobin

NO consumption

Hb-Fe(II)O_2 oxyhemoglobin	+	NO	→	Hb-Fe(III) methemoglobin	+	NO_3^- nitrate

Figure 17. Hemoglobin "regulates" the NO• use/consumption, from [38]

Two recent theories try to explain the Hb involvement in nitric oxide use/consumption in vasorelaxation process in [42].

- Stamler and colleagues originally suggested in [43] a role for a thiol (SH) group in Hb as a carrier and releaser of NO•. According to this theory, the binding (formation of *S*-nitrosohemoglobin) and release of NO• from Hb are allosterically regulated so that NO• release occurs when Hb is deoxygenated.
- Cosby, Crowford et all suggest in [44] that Hb is not a transporter of NO• but rather an "enzyme" dealing with NO• depending oxygen saturation as follows: when Hb is fully oxygenated, the primary reaction is oxidation of nitrite into biologically inert and supposed "pool" nitrate. As oxygen saturation falls along the vascular tree, Hb gradually turns into a "reductase" and starts to reduce nitrite into vasodilator NO• (figure 18). The maximal nitrite reduction is observed when Hb is approximately 50% oxygenated (P_{50}) in [45,46]. Concomitantly, vasodilation is initiated at the P_{50}, ideally suited for the regulation of hypoxic vasodilation under varied physiologic and pathologic conditions (figure 19).

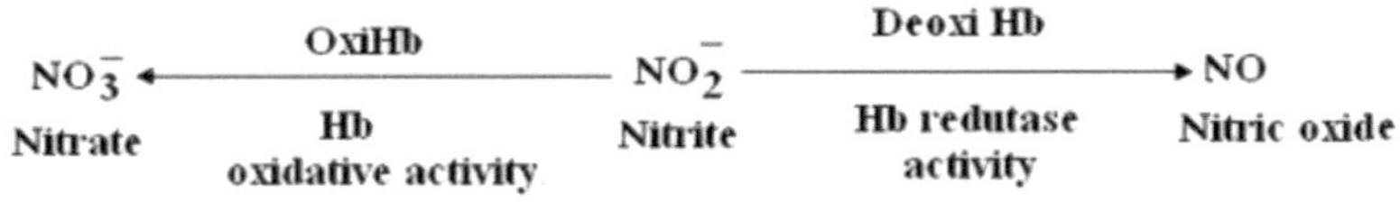

Figure 18. Hemoglobin behavior depending on oxygen saturation.

J.O.Lunderg concluded in [42] that: "in just one decade, Hb has gone from being merely a NO• scavenger to NO• carrier and now NO• generator".

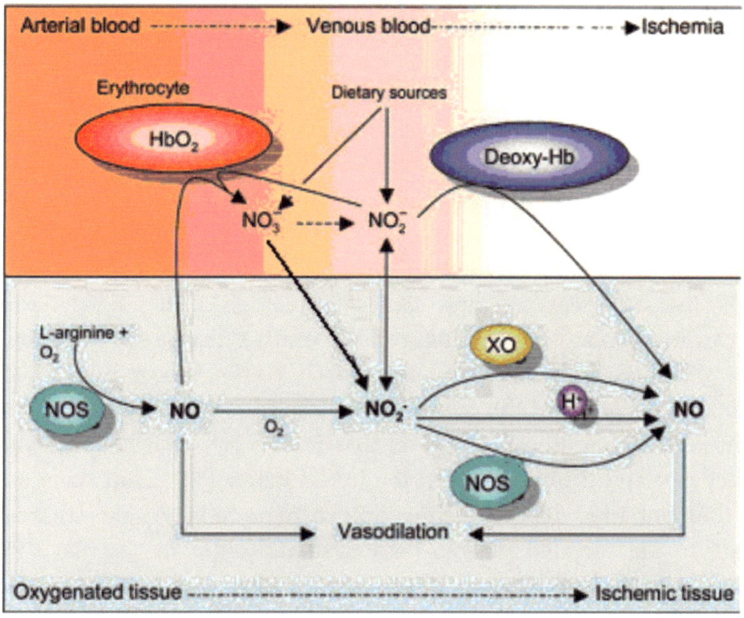

Figure 19. Hemoglobin uses NO• to generate nitrate a supposed "NO_2^-/ NO• pool" in full oxygenation and releases it with maximal activity at P_{50} oxygen saturation in hypoxia [modified from [38].

To summarize: when there is plenty of oxygen, NO• is mainly produced by endothelial NOS or by erythrocyte own NOS. Thus nitric oxide radical maintains good erythrocytes deformability and probably oxy-Hb regulates the amount of NO• by trapping its extra amount to form *S*-nitrosohemoglobin. When oxygen is scarce NO• is synthesized in low amount (as a consequence of low eNOS activity where oxygen is cofactor). In this condition NO• is saved through binding on deoxyHb which becomes a source of NO• in vascular circulation, or deoxy-Hb "catalyses" the NO• generation from nitrite. Behaving this way deoxy-Hb can maintain also red blood cell deformability in hypoxic condition. As a consequence hemoglobin may "regulates" membrane deformability along circulating branches through the way it uses/produces NO• radical. [47]

In addition two other supplementary mechanisms, endothelial xantinoxidase activity and blood pH dictate superoxid radical versus NO• generation depending on the blood oxygenation/deoxigenation status in [48,49].

2.2. Homocysteine metabolism

Homocysteine is a metabolic compound formed in methionine and betaine metabolism. The already mention metabolisms require vitamin B_{12}, B_6 and folic acid involvement and the proper activity of two main enzymes cystathionine β-synthase (CBS) and methylenetetrahydrofolate reductase (MTHFR). Every deficiency in vitamins supplies or enzymes activity triggers the onset of different disease. Megaloblastic anemia or Biermer disease affect primarily the red blood cells. Secondary to the above mentioned illnesses hyperhomocysteinemia can also install.

Hyperhomocysteinemia is considered to be involved in many diseases from cardiovascular to neurological illnesses. It is generally agreed that two general mechanisms cause hyperhomocysteinemia: one is low vitamins (B12, B6, folic acid) supplies and second the main enzymes deficiencies (cystathionine ß-synthase deficiency and methylenetetrahydrofolate reductase deficiency). Hypehomocysteinemia is today considered a severe risk factor in vascular illnesses. Many approaches envisage lowering homocysteine levels by vitamin B or oral folic acid supplementation but many recent studies show that vitamins administration fail to give a real clinical benefit and suggest that B vitamins might instead increase some cardiovascular risks in [50,51]. However not all patients with cardiovascular events or neurodegenerative diseases are enzymes deficient or poor vitamins supplied. The majority of research works report hyperhomocysteinemia associated to many diseases but the question what triggers hyperhomocysteinemia is yet to answer. An interesting hypothesis suggests that in fact hyperhomocysteinemia is more a secondary effect that amplifies in its turn the initial injury [52]. Brattström and Wilcken in [52] consider that impaired renal function due to hypertension and atherosclerosis is an important cause of the elevated plasma homocysteine found in vascular disease patients. The reasons are as follows. Atherogenesis and elevation of blood pressure commonly develop silently over many years before the emergence of clinically evident vascular events. These processes also lead to nephrosclerosis and a degree of deterioration of renal function, and this is highly relevant to the plasma clearance of homocysteine. For these reasons, the presence of vascular disease itself may contribute to an elevation in circulating homocysteine by leading to a decline in renal function. This means that because of reduced renal function, patients with either occult or clinically evident cardiovascular disease may have elevated circulating homocysteine concentrations (figure 20). This could also explain the relation between plasma homocysteine and the severity of atherosclerosis.

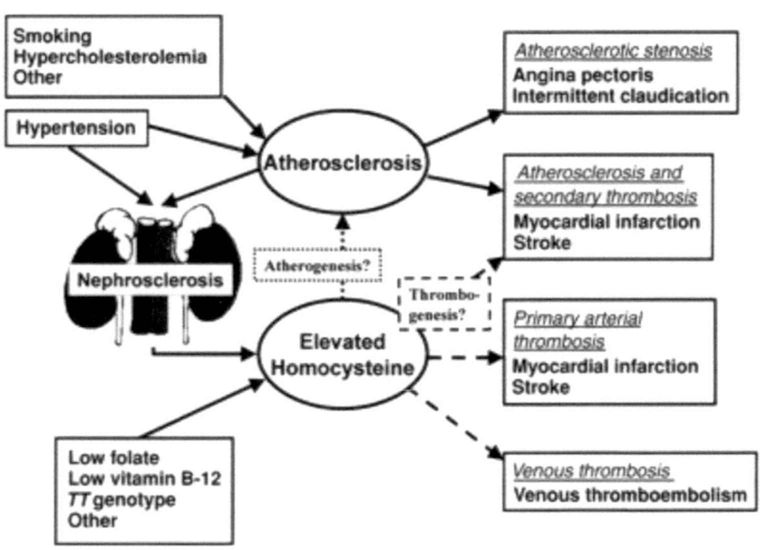

Figure 20. Proposed mechanisms for the causes of hyperhomocysteinemia (taken from [52])

2.3. Hyperhomocysteinemia a disturbing factor of the endothelial function

Homocysteine refers to all species that contain and can release homocystein including homocystine (the dimer of homocysteine) and mixed cysteine-homocysteine disulfide or homocysteine bound on proteins. In fact the major form of homocysteine in circulation, around 70% is protein bounded.

In early data normal levels of homocysteine were admitted to be around 15μM/L. It was found that homocysteine slightly increases with age in [53]. Levels of 15-30 μM/L corresponds to mild, 30-100 μM/L to moderate and more than 100 μM/L to severe hyperhomocysteinemia in [54].

Nowadays it is considered that concentrations below 9 micro mol/L are an appropriate target level for therapy in [55].

Nowadays it is generally accepted that homocysteine promotes thrombosis with simultaneously vasodilatation inhibition. It is considered that homocysteine triggers its effects by three distinct mechanisms which can possibly integrate and are not mutually exclusive; oxidative processes, decreasing NO• bioavailability and specific protein targeting (figure 21).

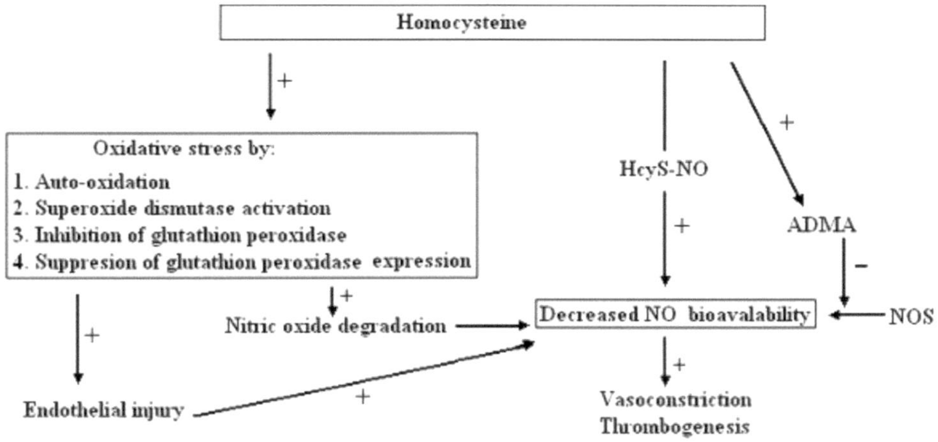

Figure 21. Homocysteine adverse effects. (+/— represent activation/inhibition processes)

Even the precise path was not yet established, it seems that Hcys inhibits some "good" factors and activates same "bad" factors that finally influence the processes of thrombosis-fibrinolysis and constriction–vasorelaxation and which are summarized in (figure 21) [56].

Amongst "good" factor can be included: NO•, GPx, eNOS, protein C, tissue Plasminogen Activator (tPA), annexin II. Amongst "bad" factor can be included: ADMA, $O_2^{\bullet -}$, H_2O_2

Homocysteine directly and indirectly influences erythrocytes metabolism. It directly affects the erythrocyte antioxidant enzyme systems promoting free radical generation. Indirectly Hcy decreases NO• bioavailability and modifies the environment where erythrocytes move and act.

2.3.1. Homocysteine pro-oxidative activity

Homocysteine is involved in reducing–oxidative processes by reacting either with itself or with different compounds. In other words homocysteine can submit auto-oxidative as well as oxidative processes.

Thiols (RSH) can auto-oxidize in the presence of transition metal catalysts and molecular oxygen, leading to the formation of reactive oxygen species (ROS). Hcy like all containing thiol group undergoes oxidation to disulfide (RS-SR) in O_2 presence at normal pH. It was found that cooper catalyses Hcy (noted with general formula RSH) auto-oxidation, even in low homocysteine concentration, yielding hydrogen peroxide and thus promoting ROS generation in both extra and intracellular compartments through reaction proposed by Starkebaum in [57]:

$$2\text{ Homocysteine (RSH)} + O_2 \rightarrow \text{Homocystine (RS-SR)}$$

$$\text{Homocystine (RS-SR)} + \text{superoxid } (O_2^{\bullet -}) \rightarrow H_2O_2$$

Hydrogen peroxide generated by the copper catalysed auto-oxidation of homocysteine was involved in the mechanism of toxicity by the demonstration of the reduction in endothelial damage with the addition of catalase in [58].

Homocysteine was proved to generate superoxide radicals which promote vasoconstriction. Lang et al. demonstrates in [59] that the inhibitory effect of homocysteine on endothelium-dependent relaxation is caused by an increase of the intracellular levels of $O_2^{\bullet -}$ in the endothelial cell and provide a possible mechanism for the endothelial dysfunction associated with hyperhomocysteinemia.

Cysteine is also a thiol circulating aminoacid related to homocysteine and its concentration is 20 to 30 times higher than Hcys one. In fact Cys is the main circulatory thiol but there was found no correlation of Cys with free radicals generation. Instead a strong association of hyperhomocysteinemia with F_2-isoprostane was found. F_2-isoprostane is an indicator of in vivo lipid-peroxidation and its association with Hcy lead to the conclusion that this amino acid is involved in free radicals generation in [60] thus pointing Hcy as pro-oxidative agent.

Hcy involvement in ROS generation was also indirectly proved in connection with antioxidant enzyme system modulation SOD and GPx.

The activity of superoxide dismutase, an important antioxidant enzyme in vascular tissue, was measured along with homocysteine in homocystinuric patients and found to be positively associated with homocysteine levels. This strong relationship can be regarded as a protective antioxidant response to homocysteine-induced oxidative action and as indirect evidence that Hcy represents a source of free radicals in [61]. In our study we found an increased superoxide dismutase activity in red blood cells lysate in experimental induced hyperhocysteinemia in rats. We consider this increased response in enzyme activity as evidence for free radicals' production in [62].

Homocysteine may affect glutathione peroxidase activity, thus altering the microenvironment in the propagation of ROS in [63]. Our study on GPx activity, in installed hyperhomocysteinemia, was consistent with these reported data. GPx activity in red blood cells lysate significantly decreases as a consequence of experimental induced hypehocysteinemia in rats. We considered that increased amount of free radicals consume the GSH enzyme cofactor which subsequently trigger the enzyme activity decay in [62]. As a consequence GPx activity is lowered in hyperhomocysteinemia thus disturbing the detoxification process of H_2O_2 within cell.

Upchurch in[63] demonstrates that homocysteine reduces mRNA levels of glutathione peroxidase, indicating that the expression of this enzyme is inhibited and/or down-regulated.

Even it was attributed to different causes such as: a decrease in enzyme activity, a down regulation from high homocysteine levels or an inappropriate gene expression of GPx, the decrease in GPx activity in Hcys presence is generally reported.

Homocysteine-induced oxidative stress was proved to be generated within vascular cells in [64]. Our data show that in installed hyperhomocysteinemia the intracellular space is more affected than the extracellular, circulatory one. We found significant changes in antioxidant enzyme systems within erythrocyte (we worked on erythrocyte lysate) as compared with total antioxidant capacity (TAC) in plasma in [62].

As a conclusion hyperhomocysteinemia by promoting free radical generation affects both erythrocytes and endothelial cells as well in [65,66].

2.3.2. Homocysteine decreases NO bioavailability

The second hypothesis considers that Hcy acts to prevent NO• bioavailability. This process is considered to have, at least partially, the same oxidative basis. In living organisms, including in human, endothelial-derived nitric oxide performs the following function: regulates vessel tone by promoting vasodilatation, inhibits platelet activation, adhesion and aggregation, limits smooth muscle proliferation and modulates endothelial–leukocyte interactions in [56]. Homoysteine was proved to limits NO bioavailability thus promoting the contrary processes: vasoconstriction, thrombosis and fibrinolysis inhibition.

There are proposed many patterns for homocysteine impairing NO• bioavailability (figure 22).

A first process that limits NO• bioavailability seems to be more a protecting mechanism than a harmful one. Homocysteine reacts with nitric oxide to form S-nitroso-homocysteine, which has some of the properties of nitric oxide. It markedly inhibits platelet aggregation, is a potent vasodilator and does not support hydrogen peroxide generation. This represents much more a protective mechanism against the adverse effects of homocysteine than a limiting process in NO• bioavailability in [56].

However prolonged exposure to high homocysteine concentrations impairs nitric oxide production. Thus in hyperhomocysteinemia the limited bioavailability of nitric oxide could be due to S-nitrosothiol formation in [67].

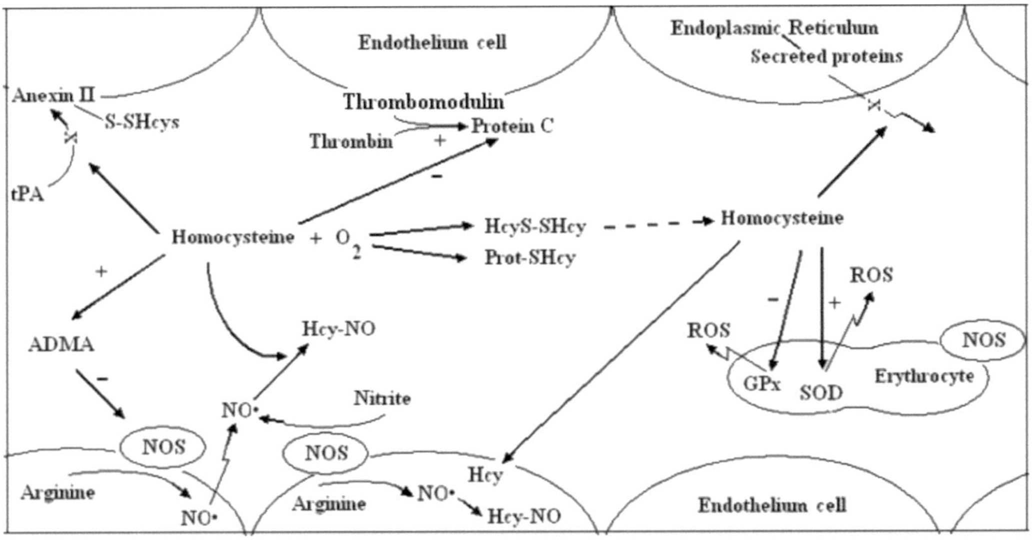

Figure 22. Proposed mechanism through which Hcy inhibits some "good" factors and activates same "bad" factors thus influencing thrombosis-fibrinolysis respectively constriction–vasorelaxation processes. tPA, ADMA represents tissue plasminogen activator/respectively asymmetrical dimethyl arginine.

A second process that limits NO• bioavailability is nitric oxide trapping/degradation by other radical species. NO• is trapped by superoxide to form peroxinitrite thus being inactivated. This mechanism was confirmed by many experimental data in [63, 68].

Nitric oxide can be alternatively degraded by hydrogen peroxide as a consequence of GPx activity inhibition through Hcy-dependent mechanism. Homocysteine seems to be the only amino acid amongst all circulating others capable to inhibit glutathione peroxidase activity in vitro. Cysteine is also capable of generating free radicals and is present in serum at concentrations four times higher than homocysteine but cysteine doesn't prove inhibiting properties on GPx activity. Experimental data show that Hcy inhibits GPx activity and also suppresses the cellular GPx expression thus promoting the increase of hydrogen peroxide concentration in [64]. Hydrogen peroxide promotes in its turn free radicals generation and peroxinitrite production thus decreasing NO• availability.

A third mechanism that limits NO• bioavailability is the decrease in NO• synthesis through Hcy-dependent asymmetrical dimethylarginine (ADMA) generation. ADMA is produced by methylation of specific arginine residues of certain cellular proteins. Most of these proteins are found in the nucleus. When the proteins are degraded, ADMA and other isomers are released to the extracellular space where especially ADMA acts as potent endogenous inhibitors of NOS enzyme in [69].

Methionine loading was proved to induce hyperhomocysteinemia. In methionine loading there is S-adenosylmethionine accumulation and as a consequence a high proteins methylation. Asymmetrical dimethylarginine (ADMA) the product of degradation from methylated proteins competitively inhibits NO-synthetase activity. Elevated ADMA levels found in hyperhomocysteinemia are supposed to inhibit NO• synthesis thus decreasing the NO availability in [70].

2.3.3. *Homocysteine own action*

A third way that homocysteine acts is targeting specific proteins which are located within cell, on cell membrane or in the extracellular space.

Two important intracellular proteins, already mentioned, targeted by Hcy are the antioxidant enzyme GPx which activity decreases and SOD which activity increases in homocysteine presence (fig22). Hcy alters other intracellular proteins disturbing the redox potential of endoplasmic reticulum and Golgi apparatus thus inhibiting the surface expression and secretion of proteins in [71,72].

Hcy targets proteins located on both membrane surface and within cell. Jacobsen considers that circulatory oxidized form of Hcy enters the cell were it is converted back to reduced Hcy, in reducing environment within cell. Under reduced form Hcy impairs the binding of tissue plasminogen activator (tPA), a protein involved in the breakdown of blood clots, to annexin II in [71] by forming a disulfide bridge with Cys9 on annexin II. Thus Hcy limits the plasminogen conversion to plasmin. This results in a decreased fibrinolysis. The circulating reduced Hcy acts in the same manner with annexin II on the membrane from the vascular endothelium. Homocysteine was found to be the only circulating thiol that impairs the binding of tissue-plasminogen activator.

The atherogenic factor lipoprotein (a) [Lp (a)] competitively inhibits the binding of plasminogen to fibrin. Fibrin is a cofactor for plasminogen activation to plasmin, an important enzyme that degrades fibrin clot. Homocysteine was found to interfere in this process. Hcy and lipoprotein (a) seems to act in the same direction: homocysteine promotes lipoprotein(a) binding to fibrin and lipoprotein(a) competitively inhibits the binding of plasminogen to fibrin. The final effect is the decrease of fibrinolysis. The combination of Lp (a) plus homocysteine is a possible mechanisms for the occurrence of thrombosis in hyperhomocysteinemia in [73].

Protein C is an example of circulating proteins whose activity is inhibited by Hcy. The protein C enzyme system appears to be one of the most important anticoagulant pathways in the blood. Its activation depends on the complex thrombomodulin-trombin. Thrombomodulin is an integral membrane protein expressed on the surface of endothelial cells where it serves as a receptor for thrombin. The complex thrombomodulin-trombin activates protein C thus raising its activity. Homocysteine inhibits the function of thrombomodulin. Both thrombomodulin and protein C contain disulfide-rich domains. Reduction of these disulfide bonds by homocysteine may disrupt important structures within these domains, resulting in impaired function in [74]. The result is the promotion of thrombotic process.

Hcy acts on both endothelial cells and smooth muscle where it generates contrasting effect. On endothelium it promotes injury and impairs DNA repair, in smooth muscle Hcy stimulates proliferation in [69]. Md S. Jamaluddin considers that Hcys promotes vascular injury through hypomethylation. When Hcys accumulates it uses adenosine, a normal constituent of all cells, to form S-adenosyl-homocysteine (SAH) a potent inhibitor of cellular methylation. By impairing methylation Hcy arrests cell growth, increases cellular SAH concentration in endothelial cells (EC) and decreased DNA synthesis thus decreasing cellular repair. This chain of events was not found in vascular smooth muscle cells in [75].

Erythrocytes are also affected by homocysteine-induced hypometilation. High intracellular SAH impairs the posttranslational methylation of membrane proteins. Reduction in membrane protein methylation was particularly observed for erythrocyte cytoskeletal component ankyrin, which is known to be involved in membrane stability and integrity. Because of hypomethylation, structural damages accumulate in erythrocyte membrane proteins, and are not adequately repaired thus affecting membrane physical properties. Erythrocyte deformability is a crucial properties for circulatory function in [76].

As a conclusion the effect of elevated homocysteine appears multifactorial affecting both the vascular wall structure and the blood coagulation system as well as erythrocytes metabolism in [77].

3. The pharmacological influences on the blood cell metabolism – Antioxidant drugs in cardiovascular risk status and roll of red blood cell antioxidant defense capacity

There are growing evidences on the role of adaptive mechanisms of erythrocyte in pathological processes: atherosclerosis, ischemic attack, bacterial infections, etc. All of this processes involve as main mechanism oxidative stress. Erythrocytes have an intracellular enzyme and non-enzyme defense system. In order to remove reactive species of oxygen, superoxide dismutase (SOD), glutathione peroxidase (GPx) and catalase act together. Glutathione (GSH) participates as a co-substrate for GPx in order to detoxify H_2O_2 generated by SOD enzyme. GSH is a critical tripeptide that oxidizes to glutathione disulphide (GS-SG) inactive form after reacting with oxygen radicals. GSH proves to be essential for reactive species detoxification as a consequence it is permanently restore in its reduced active form by glutathione reductase based on nicotinamide adenine dinucleotide phosphate-oxidase (NADPH) from Glucose-6-phosphate dehydrogenase (G6P-DH) catalysed reaction in pentose phosphate pathway. When reactive species of oxygen are quickly and intensely generated under external or internal stimulus the activity of SOD, GPx and GSH concentration are severely changed.

When erythrocytes are undergo shear stress in constricted vessels, they release ATP which causes the vessel walls to relax and dilate so as to promote normal blood flow [78].

Also, when their hemoglobin molecules are deoxygenated, erythrocytes release **S-**nitrosothiols which acts to dilate vessels, thus directing more blood to areas of the body depleted of oxygen in [35].

Using L-arginine as substrate, erythrocytes can also synthesize nitric oxide enzymatically, just like endothelial cells. The nitric oxide synthase is activated when the erythrocytes are exposure to physiological levels of shear stress, thus, nitric oxide is synthesized, exported and it may contribute to the regulation of vascular tonus [79].

Another mechanism that involves the erythrocytes in relaxing vessel walls is the production of hydrogen sulfide. It works as a signaling gas. It is believed that the cardioprotective effects of garlic are due to erythrocytes converting its sulfur compounds into hydrogen sulfide. [80]

The free radicals released by erythrocytes when they are lysed by pathogens break down the pathogen's cell wall and cell membrane, and so, they are killing them. This represents the involving of erythrocytes in the body's immune response in [81].

On the other hand, as response of injury after several stressors, including oxidative stress, energy depletion, as well as a wide variety of endogenous mediators and xenobiotics, the erythrocytes can initiate the self suicidal death (eryptosis). Eryptosis is characterized by cell shrinkage, membrane blebbing, activation of proteases, and phosphatidylserine exposure at the outer membrane leaflet. This can make the macrophages to recognized and engulf erythrocyte to be degraded. Eryptosis can be considered a mechanism of defective erythrocytes to escape hemolysis. Conversely, excessive eryptosis favors the development of anemia. Conditions with excessive eryptosis include iron deficiency, lead or mercury intoxication, sickle cell anemia, thalassemia, glucose 6- phosphate dehydrogenase deficiency, malaria, and infection with hemolysis-forming pathogens. Inhibitors of eryptosis include erythropoietin, nitric oxide, catecholamine and high concentrations of urea in [82, 83]

The red blood cell SOD activity has been found to be useful in evaluating the biochemical index of copper, zinc and manganese nutrition. The largest amount of SOD enzyme is found in liver and erythrocytes. There are two forms of SOD in human tissue. One form is present in cytosol and it is a protein containing two atoms each of copper and zinc. The other form is a much larger molecule containing four atoms of manganese and it is found in mitochondria and cytosol. Significant changes in cellular concentration of copper, manganese and zinc have the potential of altering the antioxidant activity of SOD. On the other hands, the correlation between of copper and zinc plasma level, the oxidase activity of ceruloplasmin in serum, and Cu,Zn-SOD activity in erythrocytes can be a way to investigate involvement of oxidative stress in pathological conditions, as atherosclerosis obliterans [84]

Another element involved in the function of necessary enzyme for cellular protection is selenium. Selenium functions primarily as an activator of enzymes necessary for cellular protection from oxidative damage and maintenance of normal redox potentials. A primary role of selenium in erythrocytes appears to be the activation of the enzyme glutathione peroxidase whereby glutathione (the critical tripeptide antioxidant/antitoxin for all cells) reacts with oxygen radicals. Importantly, selenium catalyzes glutathione reductase, an enzyme that maintains the glutathione in its reduced or active form [85].

Specify participation of erythrocyte enzymatic system as adaptive mechanism to different pathological processes and specify how nutritional deficiencies and oxidative drugs can interfere these systems introduces the chapter on pharmacology of erythrocyte antioxidant system.

3.1. Antioxidant drugs in cardiovascular risk status and roll of red blood cell antioxidant defense capacity

3.1.1. Probucol

Probucol has modest lipid-lowering properties. It was used for the treatment of hypercholesterolemia until more tolerable and effective cholesterol-lowering treatments, such as the HMG Co-A reductase inhibitors, or "statins," became available. Probucol lowers the level of cholesterol in the bloodstream by increasing the rate of LDL catabolism. Additionally, probucol may inhibit cholesterol synthesis and delay cholesterol absorption in [86]. Another possible mechanism of action of probucol is inhibition of ABCA1-mediated cholesterol efflux without influencing scavenger receptor class B type I–mediated efflux (ABCA1 = ATP-binding cassette transporter - member 1 of human transporter sub-family ABCA, also known as the cholesterol efflux regulatory protein is a protein which in humans is encoded by the ABCA1 gene). The inhibition of ABCA1 translocation to the plasma membrane may in part explain the reported in vivo high-density lipoprotein–lowering action of probucol in [89].

Probucol is a powerful antioxidant which inhibits the oxidation of cholesterol in LDLs; this slows the formation of foam cells, which contribute to atherosclerotic plaques.

The major mechanism by which probucol lowers LDL levels relates not to changes in the cellular mechanisms for LDL uptake or to changes in LDL production but rather to intrinsic changes in the structure and metabolism of the plasma LDL in [87]. It has been postulated that the oxidative modification of LDL might contribute to atherogenesis by facilitating lipid accumulation in macrophages (foam cells) and by inhibiting macrophage motility. LDL resists oxidative modification, however, when probucol is added to in vitro incubations or when the LDL itself is isolated from probucol-treated patients in [88]. Under the treatment with probucol xanthomatous lesions disappear which that suggest a facilitation of cholesterol transferred from tissues to the excretion or catabolic pathways. Compared with other hipolipemiants, probucol is a non hepatotoxic drug and induces a decrease of lithogenic index of bile.

In recent studies was shown that probucol protect against diabetes-associated and adriamycin-induced cardiomyopathy by enhancing the endogenous antioxidant system including glutathione peroxidase, catalase and superoxide dismutase [90].

3.1.2. The HMG Co-A reductase inhibitors, or "statins"

Specific for hypercholesterolemia status is the high production of free oxygen radicals. These can impair the endothelial function because destroying of nitric oxide (NO) and secondary affecting its beneficial and protective effects on the vessel wall. Most of the other cholesterol-lowering therapies present, also, antioxidant effects. There are two way improving antioxidant defence system in hypercolesterolemiant patients: either increasing the activities of CuZn-SOD and GSH-Px or preventing the production of the superoxide radicals.

Malone dialdehyde (MDA), more than cholesterol plasma level, is considered a marker of patients with increased risk of coronary heart disease, because MDA is a marker of lipid peroxidation. In individuals who smoke or who have diabetes are particularly prone to oxidative stress that can lead to the formation of oxidized LDL (oxLDL). Oxidatively modified LDL is considered to be highly atherogenic and can be considered a biochemical risk marker for coronary heart disease. Oxidative modification of LDL increases their ability to bind to the extracellular matrix, increasing its retention within the intima and accumulation of oxLDL in macrophages, so, it contributes to the formation of an atherosclerotic lesion.

The oxLDL accumulation within macrophages promotes the chemotaxis of monocytes into the vessel wall and initiates the various pro-inflammatory effects by different scavenger receptor pathways: CD36 class B scavenger receptors from human macrophages (activates nuclear factor kB that regulates the expression of many pro-inflammatory genes), class A scavenger receptors (modify macrophage activation), lectin-like oxidized LDL receptor - LOX-1 (the expression of endothelial cell adhesion molecule). On the other hands, the accumulation of inflammatory cells can further increase the levels of oxidative stress. Oxidative stress inactivates nitric oxide (NO) and inhibits its synthesis by endothelial nitric oxide synthase (eNOS). On this way, the vasoprotectant effect of NO (anti-inflammatory, anti-platelets, antioxidant and vasodilator) is affected [92].

Statins inhibit 3-hydroxy-3-methylglutaryl-CoA (HMG-CoA) reductase the rate-limiting enzyme in the mevalonate pathway through which cells synthesizes cholesterol. On this way, the "statins" increase the resistance of LDL to oxidation. Statins may also exert effects beyond cholesterol lowering. These “pleiotropic” vascular effects of statins are involved in restoring or improving endothelial function: by increasing the bioavailability of nitric oxide, promoting reendothelialization, reducing oxidative stress, and inhibiting inflammatory responses.

Other effects of statins that explain their involving in preserving normal vascular function and blood flow are: inhibition of the uptake and generation of Ox-LDL, decreasing the vascular and endothelial superoxide anion formation by inhibition of NADH oxidases via Rho-dependent mechanisms and preserving the relative levels of vitamin E, vitamin C and endogenous antioxidants (such as, ubiquinone and glutathione) in LDL particles. All these mechanisms explain a dual action of statins on oxidative stress, not only decreasing oxidants but also restoring antioxidants [92]. Statins reduce both extracellular LDL oxidation (by reducing substrate availability) and intracellular oxidative stress (by cholesterol-independent effects on NO and, indirectly, by reducing Ox-LDL) [91].

Statins themselves may be able to reduce levels of superoxide radicals, an effect that can only partially be explained by a reduction in LDL cholesterol. Rosuvastatin has been reported to reduce markers of oxidative stress in ApoE (−/−) mice [93] while fluvastatin treatment has been shown to decrease superoxide radical generation and to reduce the susceptibility of LDL to oxidation in cholesterol-fed rabbits [95, 96].

Atorvastatin has been demonstrated to inhibit angiotensin II-induced superoxide formation by NADPH oxidase in isolated rat vascular smooth muscle cells [96] and in rats in vivo [97]. In addition, statins have been shown to reduce NADPH-dependent superoxide formation by a monocyte-derived cell line in culture [98].

Another beneficial effect of statins is potentiation the synthesis of tetrahydrobiopterin, which may prevent the uncoupling of eNOS and shift the balance away from NOS-generated superoxide production to the generation of NO [99]. Statins may also be influence the endogenous antioxidants other than NO. Atorvastatin has been shown to increase paraoxonase activity and reduce the enhanced cellular uptake of oxLDL of monocytes differentiating into macrophages [100]. Long-term treatment with HMG-CoA reductase inhibitors (statins) appears to upregulate the expression and the activity of the vascular endothelial NO synthase (eNOS) pathway and increases nitric oxide availability, resulting in not only a downregulation of oxidative enzymes but also a direct scavenging of superoxide anion. As oxygen radical production is increased in various clinical settings such as hypercholesterolaemia, diabetes and hypertension, this statin-induced eNOS upregulation may play a foremost role in the vascular protective effects of these drugs. [119]. Moreover, sustained nitroglycerin (NTG) treatment is associated with an increased bioavailability of superoxide anion, likely playing a major role in the development of nitrate tolerance. The triggering events leading to this redox imbalance remain controversial as several cellular enzyme systems have been shown to be impaired by sustained in vivo exposure to NTG, including membrane bound oxidases in [121] endothelial NOS in [122] and arginine transporters [123].

Other effects than hipocholesterolemic of statins was described. Lovastatin or simvastatin has been shown to have anti-inflammatory properties. They reduce monocyte adhesion to endothelial cells, cytokine expression and MCP-1 production [101-103]. By limiting the influx of inflammatory cells statins may reduce the release of superoxide radicals and the oxidative modification of LDL. On this way statins increases the resistance of LDL to oxidation. Macrophage growth stimulated by oxLDL can also be inhibited by statins [92]

3.1.3. Fenofibrate

Very few data concerning the fibrates are available. In hypercholesterolemic patients, it has been shown that bezafibrate is more active than pravastatin in reducing the susceptibility of LDL oxidation [104]. Moreover, in diabetics, De Leeuw and Van Gaal have found that fenofibrate, but not pravastatin or simvastatin, can reduce the oxidizibility of LDL and of VLDL [105].

3.1.4. Beta-adrenergic blockers

Beta adrenergic blocking agents have also been shown to have beneficial effect on atherosclerosis. Several mechanisms of action have been suggested including an antioxidant action. All β-blockers have in vitro antioxidant activity which appears to be related to their degree of lipophilicity. In patients with CHD, Croft and coworkers showed that, while the lag time in patients with CHD is not significantly different from controls, in patients with CHD who are taking β-blockers, the lag time is higher than that observed in patients who are not taking β-blockers in [106]. When LDL are oxidized in vitro by copper or by macrophages, carvedilol, the most lipophilic β -blocker appears more potent than pindolol, labetolol, atenolol and propranolol and this is confirmed in vivo [107].

3.1.5. Angiotensin-converting enzyme (ACE) inhibitors

ACE inhibitors have been shown to have a beneficial effect in atherosclerosis. They reduce the progression of the disease in animals. These beneficial effects of ACE inhibitors have been related to an antioxidant activity against LDL oxidation that has been demonstrated. In vitro, the lag time was found to be clearly increased by the presence of captopril at concentrations close to those that can be achieved therapeutically with large doses. A similar effect is observed with *N*-acetylcysteine which contains like captopril, a sulfhydryl group. Quinapril, which lacks the sulfhydryl group, had no antioxidant activity [108]. In vivo, Aviram and coworkers have shown that the propensity of LDL to oxidation is increased in patients with hypertension and is positively correlated with the blood pressure. Giving captopril or enalapril for 3 weeks decreases the oxidizibility of LDL. That suggests that the sulfhydryl group, which is absent in enalapril, does not have any influence on the resistance of LDL oxidation [109]. Actually, the same group gave data suggesting that the antioxidant activity might be related to the decreased production of angiotensin-II (A-II) as A-II appears to increase the LDL oxidation by macrophages [110].

3.1.6. Calcium channel blocker

All calcium channel blocker are potent antioxidants in vitro and this property is probably related to their interaction with the lipid bilayer of the membranes. Lacidipine has the highest degree of interaction with the membrane Lacidipine inhibits the LDL oxidation produced by several oxidants. [111].

3.1.7. Metabolic medication - Trimetazidine

Trimetazidine (TMZ) is the first in a new class of metabolic agents, available for clinical use. In conditions of hypoxia or induced ischemia, TMZ maintains homeostasis and cellular functions by selectively inhibiting 3-ketoacyl-CoA-thiolase [112]. As a consequence, fatty acid b-oxidation is reduced and glucose oxidation is stimulated, resulting in decreased cellular acidosis and higher ATP production [113, 114]. In humans, TMZ has been shown to increase the ischaemic threshold and to relieve angina pectoris in patients with coronary artery disease. These benefits have been observed without any change in heart rate, blood pressure, and rate-pressure product at rest, during submaximal and peak exercise in [115,116]. There is also demonstration that TMZ has antioxidant properties. During acute and chronic ischemia, TMZ reduces the loss of intracellular K+ induced by oxygen free radicals and also the membrane content of peroxidated lipids [117]. In vivo, pre-treatment with TMZ (40–60 mg per day for 7 days) significantly decreases membrane malondialdehyde (MDA) content of red blood cells incubated with superoxide dismutase inhibitor diethyldithiocarbamate [118]. In humans, plasma levels of MDA were decreased after pre-treatment with TMZ during coronary artery bypass surgery [118].

4. Instead of conclusion

Mechanism of action of homocysteine is far from being elucidated. The big number of studies on this subject was gathered a lot of evidences about the role of Hcy as a major cardiovascular risk factor. All studied diseases: nephropathies, neurodegenerative illnesses, osteoporosis, atherosclerosis seems to be tributary to this homocysteine effect. It is widely accepted that involvement of homocysteine in the pathogenesis of these diseases activates prooxidative mechanisms. Therefore, the initiation of therapy of drug with antioxidant properties in such pathologies is justified. Moreover, there is clinical evidence to support this point of view. Thus, although the clinicians question the value of trimetazidine in the treatment of myocardial ischemia or degenerative deafness. [124-128] there are the clinical trials and basic research that support the benefits of this antioxidant metabolic medication. Scientific arguments exist regarding the use of atorvastatin [129, 130] or nimodipine [131] therapy for antiischemic effects and prevention of vascular events.

Author details

Filip Cristiana and Zamosteanu Nina
Dept. Biochemistry. Univ.Med. Pharm. "Gr.T.Popa", Iasi, Romania

Albu Elena
Dept. Pharmacology. Univ.Med. Pharm. "Gr.T.Popa", Iasi, Romania

5. Acknowledgement

Our research study to which we referred at the references was supported by grant PNCDII Idei 1225/2007 sustained by Ministry of Education and Research National Authority for Scientific Research UEFISCSU

6. References

[1] Rifkind JM, Nagababu E, Ramasamy LB. Redox Rep. Review hemoglobin redox reactions and oxidative stress, 2003, (8): 234-7

[2] Ingraham, L. L., (1966) Compressive Biochemistry 14, 424-446

[3] David E. Metzler, Biochemistry. The Chemical Reaction of Living Cells, second edition, 2001, Elsevier Academic Press

[4] Michael Lieberman, Allan D. Marks, Colleen Smith, Marks'Essentials of Medical Biochemistry. A Clinical Approach.2007, edited by Lippincott Williams&Wilkins

[5] T.McKee, J. McKee. Biochemistry: The Molecular Basis of Life. 2004. 3rd Ed *T McKee, J McKee* (McGraw Hill)

[6] Halliwell B; Plant Physiol. 2006,141, 312-322

[7] Hara P. Misra and Irwin Fridovici, The generation of superoxide radical during the autoxidation of hemoglobin, The Journal of Biological Chemistry, 1972, 247(21): 6960-6962

[8] Balagopalakrishna C . Manoharan PT, Abugo OO, Rifkind JM, Production of superoxide from hemoglobin-bound oxygen under hypoxic condition, Biochemistry, 1996, 35(20): 6393-8

[9] Koppenol, W.H. (2001). "The Haber-Weiss cycle – 70 years later". *Redox Report* 6 (4): 229–234.

[10] Mwebi N.O., Fenton&Fenton-like reaction: the nature of oxidizing intermediates involved (dissertation submitted to the Faculty of the Graduate School of the University of Maryland, Maryland 2005

[11] Bray W.C. and Gorin M.H., J. Am. Chem. Soc., 1932, 54, 2124-2125,

[12] Bogdanova A. Y. and Nikinmaa M., J. Gen. Physiol., 2001,117,181-190, Groves J.T., Inorg. Biochem., 2006, 100, 434-447

[13] Krzysztof Barbusinski, Fenton reaction-controversy concerning the chemistry, Ecological Chemistry and Engineering S, 2009, 16 (3), 347-358

[14] Prousek J., Pure Appl. Chem., 2007, 79, 2325-2338

[15] Erica Novo and Maurizio Parola , Redox mechanisms in hepatic chronic wound healing and fibrogenesis, Fibrogenesis & Tissue Repair, 2008, 1-58

[16] R.S. Richards, L. Wang, H. Jelineka, Erythrocyte Oxidative Damage in Chronic Fatigue Syndrome, Archives of Medical Research, 2007, 38, 94-98

[17] Jennifer L. Martindale, Nikki J. Holbrook, Cellular response to oxidative stress: Signaling for suicide and survival. Journal of Cellular Physiology, 2002, 192 (1):1-15

[18] Chen Z, Gibson TB, Robinson F, Silvestro L, Pearson G, Xu B, Wright A, Vanderbilt C & Cobb MH (*2001*). MAP kinases. Chem Rev, 101, 2449–2476.
[19] S. K.Powers, J. Duarte, A.N. Kavazis, E.E. Talbert, Reactive oxygen species are signalling molecules for skeletal muscle adaptation, Experimental Physiology, 2010, 95, 1-9
[20] Wulf Droge, Free Radicals in the Physiological Control of Cell Function, Physiol Rev, 2002, 82 (1):47-95
[21] Bahorun T, Soobratte MA, Luximon-Ramma V, Aruoma OI., Free Radicals and Antioxidants in Cardiovascular Health and Disease. Internet Journal of Medical Update 2006,1(2): 25-41
[22] Heinrich, Peter; Georg Löffler; Petro E. Petrides (2006). *Biochemie und Pathobiochemie (Springer-Lehrbuch) (German Edition)*. Berlin: Springer. pp. 123. ISBN 3-540-32680-4
[23] Ernst E. van Faassen et all. Nitrite as regulator of hypoxic signaling in mammalian physiology, Med Res Rev, 2009, 29(5):683-741
[24] Govers R, Rabelink TJ. Cellular regulation of endothelial nitric oxide synthase. Am J Physiol Renal Physiol. 2001;280:F193– F206
[25] N.V. Bhagavan, Medical Biochemistry, fourth edition, 2002, Harcourt/Academic Press
[26] Abu-Soud HM, Stuehr DJ. Nitric oxide synthases reveal a role for calmodulin in controlling electron transfer. *Proc Natl Acad Sci U S A.* 1993;90:10769–10772.
[27] Victor W.M. van Hinsbergh, NO or H2O2 for endothelium-dependent vasorelaxation. Tetrahidrobiopterin makes the differences. Arteriosclerosis, Thrombosis, and Vascular Biology. 2001;21:719-721
[28] Abu-Soud HM, Ichimori K, Presta A, Stuehr DE. Electron transfer, oxygen binding and nitric oxide feedback inhibition in endothelial nitric-oxide synthase. J Biol Chem. 2000;275:17349– 17357
[29] Gautier C, van Faassen E, Mikula I, Martasek P, Slama-Schwok A. Endothelial nitric oxide synthase reduces nitrite anions to NO under anoxia. Biochem Biophys Res Commun. 2006;341:816– 821
[30] Stroes E, Hijmering M, van Zandvoort M, Wever R, Rabelink T, van Faassen E. Origin of superoxide production by endothelial nitric oxide synthase. FEBS Lett. 1998;438:161–164,
[31] Stroes E, Rabelink T, van Faassen E. Vascular Protection: Molecular Mechanisms, novel therapeutic Principles and Clinical Applications. Ch. 3. Taylor and Francis; 2002. Uncoupling of endothelial nitric oxide synthase: A molecular basis for atherosclerosis;
[32] [Ana Denicola, Jose M. Souza, Rafael Radi, Diffusion of peroxinitrite across erythrocytes membrane, Proc Natl Acad of Sci U S A. 1998, 95(7):3566-3571
[33] Robert D. Guzy, Paul T. Schumacker, Oxygen sensing by mitochondria at complex III: the paradox of increased reactive oxygen species during hypoxia, Experimental Physiology, 2006, 9, 807-819,

[34] N.S.Chandel, E. Maltepe, E.Goldwasser, C.E.Mathieu, M.C.Simon, T.Schumacker, Mitochondrial reactive oxygen species trigger hypoxia induced Transcription, Proc. Natl. Acad. Sci. USA,1998, 95, 11715–11720
[35] Kleinbongard P, Schutz R, Rassaf T, et al. Red blood cells express a functional endothelial nitric oxide synthase. Blood 2006; 107(7): 2943-51
[36] Ulker P, Sati L, Celik-Ozenci C, Meiselman HJ, Baskurt OK, Mechanical stimulation of nitric oxide synthesizing mechanisms in etrytrocytes, Biorheology, 2009; 46(2):121-32
[37] Joshi MS, Ferguson TB Jr, Han TH, Hyduke DR, Liao JC, Rassaf T, Bryan N, Feelisch M, Lancaster JR Jr. Nitric oxide is consumed, rather than conserved, by reaction with oxyhemoglobin under physiological conditions. Proc Natl Acad Sci U S A. 2002; 99: 10341–10346.
[38] J.O.Lunderg, Eddie Weitzber, NO generation from nitrite and its role in vascular control, Arteriosclerosis, Thrombosis, and Vascular. 2005; 25: 915-922.
[39] Reutov VP, Sorokina EG. NO-synthase and nitrite-reductase components of nitric oxide cycle. Biochemistry. 1998; 63: 874–884;
[40] Cosby K, Partovi KS, Crawford JH, Patel RP, Reiter CD, Martyr S, Yang BK, Waclawiw MA, Zalos G, Xu X, Huang KT, Shields H, Kim-Shapiro DB, Schechter AN, Cannon RO III, Gladwin MT. Nitrite reduction to nitric oxide by deoxyhemoglobin vasodilates the human circulation. Nat Med. 2003; 9: 1498–1505.;
[41] Nagababu E, Ramasamy S, Abernethy DR, Rifkind JM. Active nitric oxide produced in the red cell under hypoxic conditions by deoxyhemoglobin-mediated nitrite reduction. J Biol Chem. 2003; 278: 46349–46356
[42] Jon O. Lundberg , No kidding. Hemoglobin makes NO, Blood, 2006, 107(2):414
[43] Jonathan S. Stamler, Li Jia, Jerry P. Eu, Timothy J. McMahon, Ivan T. Demchenko, Joseph Bonaventura, Kim Gernert, Claude A. Piantadosi, Blood Flow Regulation by S-Nitrosohemoglobin in the Physiological Oxygen Gradient, Science, 1997, 276(27): 2034-37
[44] Cosby K, Partovi KS, Crawford JH, Patel RP, Reiter CD, Martyr S, Yang BK, Waclawiw MA, Zalos G, Xu X, Huang KT, Shields H, Kim-Shapiro DB, Schechter AN, Cannon RO, Gladwin MT. Nitrite reduction to nitric oxide by deoxyhemoglobin vasodilates the human circulation, Nat. Med. 2003;9:1498–1505.
[45] Crawford JT, Scott Isbell T, Huang Z, Shiva S, Chacko B, Schechter A, Darley-Usmar V, Kerby J, Lang J, Kraus D, Ho C, Gladwin M, Patel R. Hypoxia, red blood cells, and nitrite regulate NO-dependent hypoxic vasodilation. Blood. 2006; 1007:566–574.
[46] Huang Z, Shiva S, Kim-Shapiro D, Patel R, Ringwood L, Irby C, Huang K, Ho C, Hogg N, Schechter Am Gladwin M. Enzymatic function of haemoglobin as a nitrite reductase that produces NO under allosteric control. J Clin Invest. 2005; 115:2099–2107.
[47] Mehmet Uyuklua, Herbert J. Meiselman, Oguz K. Baskurt, Role of hemoglobin oxygenation in the modulation of red blood cell mechanical properties by nitric oxide, Nitric Oxide, 2009, 21(1): 20-26

[48] Li H, Samouilov A, Liu X, Zweier JL. Characterization of the magnitude and kinetics of xanthine oxidase-catalyzed nitrate reduction: evaluation of its role in nitrite and nitric oxide generation in anoxic tissues. Biochemistry. 2003; 42, 1150–1159.

[49] Modin A, Bjorne H, Herulf M, Alving K, Weitzberg E, Lundberg JO. Nitrite-derived nitric oxide: a possible mediator of "acidic-metabolic" vasodilation. Acta Physiol Scand. 2001; 171: 9–16

[50] Lonn, E; Yusuf, S; Arnold, MJ; Sheridan, P; Pogue, J; Micks, M; McQueen, MJ; Probstfield, J et al. Homocysteine lowering with folic acid and B vitamins in vascular disease, N Engl J Med, 2006, 354 (15), 1567–77,

[51] Bonaa KH, Njolstad I, Ueland PM, Schirmer H, Tverdal A, Steigen T, Wang H, Nordrehaug JE, Arnesen E, Rasmussen K. Homocysteine lowering and cardiovascular events after acute myocardial infarction, N Engl J Med, 2006, 354 (15): 1578–88

[52] Lars Brattström and David EL Wilcken. Homocysteine and cardiovascular disease: cause or effect?, American Journal of Clinical Nutrition, (2000), 72(2): 315-323

[53] Welch G., and Loscalo,J; Homocysteine and atherosclerosis. New Engl.J.Med., 1998. 338(15),1042

[54] Alexander Boldyrev, Molecular mechanisms of homocysteine toxicity and possible protection against hyperhomocysteinemia, Recent Advances on Nutrition and the Prevention of Alzheimer's disease, 2010:127-143

[55] Spence JD. Patients with atherosclerotic vascular disease: how low should plasma homocysteine levels go?, Am J Cardiovasc Drugs. 2001; 1(2):85-9

[56] J. Thambyrajah, J.N. Townend, Homocysteine and atherothrombosis-mechanism for injury, *European Heart Journal* (2000) 21, 967–974

[57] Starkebaum G, Harlan JM, Endothelial injury due to cooper-catalyzed hydrogen peroxide generation from homocysteine, J. Clin. Invest, 1986, 77:1370-76

[58] Loscalzo J. The oxidant stress of hyperhomocyst(e)inemia. J Clin Invest 1996; 98: 5–7

[59] Lang D, Kredan MB, Moat SJ et al. Homocysteine-induced inhibition of endothelium-dependent relaxation in rabbit aorta: role for superoxide anions. Arterioscler Thromb Vasc Biol, 2000;20:422– 427

[60] Lawson JA, Rokach J, FitzGerald G A, Isoprostanes: Formation analyses and use as indices of lipid peroxidation in vivo, J.Biol. Chem., 1999, 274: 24441-44

[61] Wilcken DEL, Wang XL & Adachi T *et al*. Relationship between homocysteine and superoxide dismutase in homocystinuria. Possible relevance to cardiovascular risk. *Arterioscler Thromb Vasc Biol* 2000; 20: 1199–1202

[62] Christiana Filip, Elena Albu, Nina Zamosteanu M Jaba Irina and Mihaela Silion, Hyperhomocysteinemia's effect on antioxidant capacity on rats, Central European Journal of Medecine, 2010, 5(5) 620-6

[63] Upchurch GR, Welch G & Fabian A *et al*. Homocysteine decreases bioavailable nitric oxide by a mechanism involving glutathione peroxidase. *J Biol Chem* 1997; 272: 17012–17017.

[64] Jacobsen DW. Hyperhomocysteinemia and oxidative stress. Time for a reality check? *Arterioscler Thromb Vasc Biol* 2000; 20: 1182–1184

[65] Starkebaum G, Harlan JM, Endothelial injury due to cooper-catalyzed hydrogen peroxide generation from homocysteine, J. Clin. Invest, 1986, 77:1370-76

[66] Halverson B, Effect of homocysteine on copper ion-catalyzed, azo compound-initiated, and mononuclear cell-mediated oxidative modification of low density lipoprotein. J.Lipid. Res. 1996 Jul; 37(7):1591-600.

[67] Upchurch GR, Jr., Welch GN, Loscalzo J. Homocysteine, EDRF, and endothelial function. J Nutr 1996; 126 (4 Suppl): 1290S–4S.29

[68] Welch GN, Loscalzo J., Homocysteinei and atherothrombosis, N. Engl. J. Med, 1998, 338: 1042-50

[69] D Zakrzewicz and O Eickelberg From arginine methylation to ADMA: A novel mechanism with therapeutic potential in chronic lung diseases *BMC Pulmonary Medicine* 2009 9:5

[70] Karsten Sydow, Edzard Schwedhelm, Naoshi Arakawa, Stefanie M. Bode-Boger,Dimitrios Tsikas , Burkhard Hornig , Jurgen C. Frolich , Rainer H. Boger, ADMA and oxidative stress are responsible for endothelial dysfunction in hyperhomocyst(e)inemia: effects of L-arginine and B vitamins, Cardiovascular Research 57 (2003) 244–252

[71] Ralph Carmel, Donald W Jacobsen "Homocysteine in health and disease" Cambridge University Press, 2001 ISBN, 0 521 65319 3

[72] Austin RC, Lentz SR, Werstuck GH, . Role of hyperhomocysteinemia in endothelial dysfunction and atherothrombotic disease, Cell Death Differ. 2004; 11 Suppl1:S56-S64

[73] Harpel PC, Zhang X, Borth, Homocysteine and hemostasis: pathogenic mechanism predisposing to thrombosis, Nutr. 1996,126(4 Suppl):1285S-9S

[74] Steven R. Lentzt and J. Evan Sadler, Inhibition of Thrombomodulin Surface Expression and Protein C Activation by the Thrombogenic Agent Homocysteine, J.Clin. Invest, 1991, 88, 1906-1914

[75] Md S. Jamaluddin, Irene Chen, Fan Yang, Xiaohua Jiang, Michael Jan, Xiaomomg Liu, Andrew I Schafer, William Durante, Xiaofeng Yang, Hong Wan, Homocysteine inhibits endothelial cell growth via DNA hypomethylation of the *cyclin A*gene, *Blood* November 15, 2007 vol. 110 no. 10 3648-3655

[76] Perma AF, Ingrosso D, Zappia V, Galletti P, Capasso P, De Santo NG. Enzymatic methyl esterification of erythrocyte membrane proteins is impaired in chronic renal failure. Evidence for high levels of the natural inhibitor S-adenosylhomocysteine. J.Clin. Invest. 1993 Jun;91(6):2497-503

[77] Guilland JC, Favier A, Potier de Courcy G, Galan P, Herceberg S, Hyperhomocysteinemia: an independent risk factor or a simple marker of vascular disease?. 1. Basic data Pathol Biol (paris), 2003, ,51(2):101-10

[78] Diesen DL, Hess DT, Stamler JS (2008) Hypoxic vasodilation by red blood cells: evidence for an s-nitrosothiol-based signal, Circulation Research 103 (5): 545–53

[79] Benavides, Gloria A; Giuseppe L Squadrito, Robert W Mills, Hetal D Patel, T Scott Isbell, Rakesh P Patel, Victor M Darley-Usmar, Jeannette E Doeller, David W Kraus (2007) Hydrogen sulfide mediates the vasoactivity of garlic. Proceedings of the National Academy of Sciences of the United States of America 104 (46): 17977–17982

[80] NUS team (2007). Red blood cells do more than just carry oxygen. New findings by NUS team show they aggressively attack bacteria too., The Straits Times 1

[81] Jiang N, Tan NS, Ho B, Ding JL (2007). Respiratory protein-generated reactive oxygen species as an antimicrobial strategy. Nature Immunology 8 (10): 1114–22

[82] Lang F, Lang KS, Lang PA, Huber SM, Wieder T. (2006) Mechanisms and significance of eryptosis.Antioxid Redox Signal 8 (7-8):1183-92

[83] Florian Lang, Karl S. Lang, Philipp A. Lang, Stephan M. Huber, and Thomas Wieder. (2006) *Mechanisms and Significance of Eryptosis*, Antioxidants & Redox Signaling 8: 1183-1192

[84] Iskra M, Majewski W. (2000) Copper and zinc concentrations and the activities of ceruloplasmin and superoxide dismutase in atherosclerosis obliterans. Biol Trace Elem Res. 73(1):55-65

[85] Yakup Alicigüzel,Sebahat Nacitarhan Özdem,Sadi S Özdem, Ümit Karayalçim, Sandra L Siedlak, George Perry, Mark A Smith. (2001) Erythrocyte, plasma, and serum antioxidant activities in untreated toxic multinodular goiter patients, Free Radical Biology and Medicine Volume 30, Issue 6: 665 -670

[86] Yamamoto A (2008). A Uniqe Antilipidemic Drug - Probucol. J. Atheroscler. Thromb. 15 (6): 304–5

[87] Naruszewicz M, Carew TE, Pittman RC, Witztum JL, Steinberg D. (1984) A novel mechanism by which probucol lowers low density lipoprotein levels demonstrated in the LDL receptor-deficient rabbit.J Lipid Res. 25(11):1206-13

[88] Steinberg D. (1986) Studies on the mechanism of action of probucol. Am J Cardiol. 57(16):16H-21H

[89] Davignon J. (1986) Medical management of hyperlipidemia and the role of probucol. Am J Cardiol. 57(16):22H-28H

[90] Ebtehal El-Demerdash, Azza S. Awad, Ragia M. Taha, Asmaa M. El-Hady, Mohamed M. Sayed-Ahmed, (2005) Probucol attenuates oxidative stress and energy decline in isoproterenol-induced heart failure in rat Pharmacological Research 51: 311–318

[91] M. Ilker Yilmaz, Y. Baykal, M. Kilic, A. Sonmez,F. Bulucu, A. Aydin, A. Sayal, I. Hakki Kocar, (2004) Effects of Statins on Oxidative Stress, Biological Trace Element Research. 98:119-27

[92] Robert S. Rosenson. (2004) Statins in atherosclerosis: lipid-lowering agents with antioxidant capabilities, Atherosclerosis 173: 1–12

[93] Sanguigni V, Pignatelli P, Caccese D, et al. (2002) Atorvastatin decreases platelet superoxide anion production in hypercholesterolemic patients., Eur Heart J 4:372.
[94] Li W, Asagami T, McTaggart F, Tsao P. (2002) Rosuvastatin inhibits monocyte /endothelial interactions in APOE (–/–) mice. Int J Clin Pract. 24 (Suppl):5
[95] Rikitake Y, Kawashima S, Takeshita S, et al (2001). Anti-oxidative properties of fluvastatin, an HMG-CoA reductase inhibitor, contribute to prevention of atherosclerosis in cholesterol-fed rabbits. Atherosclerosis 154:87–96
[96] Wassmann S, Laufs U, Muller K, et al. (2002) Cellular antioxidant effects of atorvastatin in vitro and in vivo. Arterioscler Thromb Vasc Biol; 22:300–5
[97] Wassmann S, Laufs U, Baumer AT, et al. (2001) HMG-CoA reductase inhibitors improve endothelial dysfunction in normocholesterolemic hypertension via reduced production of reactive oxygen species. Hypertension 37:1450–7.
[98] Delbosc S, Morena M, Djouad F, Ledoucen C, Descomps B, Cristol JP. (2002) Statins, 3-hydroxy-3-methylglutaryl coenzyme A reductase inhibitors, are able to reduce superoxide anion production by NADPH oxidase in THP-1-derived monocytes. J Cardiovasc Pharmacol. 40:611–7
[99] Hattori Y, Nakanishi N, Kasai K. (2002) Statin enhances cytokine-mediated induction of nitric oxide synthesis in vascular smooth muscle cells., Cardiovasc Res. 54: 649–58
[100] Fuhrman B, Koren L, Volkova N, Keidar S, Hayek T, Aviram M. (2002) Atorvastatin therapy in hypercholesterolemic patients suppresses cellular uptake of oxidized-LDL by differentiating monocytes. Atherosclerosis. 164:179–85
[101] Rosenson RS. (1999) Non-lipid-lowering effects of statins on atherosclerosis. Curr Cardiol Rep. 1:225–32
[102] Ferro D, Parrotto S, Basili S, Alessandri C, Violi F. (2000) Simvastatin inhibits the monocyte expression of proinflammatory cytokines in patients with hypercholesterolemia. J Am Coll Cardiol. 36: 427–31
[103] Crisby M, Nordin-Fredriksson G, Shah PK, Yano J, Zhu J, Nilsson J. (2001) Pravastatin treatment increases collagen content and decreases lipid content, inflammation, metalloproteinases, and cell death in human carotid plaques: implications for plaque stabilization. Circulation. 103:926–33
[104] Hoffman R, Brook GJ, Aviram M. (1992) Hypolipidemic drugs reduce lipoprotein susceptibility to undergo lipid peroxidation: In vitro and ex vivo studies. Atherosclerosis 93:105–13
[105] De Leeuw I, Van Gaal L, Zhang A. (1996) Effects of lipid lowering drugs on the in vitro oxidizability of lipoproteins in diabetes. In: Gotto AM, Paoletti R, Smith LC, Catapano AL, Jackson AS, editors. Drugs Affecting Lipid Metabolism. The Netherlands: Klumer Academic Publishers and Fondazione Giovanni Lorenzini. 69–75.
[106] Croft KD, Dimmitt SB, Moulton C, Beilin LJ. (1992) Low density lipoprotein composition and oxidizability in coronary diseaseapparent favourable effect of b-blockers. Atherosclerosis 97:123–30.

[107] Maggi E, Marchesi E, Covini D, Negro C, Perani G, Bellomo G. (1996) Protective effects of Carvedilol, a vasodilating b-adrenoceptor blocker, against in vivo low density lipoprotein oxidation in essential hypertension. J Cardiovasc Pharmacol 27:532–8

[108] Godfrey EG, Stewart J, Dargie HJ, Reid JL, Dominiczak M, Hamilton CA, McMurray J. (1994) Effects of ACE inhibitors on oxidation of human low density lipoprotein. Br J Clin Pharmacol. 37:63–6

[109] Keidar S, Kaplan M, Shapira C, Brook JG, Aviram (1994) M. Low density lipoprotein isolated form patients with essential hypertension exhibits increased propensity for oxidation and enhanced uptake by macrophages: A possible role for angiotensin II. Atherosclerosis 107:71–84

[110] Keidar S, Kaplan M, Hoffman A, Aviram M. (1995) Angiotensin II stimulates macrophages-mediated oxidation of low density lipoproteins. Atherosclerosis 115: 201–15

[111] Micheli D, Ratti E, Toson G, Gavirighi (1991) G. Pharmacology of Lacidipine, a vascular-selective calcium antagonist. J Cardiovasc Pharmacol 17:S1–8

[112] Kantor PF, Lucien A, Kozak R, Lopaschuk GD. (2000) The antianginal drug trimetazidine shifts cardiac energy metabolism from fatty acid oxidation to glucose oxidation by inhibiting mitochondrial long-chain 3-ketoacyl coenzyme A tiolase. Circ Res 86:580–588

[113] Harpey C, Clauser P, Labrid C, Freyria JL, Poirier JP. (1989) Trimetazidine, a cellular anti-ischemic agent. Cardiovasc Drug Rev.6:292–312

[114] Stanley WC, Lopaschuck GD, Hall JL, Mccormack JG. (1997) Regulation of myocardial carbohydrate metabolism under normal and ischaemic conditions: potential for pharmacological interventions. Cardiovasc Res. 33: 243–257

[115] Detry JM, Sellier P, Pennaforte S, Cokkinos D, Dargie H, Mathes P. (1994). Trimetazidine: a new concept in the treatment of angina. Comparison with propranolol in patients with stable angina. Br J Clin Pharmacol. 37:279–288

[116] Szwed H, Hradec J, Preda I. (2001). Anti-ischaemic efficacy and tolerability of trimetazidine administered to patients with angina pectoris: results of three studies. Coron Artery Dis. 12 (Suppl. 1):S25–S28

[117] Guarnieri C, Muscari C. (1993) Effect of trimetazidine on mitochondrial function and oxidative damage during reperfusion of ischemic hypertrophied myocardium. Pharmacology 46:324–331

[118] Maridonneau-Parini K, Harpey C. (1985). Effects of trimetazidine on membrane damage induced by oxygen free radicals in human red cells. Br J Clin Pharmacol. 20:148–151

[119] Fabiani JN, Ponzio O, Emerit I, Massonet-Castel S, Paris M, Chevalier P, Jebara V, Carpentier A. (1992). Cardioprotective effect of trimetazidine during coronary artery graft surgery. J Cardiovasc Surg. 33:486–491

[120] Kojda, G. & Harrison, D. (1999). Interactions between NO and reactive oxygen species: pathophysiological importance in atherosclerosis, hypertension, diabetes and heart failure. Cardiovasc. Res. 43: 562–571

[121] Munzel, T., Kurz, S., Rajagopalan, S., Thoenes, M., Berrington, W.R., Thomson, J.A., Freemen, B.A, Harrison, D.G. (1996) Hydralazine prevents nitroglycerin tolerance by inhibiting activation of a membrane-bound NADH oxidase. A new action for an old drug. J. Clin. Invest. 98: 1465–1470

[122] Munzel, T., LI, H., Mollnau, H., Hink, U., Matheis, E., Hartmann, M., Oelze, M., Skatchkov, M., Warnholtz, A., Dunker, L., Meinertz, T., Forsterman, U. (2000), Effects of long-term nitroglycerin treatment on endothelial nitric oxide synthase (NOS III) gene expression, NOS III-mediated superoxide production, and vascular NO bioavailability. Circ. Res. 86: E7–E12

[123] Ogonowski, A.A., Kaesemeyer, W.H., Jin, L., Ganapathy, V., Leibach, F.H., Caldwell, R.W. (2000). Effects of NO donors and synthase agonists on endothelial cell uptake of L-Arg and superoxide production. Am. J. Physiol. Cell Physiol.278,:C136– C143

[124] Kutala VK, Khan M, Mandal R, Ganesan LP, Tridandapani S, Kalai T, Hideg K, Kuppusamy P. (2006), Attenuation of myocardial ischemia-reperfusion injury by trimetazidine derivatives functionalized with antioxidant properties. J Pharmacol Exp Ther. 317(3): 921-8

[125] Belardinelli R, Lacalaprice F, Faccenda E, Volpe L. (2008), Trimetazidine potentiates the effects of exercise training in patients with ischemic cardiomyopathy referred for cardiac rehabilitation. Eur J Cardiovasc Prev Rehabil.15(5):533-40

[126] De Leiris J., Boucher F., (2006), Rationale for trimetazidine administration in myocardial ischaemia—reperf usion syndrome, Oxford Journals Medicine European Heart Journal Volume 14, Issue suppl G: 4-40.

[127] Haguenauer JP, Bebear JP, Bordes LR, Jacquot M, Mercier J, Morgon A, Pech A, Romanet P, Thomassin JM, Wayoff M, (1990), Trimetazidine and degenerative deafness. Effect on hearing and integration Ann Otolaryngol Chir Cervicofac.;107 Suppl 1:51-6

[128] Unal OF, Ghoreishi SM, Ataş A, Akyürek N, Akyol G, Gürsel B. (2005), Prevention of gentamicin induced ototoxicity by trimetazidine in animal model. Int J Pediatr Otorhinolaryngol. ;69(2):193-9.

[129] Steven E. Nissen, E. Murat Tuzcu, Paul Schoenhagen, B. Greg Brown, Peter Ganz, Robert A. Tim Crowe, Gail Howard, Christopher J. Cooper, Bruce Brodie, Cindy L. Grines, Anthony N. DeMaria, (2004), Effect of Intensive Compared With Moderate Lipid-Lowering Therapy on Progression of Coronary Atherosclerosis A Randomized Controlled Trial, (Reprinted) JAMA, March 3, 2004—Vol 291, No. 9: 1071-1081

[130] Dunyue Lu, M.D, Asim Mahmood, Anton Goussev, Timothy Schallert, Changsheng Qu, Zheng Gang Zhang, Yi Li, Mei Lu, and Michael Chopp.,(2004), Atorvastatin reduction of intravascular thrombosis, increase in cerebral microvascular patency and integrity, and enhancement of spatial learning in rats subjected to traumatic brain injury, Journal of Neurosurgery Vol. 101(5): 813-821

[131] Edward H. Stullken, Jr., William E. Johnston, Jr.,Donald S. Prough, Francis J. Balestrieri, and Joe M. McWhorter, (1985), Implications of nimodipine prophylaxis of cerebral vasospasm on anesthetic management during intracranial aneurysm clipping, Journal of Neurosurgery February, Vol. 62 (2):200-205

Chapter 4

Pluripotent Stem Cells in Bone Marrow and Cord Blood

Ambreen Shaikh and Deepa Bhartiya

Additional information is available at the end of the chapter

http://dx.doi.org/10.5772/48133

1. Introduction

In a short span of few years, the possibility that the human body contains cells that can repair and regenerate damaged and diseased tissue has become a reality. Adult stem cells have been isolated from numerous adult tissues, umbilical cord, and other non-embryonic sources, and have demonstrated a surprising ability for transformation into other tissue and cell types and for the repair of damaged tissues.

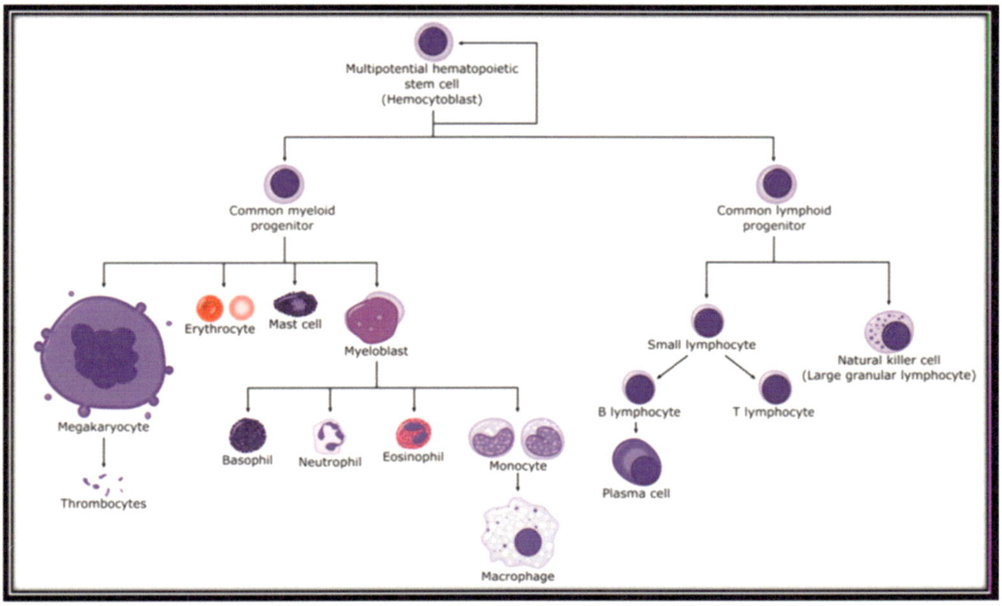

(Image: Hematopoiesis_ (human) _diagram.png by A. Rad)

Figure 1. Hematopoiesis in Bone Marrow

In the 1950s, researchers discovered that the bone marrow contains stem cells i.e. hematopoietic stem cells (HSC) with the ability to self-renew and give rise to cell types in the blood and immune system (Figure1). Multipotent HSCs reside at the apex of hematopoietic hierarchy and they are connected to mature cells by a complex roadmap of progenitor intermediates. The HSC differentiate into two different kinds of progenitors viz. Common Myeloid Progenitors (CMP) and Common Lymphoid Progenitors (CLP), which further differentiate to various blood cells including platelets, granulocytes, lymphocytes and macrophages. As a result, bone marrow transplantation became the standard method of care for most hematopoietic malignancies whereby the HSCs were able to repopulate bone marrow after any kind of hematopoietic failure. A recent review by Doulatov et al [1] describes the knowledge gathered over the years on Hematopoiesis.

Besides HSC, another stem cell population, the mesenchymal stem cells (MSC) was identified in the bone marrow about 40 years ago [2]. MSCs comprise of the adherent stem cell population with immune-modulatory properties. Besides bone marrow, MSCs can also be extracted from virtually all post-natal as well as extra-embryonic tissues such as amniotic membrane, placenta and umbilical cord. They can differentiate along multiple lineages and exhibit significant expansion capability *in vitro*. Co-transplantation with MSCs improves engraftment of HSCs after autologous intra-bone marrow transplantation [3]. MSCs are also considered useful as vehicles for emerging cell and gene therapies in the field of tissue engineering [4]. Recently it has been postulated that MSC provide the conducive microenvironment for HSCs and thus maintain the stemness and proliferation of HSCs and support HSC transplantation [3].

2. Trans-differentiation of bone marrow stem cells

Blood is one of the most highly regenerative tissues in our body with almost one trillion cells arising daily. Over the last decade several investigators have demonstrated that BM stem cells not only contribute to development of blood cells but also to the regeneration of various organs and tissues [5, 6]. MSC isolated from various sources can differentiate into diverse cell types, showing a unique ability to cross lineage borders (i.e. are able to differentiate towards ectoderm-, mesoderm- and endoderm-derived cell types) and do not express the major histocompatibility complex (MHC) class II Human Leukocyte Antigen (HLA-DR) antigens. This, together with their *in vitro* proliferative potential and their immunoregulatory properties, renders them extremely promising for regenerative medicine applications in several diseases [7].

These observations were mainly explained by the hypothesis that the BM stem cells are 'plastic' and thus could dedifferentiate into various cell types of non-hematopoietic organs and tissues [8]. The possibility that HSC/MSC are plastic and able to trans-differentiate raised hope that HSC/MSC isolated from BM, mobilized into the peripheral blood (mPB) or cord blood (CB) could become a universal source of stem cells for tissue/ organ repair. This was supported by several demonstrations of the remarkable regenerative potential of HSC in animal models, for example after heart infarct [5], stroke [9], spinal cord injury [10], and liver damage [11] and of MSC in skeletal regeneration [12], cardiac regeneration [13], diabetes [14] and osteogeneis imperfect [15]. The potential of adult stem cells also resulted in slow growth of research and funding restrictions on ES cells during President Bush regime in USA – based on the argument that destroying embryos to derive human ES cell lines was not essential, when better alternatives including adult stem cells are available for regenerative medicine (http://en.wikipedia.org/wiki/Stem_cell_controversy). However the excitement over plasticity of HSC reduced when their role in repair of damaged organs became controversial [16, 17].

Several alternative mechanisms were proposed to explain the trans-differentiation of bone marrow stem cells [18] including (i) epigenetic changes i.e. factors present in the environment of damaged organs may induce epigenetic changes in the genes that regulate pluripotency of HSCs (ii) cell fusion during which infused HSCs may fuse with cells in damaged tissues and form heterokaryons which express markers of both donor and recipient cells (iii) paracrine effect i.e. HSCs are source of different trophic and angiopoietic factors that may promote tissue/organ repair (iv) microvesicles- dependent transfer of molecules like receptors, proteins and mRNA between HSC and damaged cells and (iv) **presence of pluripotent stem cell population in the bone marrow in addition to HSC & MSC that may contribute to regeneration**. Presence of other stem cells in the BM may also explain the loss of contribution of BM cells to organ regeneration with the use of highly purified population of HSC [16]. Of these various possibilities (i) and (ii) are extremely rare and most likely the fact that BM houses heterogeneous and perhaps pluripotent stem cells may explain transdifferentiation potential of bone marrow. It has been demonstrated that there are heterogeneous stem cell populations in adult bone marrow compartment. Under appropriate experimental conditions, a certain type of bone marrow stem cells appears to differentiate (or transdifferentiate) into a variety of non-haemopoietic cells of ectodermal, mesodermal and endodermal origins (such as myocytes, neural cells and hepatocytes) [67].Various investigators have reported pluripotent stem cells in the bone marrow by using varied approaches to demonstrate their presence and are listed in Table 1.

The potential relationship of the BM-derived pluripotent stem cells reported by various investigators and compiled in Table1 is not clear. It is possible that these are overlapping populations of cells identified by slightly different isolation/ expansion strategies and likely that all of these versatile BM-derived Oct-4+ non-hematopoietic stem cells, which were given different names, are in fact very closely related to the same type of BM-residing Pluripotent Stem Cells (PSC). This overlap was elegantly described earlier by Ratajczak and his group [25] that various investigators are looking from different "keyholes" at the same population of stem cells that are hiding in a "darkroom" of the bone marrow environment. They further suggested that a 'founder cell' may exist in the bone marrow which is responsible for multi-lineage differentiation. Table 2 is a compilation of various markers reported on these differently described PSCs in the bone marrow responsible for their mobility (CXCR4), pluripotency (Oct-4, Nanog, Rex, Tert), non-hematopoietic lineage (CD45), immune status (MHC-1) and their developmental migration similarity to PGCs (SSEA1).

Stem Cell	Functional attributes (in brief)
MAPCs Multipotent Adult Progenitor Cells	Described first by Verfailles and her group [19] Extracted from bone marrow in mouse, rat and human Plastic in nature and give rise to multiple cell types Single MAPC in early mouse embryo can contribute to all body tissues Ability to transdifferentiate Do not form teratomas SSEA-1+, CD13+, Flk-1low, Thy-1low, CD34–, CD44–, CD45–, CD117(c-kit)–, MHC I–, MHC II–m SSEA1+, OCT-4+ Can reconstitute bone marrow and also give rise to HSCs Many characteristics like ES cells MAPCs maintain telomere length Pluripotent properties even after 50 doublings
MIAMI Marrow Isolated Adult Lineage Inducible Cells	Bone marrow derived adult stem cells isolated in humans aged 3- 72 years [20] Pluripotent by nature Capable of differentiating into cells from all three germ layers Positive for OCT-4, REX-1 and telomerase >50 population doublings with no sign of senescence Express markers typically associated with embryonic stem cells
RS cells Recycling Stem Cells	Are a sub-population of cells present amongst the MSCs [21] Small in size Proliferate rapidly $CD45^-$
MACS Multipotent Adult Progenitor Cells	Express pluripotent-state-specific transcription factors (OCT-4, Nanog and Rex1[22] Cloned from human liver, heart, and BM-isolated mononuclear cells High telomerase activity Wide range of differentiation potential.
MPCs Mesodermal Progenitor Stem Cells	Detected in bone marrow and cord blood [23] Exist as a sub-population in MSC culture Fail to divide in culture thus quiescent Multi- to pluripotent by nature Express SSEA-4, OCT-4, Nanog by IF and RT-PCR
VSELs Very Small Embryonic-like Stem Cells	Homogenous population of rare (~0.01% of BM mononuclear cells) Sca-1+ Lin– $CD45^-$ cells identified in murine BM [24] Express SSEA-1, OCT- 4, Nanog and Rex-1 & Rif-1 telomerase protein Small size (~3.5 μm in diameter) Large nucleus surrounded by a narrow rim of cytoplasm Open-type chromatin (euchromatin) Differentiate into three lineages Do not form teratoma Quiescent population of cells

Table 1. Pluripotent Stem Cells Reported in the Bone Marrow

Characteristics Markers	MAPC	MIAMI	MACS	RS	VSEL
Shape and size	Form small colonies in culture	Form small colonies in culture	Small	Small	Small
CXCR4	+	+	+	+	+
CD 133	ND	ND	-	-	+
Sca 1	ND	ND	ND	ND	+
CD 45	-	-	-	-	-
OCT-4	+	+	+	ND	+
REX-1	ND	+	+	ND	+
Nanog	+	+	+	+	+
TERT	+	+	ND	+	+
SSEA 1	+	ND	ND	ND	+
MHC-1	-	ND	+	ND	-
Quiescent by nature	No data available	No data available	No data available	No data available	+
Teratoma formation	Do not form teratoma	Do not form teratoma	Do not form teratoma	Do not form teratoma	Do not form teratoma

ND-experiment not done; + positive; - negative

Table 2. Compilation of Various Markers on BM Pluripotent Stem Cells

Besides these pluripotent stem cells, BM also houses Tissue Committed Stem Cells (TCSCs) including Epithelial Progenitor Cells (EPCs). Available literature suggests that postnatal neovascularization does not rely on formation of new blood vessels from pre-existing ones (angiogenesis) rather on EPCs migrating from the BM to induce neovascularization. EPCs and HSCs share certain markers like Flk-1, Tic2, Sca-1, and CD34. As a result it has been suggested that they both may arise from a common precursor [26].

Interestingly the trans-differentiation ability of adult BM cells into various TCSCs like hepatocytes, cardiomyocytes, vascular endothelial cells, neuronal cells etc. occurs only when there is a need i.e. into hepatocytes when damage is inflicted on the liver by radiation or chemical damage [27], into cardiomyocytes when myocardial infarction is induced [28], into endothelial cells on inducing ischemia [29] and into neural stem cells on inducing stroke [30]. In the same manner, the BM stem cells have also been shown to trans-differentiate into germ cells when gonadal function is compromised e.g. by treating with busulphan in female [31] and male [32] mice. Freshly prepared BM may also exhibit early tissue-specific markers but are up-regulated several folds when the function of organ is compromised [33].

Pluripotent stem cells are expected to be more primitive to TCSCs based on their developmental hierarchy (totipotent - pluripotent - multipotent– unipotent stem cells). This is also supported by various observations shown below.

- Freshly isolated TCSC from the BM express tissue committed markers
- PSCs in BM acquire these markers after many days in culture
- TCSCs express c-Kit which is a more differentiated marker not expressed by PSCs.

Thus we propose following developmental hierarchy of stem cells in bone marrow (Figure:2) as opposed to the existing notion that HSC sit at the apex of hematopoietic system [1].

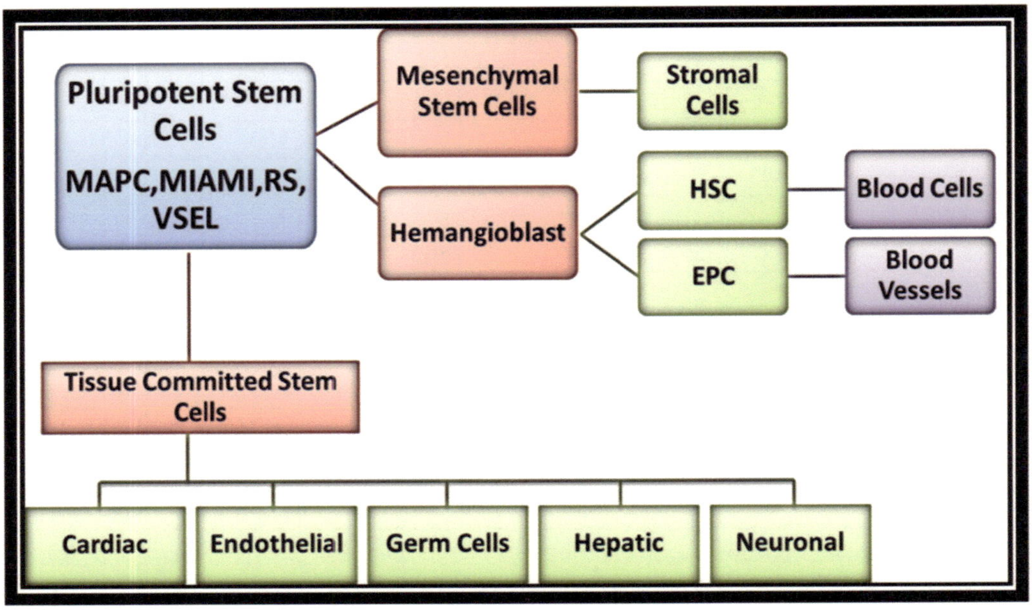

Figure 2. Developmental hierarchy of stem cells in bone marrow

The existing controversial literature that HSCs and MSCs can trans-differentiate into various lineages can be alternatively explained by the presence of these pluripotent stem cells. These PSCs interact closely with the MSCs by a process defined as emperipolesis [34]. The MSCs secrete SDF-1(Stromal Derived Factor-1) and other chemo-attractants thereby creating a homing environment for these pluripotent stem cells (express CXCR4). Thus isolated BM stem cells have always been contaminated with these PSCs which may have resulted in trans-differentiation and that HSCs/MSCs (being lineage restricted themselves) possibly do not account for the observed plasticity.

3. Origin & deposition of hematopoietic and non-hematopoietic stem cells in bone marrow

Early embryogenesis is the most active period for the developmental migration/trafficking of stem cells. With the beginning of gastrulation and organogenesis, stem cells migrate to places where they establish rudiments for new tissues and organs. At certain points, of development stem cells colonize tissue specific niches, where they reside as a population of self renewing cells supplying new cells that effectively replace senescent ones or those undergoing apoptosis.

In mammals the first primitive HSC are found in the yolk sac and first definitive HSC a few days later in the aorta-gonadmesonephros (AGM) region [35]. From the yolk sac and/or AGM region HSC migrate to the fetal liver (FL), which during the second trimester of gestation becomes the major mammalian hematopoietic organ. By the end of the second trimester of gestation, HSC leave the fetal liver and colonize BM tissue. Signals for the translocation of HSC from the fetal liver to BM are provided by the alpha chemokine – SDF-1 that is secreted by osteoblasts lining the developing marrow cavities, marrow fibroblasts and endothelial cells. In response to SDF-1, HSC that expresses, SDF-1 receptor-a seven transmembrane-spanning G protein coupled CXCR4 receptor, leave the fetal liver and begin to home into BM where they finally establish adult haematopoiesis.

It is very likely that at this point BM is also colonized by several other nonhematopoietic stem cells that may circulate during organogenesis and rapid foetal growth/expansion. In support of this stem cells for different tissues express CXCR4 on their surface and follow an SDF-1 gradient. Thus the SDF-1-CXCR4 axis alone or in combination with other chemoattractants plays a crucial role in the accumulation of non-hematopoietic stem cells in developing BM [36, 37]. These cells find a permissive environment to survive in BM, and may play an underappreciated role as a reserve pool of stem cells for organ/tissue regeneration during postnatal life.

The presence of these various populations of stem cells in the BM (Table 1) is a result of the 'developmental migration' of stem cells during ontogenesis and the presence of the permissive environment that attracts them to the BM tissue. HSC and other non-hematopoietic stem cells are actively chemoattracted by factors secreted by BM stromal cells and osteoblasts (e.g. SDF-1), hepatocyte growth factor (HGF)) and colonize marrow by the end of the second and the beginning of the third trimester of gestation [24].

It is assumed that these non-hematopoietic pluripotent stem cells are deposited in the BM during early embryogenesis and subsequently may be mobilized in stressed situations and circulate in the peripheral blood. Similarly due to the stress of delivery these cells may also be present in cord blood [18].

Interestingly various terminologies like MAPCs, MIAMI, RS cells etc. (Table 1) disappeared from the literature after initial publications and excitement except VSELs. Ratajczak and group have made tremendous contribution to the field of VSELs biology. At present various laboratories across the world are providing evidence to support the pluripotent property and potential of VSELs isolated from cord blood and bone marrow [38]. Possible reason being the method to isolate VSELs by flow cytometry described by Ratajczak and group could easily be replicated in various labs across the world.

4. Very small embryonic like stem cells (VSELs)

VSELs were identified by Ratajczak and group in 2006 by multi parameter sorting in adult murine BM. They express several morphological (e.g., relatively large nuclei containing euchromatin) and molecular (e.g. expression of SSEA-1, Oct4, Nanog, Rex1) markers characteristic for embryonic stem cells (ESCs) [33]. The morphology of the cells was investigated using transmission electron microscopy which showed their distinctive morphology and size differentiating VSELs from HSC in particular in terms of size (3–6 μm vs. 6–8 μm for HSC), chromatin structure and nucleus/cytoplasm ratio. Based on their small size, presence of PSC markers, distinct morphology (open-type chromatin, large nucleus, narrow rim of cytoplasm with multiple mitochondria) and ability to differentiate into all three germ layers, including mesoderm-derived cardiomyocytes, these cells were named very small embryonic-like stem cells. The true expression of Oct-4 and Nanog in BM-derived VSELs (BM-VSELs) was recently confirmed by demonstrating transcriptionally active chromatin structures of Oct4 and Nanog promoters. A mechanism based on parent-of-origin-specific reprogramming of genomic imprinting that keeps VSELs quiescent in a dormant state in tissues has been described. VSELs highly express Gbx2, Fgf5, and Nodal, but express less Rex1/Zfp42 transcript as compared to ESC-D3s what suggests that VSELs are more differentiated than ICM-derived ESCs and share several markers with more differentiated EpiSCs. VSELs also highly express Dppa2, Dppa4, and Mvh, which characterize late migratory PGCs. The expression of germ line markers (Oct4 and SSEA-1) and modulation of somatic imprints suggest a potential developmental similarity between VSELs and germ line-derived primordial germ cells (PGCs) [39, 40].

Developmental Origin of VSELs: VSELs are epiblast-derived PSCs deposited early during embryonic development in developing organs as a potential reserve pool of precursors for TCSCs and thus this population has an important role in tissue rejuvenation and regeneration. VSELs originate from or are closely related to a population of proximal epiblast migratory Stem Cells (EpiSCs) that approximately at embryonic day (E)7.25 in mice, become specified to PGCs, and egress from the epiblast into extra-embryonic tissues (extra-embryonic mesoderm) [41]. VSELs follow developmental route of HSCs colonizing together with HSCs first fetal liver and subsequently BM [37].

Thus PGCs, HSCs, and VSELs form all together a unique highly migratory population of interrelated Stem Cells (SCs) that could be envisioned to be a kind of "fourth highly migratory germ layer." [37]

Self-renewal and in vitro differentiation of VSELs: VSELs exist in various mouse organs [42], have been well-characterized and are capable of differentiating into all three lineages, supporting their true pluripotent character. Murine VSELs form embryoid body-like structures in co-cultures over C2C12 supportive cell line [24] and could become specified into HSCs after co-culture over OP-9 stroma cells. VSELs-derived HSCs harvested from these co-cultures reconstitute murine bone marrow after total body irradiation [43]. The Umbilical Cord Blood (UCB)-purified VSELs have also been reported to differentiate into neural cells [44] and after co-culture over OP-9 stroma cells were specified into HSCs similar to murine BM-derived VSELs [45]. Apart from umbilical cord blood and bone marrow, VSELs have also been reported in Wharton's jelly and gonadal tissue [46- 51]. Their presence amongst the MSCs in the Wharton's jelly is in agreement with observations made by other groups that MSCs contain a sub-population of more primitive stem cells [52] or even as postulated by Taichman and group [53] that VSELs are precursors of MSCs. Various studies have also reported that VSELs are mobilized into peripheral blood in response to injury/ stress in animal models [27,54-56] as well as in humans [28-30,57] – thus suggesting a role in regeneration and homeostasis.

5. Our studies on VSELs in cord blood and bone marrow

We studied the VSELs in UCB and discarded fraction of BM [46]. Usually the 'buffy coat' obtained after Ficoll-Hypaque centrifugation is considered to be rich in stem cells and used for various studies over several decades. **However, we reported that VSELs settle along with the RBCs rather than getting enriched in the 'buffy coat (Figure:3). Similarly we found that the 'discarded' RBC pellet obtained during initial processing of bone marrow was also rich in VSELs. These results were explained on the basis of buoyancy. The adult stem cells have abundant cytoplasm, are relatively larger and thus observed in the buffy layer whereas the VSELs are the pluripotent stem cells, with high nucleo-cytoplasmic ratio, minimal cytoplasm and thus sink to the bottom of the tube along with the RBCs.** These VSELs exhibited various pluripotent markers, like $CD45^-$, $CD133^+$ $SSEA\text{-}4^+$. They also exhibit other primordial germ cell markers like Stella and Fragillis, thus supporting their origin from the epiblast stage embryo at the same time when PGCs migrate via the dorsal mesentry to the gonadal ridges to become a source of germ cells.

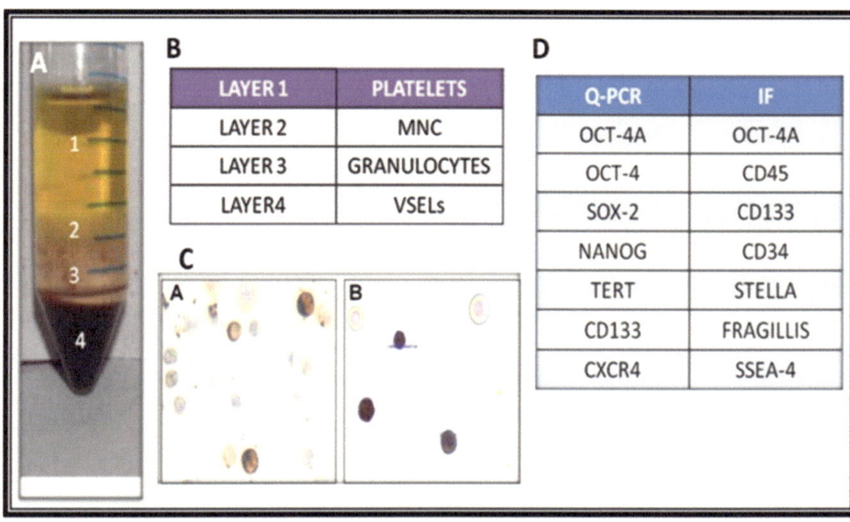

Figure 3. Isolation and characterization of VSELs from Cord Blood: A-Separation of cord blood into four layers on Ficoll-Hypaque; B-Description of cells observed in each layer separated; C-Immunolocalization studies on MNC (A) and VSEL (B) using polyclonal Oct-4 (40X); D-Markers characterized on VSELs using Quantitative PCR and immunofluorescence

These studies have several implications e.g. the stem cell biologists should ask themselves what is getting banked in the cord blood banks. VSELs unknowingly get discarded and only adult stem cells (and progenitors) including HSCs and MSCs get banked. Similarly autologus stem cell therapy for various indications other than blood related diseases have resulted in minimal improvement. This may be explained since fate restricted progenitors HSC and MSC may have limited trans-differentiation ability. The pluripotent VSELs have maximum 'plasticity' and regenerative potential but are getting discarded unknowingly. This raises a valid question on the success of BM transplantation to treat blood related diseases. This success could be accounted for by the differentiation ability of progenitor cells into blood cells.

While doing immunolocalization studies to detect OCT-4 positive cells, we found the VSELs express nuclear OCT-4 whereas a slightly bigger cell in the 'buffy coat' collected from both the cord blood and bone marrow exhibited cytoplasmic OCT-4 (Figure:4). These are possibly the most immediate progenitors 'descendants' from VSELs. We also conducted immunolocalization studies on umbilical cord tissue in the region of Wharton's jelly which is rich in MSCs. Results show that the MSCs had cytoplasmic OCT-4 like HSCs and that there was a distinct subpopulation of small cells with nuclear OCT-4 and were the VSELs, based on their size (Figure:4). On a similar note, when we did immunolocalization of mouse bone marrow stem cells, we observed that the MSCs with typical fibroblast like morphology have cytoplasmic OCT-4 along with VSELs with nuclear OCT-4. The MSCs showed a very heterogeneous staining pattern. Only a sub population of MSCs were positive whereas other MSCs totally lacked cytoplasmic OCT-4. This possibly shows different differentiation state since as the cell gets more committed, cytoplasmic OCT-4 is no longer required.

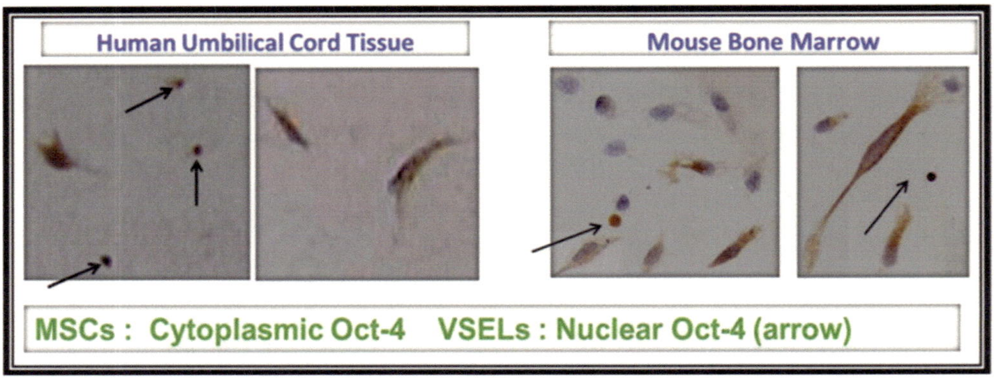

Figure 4. Immunolocalization of Oct-4 in umbillical cord tissue

Thus we concluded that the bone marrow compartment comprises of pluripotent VSELs and their immediate descendants like HSCs and MSCs. Also that the most primitive stem cell in the bone marrow is a pluripotent VSEL as shown in Figure 2. Being the most primitive stem cell in the BM, we hypothesize that VSEL will show best engraftment post transplantation and also will be best vehicle for gene therapy.

VSELs possibly undergo asymmetric cell division to self- renew and give rise to progenitors which further expand and differentiate to committed cell types. VSELs remain relatively quiescent throughout life, maintain long telomeres and are possibly the normal body stem cells which give rise to cancer stem cells (CSC) under certain unfavourable conditions. We propose that this transformation of a VSEL into CSC occurs due unidentified changes in the microenvironment. Recently it has also been reported that VSELs resist radiotherapy (because of their quiescent nature) that destroys all actively dividing stem cell population in the bone marrow [43]. The somatic microenvironment is also compromised by the radiotherapy. Thus although the VSELs persist, they are unable to reconstitute the bone marrow.

Existence of two stem cell populations in various adult body tissues is an interesting concept put forth by Li and Clevers [58]. They proposed that both quiescent (out of cell cycle and in a lower metabolic state) and active (in cell cycle and not able to retain DNA labels) stem cell subpopulations may coexist in several tissues like gut epithelium, hair follicle, bone marrow etc. We have generated data to show that similar two distinct populations of stem cells exist in mammalian gonads also. Interestingly similar stem cell biology persists in the mammalian gonads irrespective of sex and is possibly an evolutionarily conserved phenomenon as we have reported the same in mice, rabbits, sheep, monkey and humans [48, 50].

6. VSELs in mammalian testis

We have reported for the first time the presence of a distinct population of VSELs with nuclear OCT-4 in adult mouse [48] and human [47] testis, located towards the basement membrane of the seminiferous tubules. Besides, we also detected a progenitor stem cell population with cytoplasmic OCT-4, which was slightly bigger and had abundant cytoplasm. These cells showed extensive proliferation with cytoplasmic bridges as cords. As these cells differentiated further, the cytoplasmic OCT-4 was gradually lost. Interestingly the VSELs were found resistant to busulphan treatment which otherwise destroyed the dividing progenitors, haploid cells and damaged the somatic niche. Thus, it is evident that like the earlier report on bone marrow VSELs, gonadal VSELs are also resistant to oncotherapy. VSELs possibly undergo asymmetric cell division to give rise to progenitors, which undergo clonal expansion and may further differentiate into sperm (Figure:5)

7. VSELs in mammalian ovary

A gentle scraping of the adult ovary surface (mouse, rabbit, sheep, monkey and human) with a sterile blade releases stem cells in a Petri dish [50]. On H & E staining, two distinct stem cell populations can be easily detected based on their size and differential OCT-4 staining pattern. The smaller stem cell population are smaller than the RBCs and exhibit nuclear OCT-4 whereas the slightly bigger population exhibits cytoplasmic OCT-4. Like cords in the testis, in the ovary we observed the presence of germ cell nests with cytoplasmic continuity representing extensive proliferation of progenitor stem cells. These stem cells were present in peri- menopausal human ovary and also persisted in mouse ovary after busulphan treatment. Like in the testis, the functionality of ovarian stem cells is also affected by a compromised niche.

Three weeks culture of peri-menopausal ovarian stem cells produces oocyte-like structures, embryo-like structures *in vitro* [50]. Thus the stem cells retain their functionality but are unable to differentiate because of a non-supportive niche.

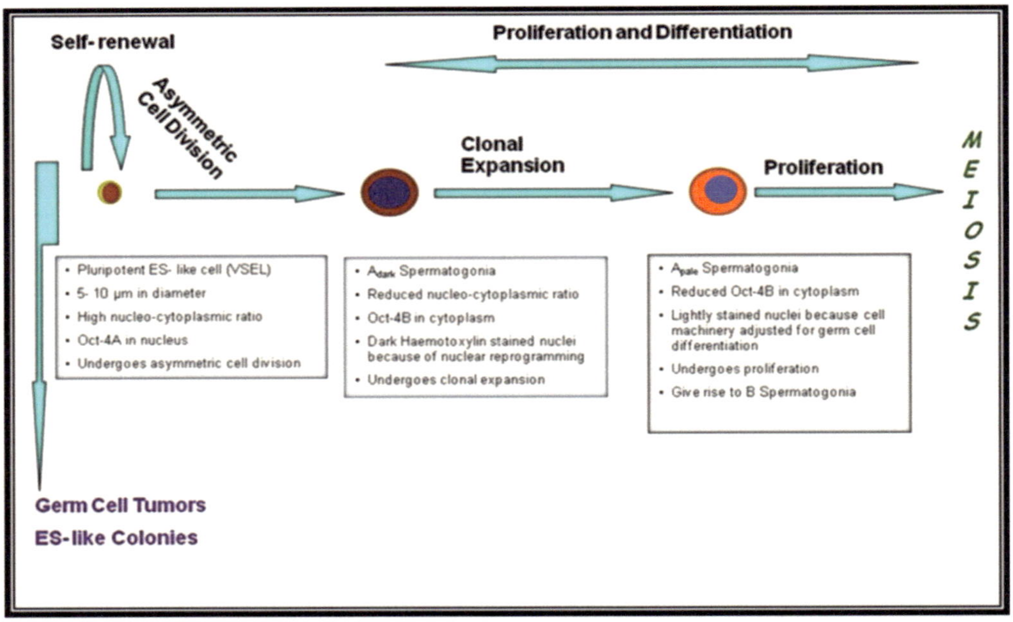

Figure 5. Revised scheme for premeiotic development of germ cells in adult human testis

8. Significance of somatic microenvironment 'Niche' on VSELs functionality

A relatively quiescent VSEL and actively dividing progenitor model that possibly exists in ovary, testis, bone marrow, cord blood and Wharton's jelly ensures that the 'master stem cell' undergoes very few rounds of DNA replication to prevent its genome from age-related changes and acquisition of errors during DNA replication.

Table 3 highlights the importance of the somatic niche in controlling the stem cell fate. It is the same VSEL that exists in different body organs but the niche dictates its fate [46].

Sr.no	Tissue	VSEL with nuclear Oct-4	Progenitor stem cells with cytoplasmic Oct-4 (tissue-specific progenitor stem cells)
1	Testis	✓	Adark spermatogonia stem cells SSCs (Adark)
2	Ovary	✓	Ovarian germ stem cells (OGSCs)
3	Bone marrow, Umbilical cord blood and tissue	✓	Hematopoietic stem cells (HSC) Mesenchymal stem cells (MSC)

Table 3. Details of Very Small Embryonic-Like Stem Cell–Derived Progenitors in Adult Human Tissues

The possible reason why extensive plasticity of VSELs is evident in bone marrow and cord blood (so many different kind of TCSCs have been described) in contrast to testis or ovary may be because the bone marrow niche is more permissive as compared to a 'gonadal' niche which is more specialized and thus restricted in nature.

9. VSELs and cancer

Several years of cancer research suggests that cancers begin with genetic changes that occur over a period of 15 to 20 years and in few cases a link to chronic inflammation has been proposed e.g. in case of ovarian cancers, Barrett's esophagus etc. However, emerging literature suggests that quiescent VSELs distributed in various organs may be a cellular origin of cancer development. In 1855 Virchow proposed the embryonal rest hypothesis of tumor formation, based on histological similarities between tumors and embryonic tissues. This theory was later expanded by other pathologist including Julius Conheim, who suggested that tumors develop from residual embryonic remnants lost during developmental organogenesis [59]

Recently identified VSELs in various adult body tissues display morphology and markers characteristics as the pluripotent embryonic stem cells. These cells could support Virchow's concept of an embryonic origin of cancer. Possibly the somatic niche, which keeps the VSELs in a quiescent stage under normal circumstances, undergoes some changes which push the quiescent VSELs to an actively dividing state i.e. the tumor.

Wang et al [60] recently reported that persisting embryonic cells in adult mice and humans at the squamo-columnar junction are possibly the source of Barrett's metaplasia and that it does not arise from mutant cells. They proposed that certain precancerous lesions, such as Barrett's, initiate not from genetic alterations but from competitive interactions between cell lineages driven by opportunity. Similarly, almost 90% of ovarian cancers arise from the ovary surface epithelium which is also the niche for ovarian stem cells. It is being proposed that ovarian niche gets compromised with age leading to menopause [61, 62] and also to cancer. It is essential to dissect out age related changes which lead to menopause and how they differ from those which lead to cancer. OCT-4, characteristic marker of VSELs is also a very good marker with high sensitivity and specificity for testicular germ cell tumors as well [63].

Cancer stem cells and VSELs with embryonic characteristics have a lot of similarities in terms of markers, telomere length, and resistance to radiotherapy; thus it may be proposed that VSELs transform into CSCs when certain not so well understood changes occur in the microenvironment. It is possible that inflammation may alter the niche where the VSELs reside. It is highly unlikely that a somatic cell which is relatively senescent and has short telomeres will dedifferentiate and acquire long telomeres to transform into a cancer stem cell. Keeping this in mind, because of a defect in stem cell in the bone marrow due to an altered niche – defective stem cell divisions occur and differentiation of such altered cells results in appearance of chromosomal defects in mononuclear cells picked by standard cytogenetic studies.

Identification of VSELs in adult tissues also opens new areas of investigation to elucidate how these cells contribute to the development of poorly differentiated tumors. Studying the biology of normal stem cells may help us to better understand the biology of cancer, and explain its resistance to radio-chemotherapy, ability to an unlimited proliferation and establishment of distant metastases.

10. Conclusions

The field of BMT also stands to greatly benefit once VSELs potential are realized. A review article by Takizawa et al [64] makes an interesting reading and that despite advances in the field, timely availability of HLA matched BM is still problematic for patients including those who require multiple transplantations. In this context, *in vitro* expansion of HSC is crucial but not yet achieved. It is still hoped that a single HSC may suffice to induce long-term multilineage engraftment. Notta et al [65] reported the possibility of CD49f as a specific marker to isolate HSC. In the chapter we are proposing that VSELs possibly give rise to HSC and may be better cell source to induce engraftment. Using cell surface markers to identify cell types always has associated issues since surface phenotype of a cell can change depending on the activation status of the precursor cells. Danova-Alt et al [66] recently concluded that UCB VSELs neither have embryonic nor adult stem cell-like phenotype, are not equivalent to mouse VSELs, have aneuploid karyotype and should not be regarded as a stem cell population. However, they have studied Lin-/CD45-/CD34+ cells and not Lin-/CD45-/CD133+ cells, which are the VSELs as described by Ratacjzak and group [38]. Further it remains to be confirmed whether the aneuploidies they report are a technical artefact, since no cell lineage is expected to be aneuploid.

VSELs could potentially be a real therapeutic alternative to the use of human ES cells since they do not form teratomas, are relatively quiescent and can be isolated from an autologous source. The fact that VSELs may differentiate *in vitro* into cells from all three germ layers makes these cells potential candidates in regenerative medicine. Finally, the mechanism by which VSELs could contribute to development of some malignancies could shed more light on origin of tumours. In conclusion it is of vital importance to evaluate if VSELs could be efficiently employed in the clinic. The work on VSELs is on the verge of development and in coming years will bring more answers to the potential of these cells.

11. Key points of the Chapter

- The trans-differentiation potential of the HSC or MSC from bone marrow is controversial and can be alternatively explained by the presence of pluripotent stem cells in the bone marrow.
- MAPC, MIAMI, VSELs, RS are possibly the same pluripotent stem cells, described differently by various investigators. All of these terminologies have disappeared over time in published literature except VSELs that are being widely studied by various groups across the world.
- VSELs are epiblast derived stem cells expressing pluripotent markers with high nucleo-cytoplasmic ratio and transcriptionally active chromatin. They have been isolated from various murine organs as well as from human organs including gonadal tissues, cord blood, bone marrow and Wharton's jelly.
- VSELs (with nuclear OCT-4) possibly are the most primitive cell type in BM and umbilical cord and give rise to HSC and MSC (with cytoplasmic OCT-4).

- The quiescent nature of VSEL prevent it from tumor formation *in vivo* but an altered somatic niche may lead to transformation of VSEL to cancer stem cell – resulting in cancer.

Author details

Ambreen Shaikh and Deepa Bhartiya*
Stem Cell Biology Department, National Institute for Research in Reproductive Health (ICMR), Mumbai, India

12. References

[1] Doulatov S, Notta F, Laurenti E, Dick J (2012) Haematopoiesis: A Human Perspective. Cell Stem Cell.10:120-136.

[2] Friedenstein AJ, Chailakhjan RK, Lalykina KS (1970) The Development of Fibroblast Colonies in Monolayer Cultures of Guinea-Pig Bone Marrow and Spleen Cells. Cell Tissue Kinet.3:393-403.

[3] Li T and Wu Y (2011) Paracrine Molecules of Mesenchymal Stem Cells for Hematopoietic Stem Cell Niche. Bone Marrow Research doi:10.1155/2011/353878.

[4] Karagianni M, Schulze T, Bieback K (2012) Towards Clinical Application of Mesenchymal Stromal Cells: Perspectives and Requirements for Orthopaedic Applications .In: Davies J, editor. Tissue Regeneration - From Basic Biology to Clinical Application. InTech. ISBN: 978-953-51-0387-5.

[5] Orlic D, Kajstura J, Chimenti S, Jakoniuk I, Anderson SM, Li B, Pickel J, McKay R, Nadal-Ginard B, Bodine DM, Leri A, Anversa P (2001) Bone Marrow Cells Regenerate Infarcted Myocardium. Nature.6829:701-5.

[6] Lagasse E, Connors H, Al-Dhalimy M, Reitsma M, Dohse M, Osborne L, Wang X, Finegold M, Weissman IL, Grompe M (2000) Purified Hematopoietic Stem Cells Can Differentiate into Hepatocytes *In Vivo*. Nature Medicine.11:1229-34.

[7] Anzalone R, Lo Iacono M, Loria T, Di Stefano A, Giannuzzi P, Farina F, La Rocca G (2011) Wharton's Jelly Mesenchymal Stem Cells As Candidates for Beta Cells Regeneration: Extending the Differentiative and Immunomodulatory Benefits of Adult Mesenchymal Stem Cells for the Treatment of Type 1 Diabetes. Stem Cell Rev.2:342-63.

[8] Mezey E, Chandross KJ, Harta G, Maki RA, McKercher SR (2000) Turning Blood into Brain: Cells Bearing Neuronal Antigens Generated *In Vivo* from Bone Marrow. Science.5497:1779-82.

[9] Hess DC, Abe T, Hill WD, Studdard AM, Carothers J, Masuya M, Fleming PA, Drake CJ, Ogawa M (2004) Hematopoietic Origin of Microglial and Perivascular Cells in Brain. Exp Neurol. 2:134-44.

[10] Corti S, Locatelli F, Donadoni C, Strazzer S, Salani S, Del Bo R, Caccialanza M, Bresolin N, Scarlato G, Comi GP (2002) Neuroectodermal and Microglial Differentiation of Bone

* Corresponding Author

Marrow Cells in the Mouse Spinal Cord and Sensory Ganglia. J Neurosci Res. 70(6):721-33.
[11] Petersen BE, Bowen WC, Patrene KD, Mars WM, Sullivan AK, Murase N, Boggs SS, Greenberger JS, Goff JP (1999) Bone Marrow as a Potential Source of Hepatic Oval Cells. Science.284(5417):1168-70.
[12] Xu Y, Malladi P, Wagner DR, Longaker MT (2005) Adipose-Derived Mesenchymal Cells as a Potential Cell Source for Skeletal Regeneration. Curr Opin Mol Ther.4:300-5.
[13] Minguell JJ, Erices A (2006) Mesenchymal Stem Cells and the Treatment of Cardiac Disease. Exp Biol Med (Maywood). 231(1):39-49.
[14] Lee RH, Seo MJ, Reger RL, Spees JL, Pulin AA, Olson SD, Prockop DJ (2006) Multipotent Stromal Cells from Human Marrow Home to and Promote Repair of Pancreatic Islets and Renal Glomeruli in Diabetic NOD/SCID Mice. Proc Natl Acad Sci U S A.103(46):17438-43.
[15] Horwitz EM, Gordon PL, Koo WK, Marx JC, Neel MD, McNall RY, Muul L, Hofmann T (2002) Isolated Allogeneic Bone Marrow-Derived Mesenchymal Cells Engraft and Stimulate Growth in Children with Osteogenesis Imperfecta: Implications for Cell Therapy of Bone. Proc Natl Acad Sci U S A.99(13):8932-7.
[16] Orkin SH, Zon LI (2002) Hematopoiesis and Stem Cells: Plasticity Versus Developmental Heterogeneity. Nat Immunol.3(4):323-8.
[17] Wagers AJ, Sherwood RI, Christensen JL, Weissman IL (2002) Little Evidence for Developmental Plasticity of Adult Hematopoietic Stem Cells. Science.297(5590):2256-9.
[18] Ratajczak MZ, Zuba-Surma EK, Wojakowski W, Ratajczak J, Kucia M (2008) Bone Marrow- Home of Versatile Stem Cells. Transfus Med Hemother. 35(3):248-259.
[19] Jiang Y, Vaessen B, Lenvik T, Blackstad M, Reyes M, Verfaillie CM (2002) Multipotent Progenitor Cells can be Isolated from Postnatal Murine Bone Marrow, Muscle, and Brain. Exp Hematol.30: 896-904.
[20] D'Ippolito G, Diabira S, Howard GA, Menei P, Roos BA, Schiller PC (2004) Marrow-Isolated Adult Multilineage Inducible (MIAMI) Cells, a Unique Population of Postnatal Young and Old Human Cells with Extensive Expansion and Differentiation Potential. J Cell Sci. 117:2971-2981.
[21] Colter DC, Sekiya I, Prockop DJ (2001) Identification of a Subpopulation of Rapidly Self-Renewing and Multipotential Adult Stem Cells in Colonies of Human Marrow Stromal Cells. Proc Natl Acad Sci U S A. 98:7841-7845.
[22] Pacini S, Carnicelli V, Trombi L, Montali M, Fazzi R, Lazzarini E, Giannotti S, Petrini M (2010) Constitutive Expression of Pluripotency-Associated Genes in Mesodermal Progenitor Cells (MPCs). PLoS ONE 5(3): e9861. doi:10.1371/journal.pone.0009861.
[23] Beltrami AP, Cesselli D, Bergamin N, Marcon P, Rigo S, Puppato E, D'Aurizio F, Verardo R, Piazza S, Pignatelli A, Poz A, Baccarani U, Damiani D, Fanin R, Mariuzzi L, Finato N, Masolini P, Burelli S, Belluzzi O, Schneider C, Beltrami CA (2007) Multipotent Cells can be Generated *In Vitro* from Several Adult Human Organs (Heart, Liver And Bone Marrow). Blood.110:3438-3446.

[24] Kucia M, Reca R, Campbell FR, Zuba-Surma E, Majka M, Ratajczak J, Ratajczak MZ (2006) A Population of Very Small Embryonic-Like (VSEL) CXCR4(+)SSEA-1(+)Oct-4+ Stem Cells Identified in Adult Bone Marrow. Leukemia 20:857-869.

[25] Ratajczak MZ, Kucia M, Reca R, Majka M, Janowska- Wieczorek A, Ratajczak J (2004) Stem Cell Plasticity Revisited: CXCR4-Positive Cells Expressing mRNA for Early Muscle, Liver and Neural Cells 'Hide Out' in the Bone Marrow. Leukemia. 18:29-40.

[26] Asahara T and Kawamoto A (2004) Endothelial progenitor cells for postnatal vasculogenesis. Am J Physiol Cell Physiol 287:C572–C579.

[27] Kucia MJ, Wysoczynski M, Wu W, Zuba-Surma EK, Ratajczak J, Ratajczak MZ (2008) Evidence that Very Small Embryonic-Like Stem Cells are Mobilized into Peripheral Blood. Stem Cells. 26(8):2083-2092.

[28] Wojakowski W, Tendera M, Kucia M, Zuba-Surma E, Paczkowska E, Ciosek J, Hałasa M, Król M, Kazmierski M, Buszman P, Ochała A, Ratajczak J, Machaliński B, Ratajczak MZ (2009) Mobilization of Bone Marrow-Derived Oct-4+ SSEA-4+ Very Small Embryonic-Like Stem Cells in Patients with Acute Myocardial Infarction. J Am Coll Cardiol. 53(1):1-9.

[29] Abdel-Latif A, Zuba-Surma EK, Ziada KM, Kucia M, Cohen DA, Kaplan AM, Van Zant G, Selim S, Smyth SS, Ratajczak MZ (2010) Evidence of Mobilization of Pluripotent Stem Cells into Peripheral Blood of Patients with Myocardial Ischemia. Exp Hematol.38(12):1131-1142.

[30] Paczkowska E, Kucia M, Koziarska D, Halasa M, Safranow K, Masiuk M, Karbicka A, Nowik M, Nowacki P, Ratajczak MZ, Machalinski B (2009) Clinical Evidence that Very Small Embryonic-Like Stem Cells are Mobilized into Peripheral Blood in Patients after Stroke. Stroke. 40(4):1237-1244.

[31] Johnson J, Bagley J, Skaznik-Wikiel M, Lee HJ, Adams GB, Niikura Y, Tschudy KS, Tilly JC, Cortes ML, Forkert R, Spitzer T, Iacomini J, Scadden DT, Tilly JL (2005) Oocyte Generation in Adult Mammalian Ovaries by Putative Germ Cells in Bone Marrow and Peripheral Blood. Cell.122(2):303-15.

[32] Nayernia K, Lee JH, Drusenheimer N, Nolte J, Wulf G, Dressel R, Gromoll J, Engel W (2006) Derivation of Male Germ Cells from Bone Marrow Stem Cells. Laboratory Investigation 86:654–663.

[33] Ratajczak MZ, Liu R, Marlicz W, Blogowski W, Starzynska T, Wojakowski W, Zuba-Surma E (2011) Identification of Very Small Embryonic/Epiblast-Like Stem Cells (Vsels) Circulating in Peripheral Blood During Organ/Tissue Injuries. Methods Cell Biol.103:31-54.

[34] Kucia M, Wysoczynski M, Ratajczak J, Ratajczak MZ (2008) Identification of Very Small Embryonic Like Stem Cells (VSEL) in Bone Marrow. Cell Tissue Res.331(1):125-34.

[35] Ivanovs A, Rybtsov S, Welch L, Anderson RA, Turner ML, Medvinsky A (2011) Highly Potent Human Hematopoietic Stem Cells First Emerge in the Intraembryonic Aorta-Gonad-Mesonephros Region. J Exp Med. 208(12):2417-27.

[36] Kucia M, Zuba-Surma E,Wysoczynski ,Dobrowolska H, Reca R, Ratajczak J, Ratajczak MZ (2006) Physiological and Pathological Consequences of Identification of Very Small

Embryonic Like (Vsel) Stem Cells in Adult Bone Marrow J Physiol Pharmacol.57 Suppl 5:5-18.

[37] Zuba-Surma EK, Kucia M, Rui L, Shin DM, Wojakowski W, Ratajczak J, Ratajczak MZ (2009) Fetal Liver Very Small Embryonic/Epiblast Like Stem Cells Follow Developmental Migratory Pathway of Hematopoietic Stem Cells. Ann N Y Acad Sci. 1176:205-18.

[38] Ratajczak MZ, Shin DM, Liu R, Mierzejewska K, Ratajczak J, Kucia M, Zuba-Surma EK (2012) Very Small Embryonic/Epiblast-Like Stem Cells (Vsels) and their Potential Role in Aging and Organ Rejuvenation - An Update and Comparison to Other Primitive Small Stem Cells Isolated from Adult Tissues. Aging (Albany NY). [Epub ahead of print].

[39] Shin DM, Zuba-Surma EK, Wu W, Ratajczak J, Wysoczynski M, Ratajczak MZ, Kucia M (2009) Novel Epigenetic Mechanisms that Control Pluripotency and Quiescence of Adult Bone Marrow Derived Oct4(+) Very Small Embryonic-Like Stem Cells. Leukemia. 23:2042-2051.

[40] Shin DM, Liu R, Klich I, Wu W, Ratajczak J, Kucia M, Ratajczak MZ (2010) Molecular Signature of Adult Bone Marrow-Purified Very Small Embryonic-Like Stem Cells Supports their Developmental Epiblast/Germ Line Origin. Leukemia. 24:1450–1461.

[41] Hayashi K, de Sousa Lopes SM, Surani MA (2007). Germ Cell Specification in Mice. Science 316:394–396.

[42] Zuba-Surma EK, Kucia M, Wu W, Klich I, Lillard JW Jr, Ratajczak J, Ratajczak MZ. (2008). Very Small Embryonic-Like Stem Cells Are Present in Adult Murine Organs: Imagestream-based Morphological Analysis and Distribution Studies. Cytometry A 73A(12):1116-1127.

[43] Ratajczak J, Wysoczynski M, Zuba-Surma E, Wan W, Kucia M, Yoder MC, Ratajczak MZ (2011). Adult Murine Bone Marrow-Derived Very Small Embryonic-Like Stem Cells Differentiate into the Hematopoietic Lineage after Coculture over OP9 Stromal Cells. Exp Hematol 39(2):225-237.

[44] McGuckin C, Forraz N, Baradez MO, Basford C, Dickinson AM, Navran S, Hartgerink JD (2006). Embryonic-Like Stem Cells from Umbilical Cord Blood and Potential for Neural Modeling. Acta Neurobiol Exp (Wars) 66(4):321-329.

[45] Ratajczak J, Zuba-Surma E, Klich I, Liu R, Wysoczynski M, Greco N, Kucia M, Laughlin MJ, Ratajczak MZ (2011) Hematopoietic Differentiation of Umbilical Cord Blood-Derived Very Small Embryonic/Epiblast-Like Stem Cells Leukemia 25(8):1278-85.

[46] Bhartiya D, Shaikh A, Nagvenkar P, Kasiviswanathan S, Pethe P, Pawani H, Mohanty S, Rao SG, Zaveri K, Hinduja I (2012) Very Small Embryonic-Like Stem Cells with Maximum Regenerative Potential get Discarded during Cord Blood Banking and Bone Marrow Processing for Autologous Stem Cell Therapy. Stem Cells Dev 21(1):1-6.

[47] Bhartiya D, Kasiviswanathan S, Unni SK, Pethe P, Dhabalia JV, Patwardhan S, Tongaonkar HB (2010) Newer Insights into Premeiotic Development of Germ Cells in Adult Human Testis using Oct-4 as a Stem Cell Marker. J Histochem Cytochem 58(12):1093-1106.

[48] Bhartiya D, Sriraman K, Parte S (2012) Stem Cell Interaction with Somatic Niche may hold the Key to Fertility Restoration in Cancer Patients. Obstet and Gynec Intl. doi:10.1155/2012/921082.

[49] Bhartiya D, Kasiviswanathan S, Shaikh A (2012) Cellular Origin of Testis derived Pluripotent Stem Cells: A Case for VSELs. Stem Cells Dev. 21(5):670-674.

[50] Parte S, Bhartiya D, Telang J, Daithankar V, Salvi V, Zaveri K, Hinduja I (2011) Detection, Characterization, and Spontaneous Differentiation *In Vitro* of Very Small Embryonic-Like Putative Stem Cells in Adult Mammalian Ovary. Stem Cells Dev 20(8):1451-64.

[51] Virant-Klun I, Zech N, Rozman P, Vogler A, Cvjeticanin B, Klemenc P, Malicev E, Meden-Vrtovec H (2008) Putative stem cells with an embryonic character isolated from the ovarian surface epithelium of women with no naturally present follicles and oocytes. Differentiation 76(8):843-856.

[52] Anjos-Afonso F, Bonnet D (2007) Nonhematopoietic/Endothelial SSEA-1+ Cells Define the most Primitive Progenitors in the Adult Murine Bone Marrow Mesenchymal Compartment. Blood 109(3):1298-1306.

[53] Taichman RS, Wang Z, Shiozawa Y, Jung Y, Song J, Balduino A, Wang J, Patel LR, Havens AM, Kucia M, Ratajczak MZ, Krebsbach PH (2010) Prospective Identification and Skeletal Localization of Cells Capable of Multilineage Differentiation *In Vivo*. Stem Cells Dev 19(10):1557-1570.

[54] Dawn B, Tiwari S, Kucia MJ, Zuba-Surma EK, Guo Y, Sanganalmath SK, Abdel-Latif A, Hunt G, Vincent RJ, Taher H, Reed NJ, Ratajczak MZ, Bolli R (2008) Transplantation of Bone Marrow-Derived Very Small Embryonic-Like Stem Cells Attenuates Left Ventricular Dysfunction and Remodeling after Myocardial Infarction.Stem Cells 26(6):1646-1655.

[55] Huang Y, Kucia M, Hussain LR, Wen Y, Xu H, Yan J, Ratajczak MZ, Ildstad ST (2010) Bone Marrow Transplantation Temporarily Improves Pancreatic Function in Streptozotocin-Induced Diabetes: Potential Involvement of Very Small Embryonic-Like Cells. Transplantation 89(6):677-685.

[56] Zuba-Surma EK, Kucia M, Dawn B, Guo Y, Ratajczak MZ, Bolli R (2008) Bone Marrow-Derived Pluripotent Very Small Embryonic-Like Stem Cells (VSELs) are Mobilized after Acute Myocardial Infarction. J Mol Cell Cardiol 44(5):865-873.

[57] Sovalat H, Scrofani M, Eidenschenk A, Pasquet S, Rimelen V, Hénon P (2011) Identification and Isolation from either Adult Human Bone Marrow or G-CSF-Mobilized Peripheral Blood of CD34(+)/CD133(+)/CXCR4(+)/ Lin(-)CD45(-) Cells, featuring Morphological, Molecular, and Phenotypic Characteristics of Very Small Embryonic-Like (VSEL) Stem Cells. Exp Hematol 39(4):495-505.

[58] Li L, Clevers H (2010) Coexistence of Quiescent and Active Adult Stem Cells in Mammals. Science 327(5965):542-5.

[59] Kucia M, Ratajczak MZ (2006) Stem Cells as a Two Edged Sword-From Regeneration to Tumor Formation. J Physiol Pharmacol 57 Suppl 7:5-16.

[60] Wang X, Ouyang H, Yamamoto Y, Kumar PA, Wei TS, Dagher R, Vincent M, Lu X, Bellizzi AM, Ho KY, Crum CP, Xian W, McKeon F (2011) Residual Embryonic Cells as Precursors of a Barrett's-Like Metaplasia. Cell 145:1023-1035.

[61] Massasa E, XS Costa and HS Taylor (2010) Failure of the Stem Cell Niche rather than Loss of Oocyte Stem Cells in the Aging Ovary. Aging 2:1–2.

[62] Niikura Y, T Niikura and JL Tilly (2009) Aged Mouse Ovaries Possess Rare Premeiotic Germ Cells that can Generate Oocytes Following Transplantation into a Young Host Environment. Aging 1:971–978.

[63] Gillis AJ, Stoop H, Biermann K, van Gurp RJ, Swartzman E, Cribbes S, Ferlinz A, Shannon M, Oosterhuis JW, Looijenga LH (2011) Expression and Interdependencies of Pluripotency Factors LIN28, OCT3/4, NANOG And SOX2 in Human Testicular Germ Cells and Tumours of the Testis. Int J Androl 34e160-74.

[64] Takizawa H, Schanz U, Manz MG (2011) *Ex Vivo* Expansion of Hematopoietic Stem Cells:Mission Accomplished? Swiss Med Wkly 141:w13316

[65] Notta F, Doulatov S, Laurenti E, Poeppl A, Jurisica I, Dick JE (2011) Isolation of Single Human Hematopoietic Stem Cells Capable of Long-term Multilineage Engraftment. Science 333(6039):218-21.

[66] Danova-Alt R, Heider A, Egger D, Cross M, Alt R (2012) Very Small Embryonic-Like Stem Cells Purified from Umbilical Cord Blood Lack Stem Cell Characteristics. PLoS ONE 7(4): e34899. doi:10.1371/journal.pone.

[67] Tao H, Ma DD (2003) Evidence for transdifferentiation of human bone marrow-derived stem cells: recent progress and controversies. Pathology 35(1):6-13.

Chapter 5

C-Reactive Protein

Moneer Faraj and Nihaya Salem

Additional information is available at the end of the chapter

http://dx.doi.org/10.5772/47735

1. Introduction

C- reactive protein (CRP) was so named because it was first discovered as a substance in the serum of patients with acute inflammation that reacted with the C- (capsular) polysaccharide of pneumococcus [1].

Discovered by *Tillett* and *Francis* in 1930[2], it was initially thought that CRP might be a pathogenic secretion as it was elevated in people with a variety of illnesses including cancer [3], however, the discovery of hepatic synthesis demonstrated that it is a native protein [4][5][6][7].

CRP is phylogenetically a highly conserved plasma protein, with homolog in vertebrates and many invertebrates that participates in the systemic response to inflammation. Its plasma concentration increases during inflammatory states, a character that has long been employed for clinical purposes. CRP is a pattern recognition molecule, binding to specific molecular configurations that are typically exposed during cell death or found on the surfaces of pathogens. Its rapid increase in synthesis within hours after tissue injury or infection suggests that it contributes to host defense and that it is part of the innate immune response [8].

2. Molecular structure of CRP

Entrez Gene summary for CRP the protein encoded by this gene belongs to the pentaxin family. It is involved in several host defense related functions based on its ability to recognize foreign pathogens and damaged cells of the host and to initiate their elimination by interacting with humoral and cellular effector systems in the blood. Consequently, the level of this protein in plasma increases greatly during acute phase response to tissue injury, infection, or other inflammatory stimuli[12]. It is induced by IL1/interleukin-1 and IL6//interleukin-6

UniProtKB/Swiss-Prot: CRP_HUMAN, P02741
Size: 224 amino acids; 25039 Da
Cofactor: Binds 2 calcium ions per subunit
Subunit: Homopentamer. Pentaxin (or pentraxin) have a discoid arrangement of 5 non-covalently bound subunits
Subcellular location: Secreted
Mass spectrometry: Mass=23028; Method=MALDI; Range=19-224; Source=Ref.15;
Mass spectrometry: Mass=22930; Method=MALDI; Range=19-223; Source=Ref.15;

Function: Displays several functions associated with host defense it promotes agglutination, bacterial capsular swelling, phagocytosis (CRP initiates the activation of the complement cascade and binds Fc gamma RI (CD64) and Fc gamma RIIA (CD32a) on phagocytes to activate phagocytic responses) and complement fixation through its calcium-dependent binding to phosphorylcholine. It can interact with DNA and histones and may scavenge nuclear material released from damaged circulating cells [13].

The CRP Entrez gene cytogenetic band located on the first chromosome: 1q21-q23

Ensemble cytogenetic band: 1q23.2
HGNC cytogenetic band: 1q21-q23.

CRP is a 224-residue protein with a monomer molar mass of 25106 Da. The protein is an annular pentameric disc in shape [14][15].

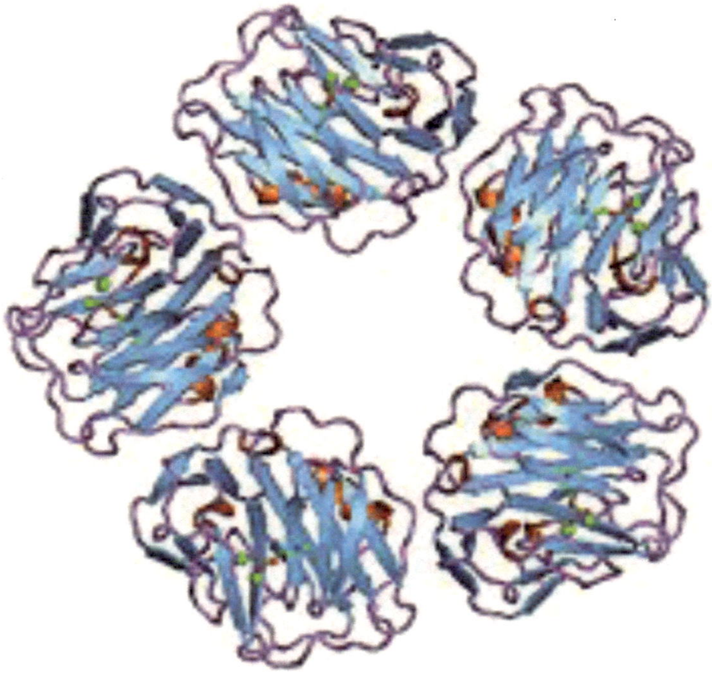

Figure 1. Pentameric structure of CRP viewed down the 5-fold symmetry axis. The effector face of the molecule is on the top, while the calcium- and PCh-binding sites are on the opposite 'recognition' face [1]

3. Methodology and clinical applications

CRP is used mainly as a marker of inflammation. Apart from liver failure, there are few known factors that interfere with CRP production

Measuring and charting CRP values can prove useful in determining disease progress or the effectiveness of treatments.

Blood, usually collected in a serum-separating tube, is analyzed in a medical laboratory or at the point of care. Various analytical methods are available for CRP determination, such as ELISA (Enzyme-linked immunosorbent assay ELISA can perform other forms of ligand binding assays instead of strictly "immuno" assays, though the name carried the original "immuno" because of the common use and history of development of this method. The technique essentially requires any ligating reagent that can be immobilized on the solid phase along with a detection reagent that will bind specifically and use an enzyme to generate a signal that can be properly quantified. In between the washes only the ligand and its specific binding counterparts remain specifically bound or "immunosorbed" by antigen-antibody interactions to the solid phase, while the nonspecific or unbound components are washed away. Unlike other spectrophotometric wet lab assay formats where the same reaction well (e.g. a cuvette) can be reused after washing, the ELISA plates have the reaction products immunosorbed on the solid phase which is part of the plate and thus are not easily reusable)[19], immunoturbidimetry (Immunoturbidimetric Method This reagent is intended for the in vitro quantitative determination of CRP concentration in serum or plasma on automated clinical chemistry analyzers)[20], rapid immunodiffusion(is a diagnostic test which involves diffusion through a substance such as agar.Two commonly known forms are Ouchterlony double immunodiffusion and radial immunodiffusion) [21], and visual agglutination [22][23] (quantitative slide method and semi quantitative diluted method)

There are two different tests for CRP. The standard test measures a much wider range of CRP levels but is less sensitive in the lower ranges. The high-sensitivity CRP (hs-CRP) test can more accurately detect lower concentrations of the protein (it is more sensitive), which makes it more useful than the CRP test in predicting a *healthy* person's risk for cardiovascular disease [24].

(hs-CRP) test measures using laser nephelometry. The test gives results in 25 minutes with sensitivity down to 0.04 mg/L [26]. hs-CRP usually is ordered as one of several tests in a cardiovascular risk profile, often along with tests for cholesterol and triglycerides. Some experts say that the best way to predict risk is to combine a good marker for inflammation, like hs-CRP, along with the lipid profile [27].

CRP is one of several proteins that are often referred to as acute phase reactants and is used to monitor changes in inflammation associated with many infectious and autoimmune diseases [28].

We should be healthy at the time of the sample collection, without any recent illnesses, infections, inflammation, or other tissue injuries. Since the hs-CRP and CRP tests measure the same molecule, people with chronic inflammation, such as those with arthritis, should not have hs-CRP levels measured. Their CRP levels will be very high due to the arthritis often too high to be measured or meaningful using the hs-CRP test [29].

Normal concentration in healthy human serum is usually lower than 4.9 mg/L, slightly increasing with aging. Higher levels are found in late pregnant women, active inflammation, bacterial infection, severe bacterial infections, tissue injury (postoperation), trauma and burns.

CRP is a more sensitive and accurate reflection of the acute phase response than the ESR[30] another blood test often ordered in conjunction with CRP (erythrocyte sedimentation rate or sed rate known as ESR) both CRP and ESR give similar information about non-specific inflammation.

CRP appears and disappears more quickly than changes in ESR. Therefore, your CRP level may drop to normal following successful treatment [31] , whereas ESR may remain elevated for a longer period.

The half-life of CRP is constant. Therefore, CRP level is mainly determined by the rate of production (and hence the severity of the precipitating cause). In the first 24 h, ESR may be normal and CRP elevated [32]. CRP and ESR have been used to diagnose postoperative infections after spinal surgery. We did a prospective study in Baghdad [33]. The aim of the study was to determine the duration of the physiological rise in the serum CRP without the development of infection following lumbar laminectomy. Forty patients (19 women, 21 men) mean age 44.2, age range 27-60 yrs were included in the study.

All patients underwent laminectomy. Additional clinical data relevant to the study included body temperature, duration of surgery & blood transfusion.

The indication of surgery established several days to weeks before the surgical procedure. Pathologic findings included:

27 lumber spinal canal stenosis
2 reoperation for stenosis
1 spinal canal hydrated cyst
10 lumber disc herneation.

Preoperatively, a single – shot antibiotic prophylaxis with cefotaxime 1 gram was give to all cases. All patients were operated under general anesthesia. Duration of surgery varied from 60-180 min. (average 80.5 min.). Before surgery no patient received steroids. Blood samples were taken on the day of surgery and on each consecutive day after surgery for10 days.

The parameters taken were CRP, ESR, Total white blood cell count. On 1st post operative day the CRP started to increase in 34 patients (range 12- 96, average 27). In the 2nd and 3rd post operative day all the patients had high CRP with an average of 39 &38 respectively. This increase was highly significant (P<0.001). A dramatic decline in the CRP level was noticed to start in the 5th post operative day (average 27), then gradual reduction was noticed until a normal ranges at day 9th post operatively (average 4.8) as shown in figure -2.

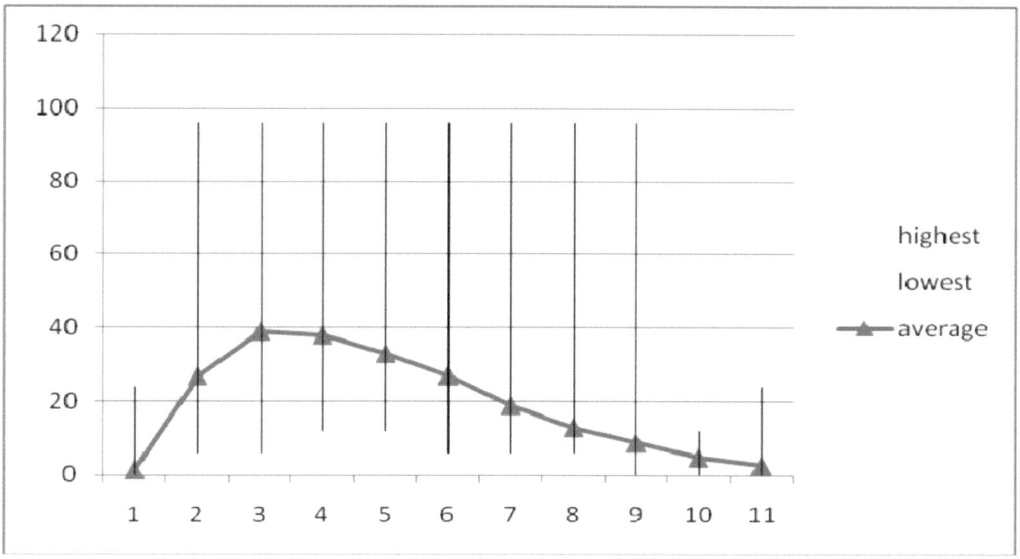

Figure 2. The CRP level of all patients from day one which is here is the operation day to day 11, the average values plotted together [34]

Increased CRP values during the first 5 post-operative days did not indicate that an infection is ongoing. An infection should be considered with prolonged CRP elevation (more than 5 days) as noticed is one of our patients or when a second rise occurs. Although we did not use steroids or non steroidal anti inflammatory drugs post operatively, but these medications seems to effect on the level of CRP. *Munoz m. et al* [35] revealed that pre-operative treatment with *naproxane* and *famotidine* was well tolerated and reduced the acute phase response after instrumented spinal surgery. In this study we could not find any correlation of the raised CRP level they age , sex , ESR , WBC count , body temperature duration of surgery blood transfusion[36] with exception of *Orrego LM et al*[37] who noticed that more complex surgical procedure had higher CRP level and explained due to the amount of tissue trauma. *Sugimorik et al* [38] showed no correlation between the high CRP concentration and the level, type of lumbar disc herneation or the preoperative clinical data. *Thelander et al* [39] noticed that peak levels were not related to bleeding, transfusion, operation time, administered drugs, age or sex However, it has not been demonstrated if resolution of the signs and symptoms of postoperative spinal wound infections in patients who are being treated with intravenous antibiotics correlates with these markers. CRP is a sensitive marker of pneumonia. A persistently high or rising CRP level suggests antibiotic treatment failure or the development of an infective complication. These results suggest that CRP, rather than TNF-α or IL-6, may have a role as a clinical marker in pneumonia [40]. Most recently CRP has made headlines as it relates to heart disease an association between minor CRP elevation and future major cardiovascular events has been recognized, leading to the recommendation by the Centers for Disease Control and the American Heart Association that patients at intermediate risk of coronary heart disease might benefit from measurement of CRP. It is yet to be determined if CRP serves as a marker of heart disease or whether it plays apart in causing atherosclerotic disease (hardening the arteries)[41]. CRP has been shown to have a close relationship with vascular diseases. CRP is a powerful independent risk factor for atherosclerosis and atherosclerosis-related diseases (Lusic et al., 2006 [42]; Verma et al., 2006)[43]. Elevated high-sensitivity CRP (hsCRP) has been measured in the blood of patients with essential hypertension (Li et al., 2005) [44] or abdominal aortic aneurysms (Vainas et al., 2003 [45]; Tambyraja et al., 2007 [46]) with enhanced systemic or local arterial strain. Elevated serum hsCRP independently correlates with blood pressure (Sung et al., 2003)[47], arterial stiffness (Kim et al., 2007) [48], and aneurysmal size (Vainas et al., 2003) [49]. Although several investigations have demonstrated that aneurysmal tissues and diseased coronary artery venous bypass grafts (Jabs et al., 2003)[50] produce CRP, little is known about its mechanism. Blood vessels are dynamically subjected to mechanical strain in the forms of stretch and shear stress that result from blood pressure and blood flow. Mechanical strain on the vessel wall can increase from 15 to 30% in hypertensive individuals (Safar et al., 1981[51]; Shaw and Xu, 2003)[52][53].

CRP testing is not precise enough to diagnose specific diseases but serves more as a general indicator that more testing may be needed if inflammation or infection is found. The CRP test is therefore useful in assessing patients with the following list[54]:

- Swelling and bleeding of the intestines (inflammatory bowel disease).
- Painful swelling of the tissues that line the joints (rheumatoid arthritis).
- Diseases of the immune system, such as lupus.
- Pelvic inflammatory disease (PID)
- Painful swelling of the blood vessels in the head and neck (giant cell arteritis).
- Cancer of the lymph nodes (lymphoma).
- Infection of a bone (osteomyelitis).
- Connective tissue disease
- Heart attack
- Infections
- Pneumococcal pneumonia
- Rheumatic fever
- Tuberculosis

4. Factors that effects on high levels of CRP

Many doctors will prescribe taking non steroidal anti-inflammatory drugs ((NSAIDs like aspirin, ibuprofen, and naproxen) or statins may reduce CRP levels in blood. Both anti-inflammatory drugs and statins may help to reduce the inflammation, thus reducing CRP. However, there are natural treatments that can help reduce inflammation in the blood.

Following are some of the natural treatments for lowering C - reactive protein levels and inflammation in the blood:

Fish Oil Omega 3 Fatty Acids Doctors and nutritionists have recommended Omega 3's for years, and recently fish oil has been the most recommended source for Omega 3 Fatty Acids. Fish oil contains two of the most therapeutic Omega 3 Fatty Acids the DHA and EPA. These two fatty acids are the most readily absorbed by the body (much more so than the ALA found in flax seed oil), and can help reduce inflammation in the blood among other benefits.

Ginger - Ginger root extract has long been used in Asian cooking, and has been used for centuries as a digestive aid and motion sickness cure, and more recently to lower cholesterol. Ginger can also help reduce inflammation, as it relaxes the muscles surrounding blood vessels and facilitates blood flow throughout the body.

MSM - Methyl Sulfonyl Methane, commonly known as MSM, is a naturally occurring sulfur compound found in some vegetables. MSM is found in many arthritis formulas, and has strong anti-inflammatory properties.

These three nutrients may help reduce CRP levels in your blood. All three are important for maintaining heart health as well as general health and wellbeing [55].

There was a study found a significant effect of treatment for 2 months with 1000 mg/day vitamin C on plasma CRP, in non diseased moderately overweight nonsmokers with baseline CRP ≥1.0 mg/L. The magnitude of the effect was similar to that of statins. There was no significant effect of vitamin E. These data represent the largest study to date on the effects of vitamins C and E on CRP and extend our previous findings in overweight active and passive smokers. They indicate that vitamin C should be further investigated for its potential for reducing chronic inflammation and its consequences. And they identify a threshold concentration above which there is a potential for reduction in CRP. Future studies to determine whether vitamin C can reduce some of the inflammation-related adverse consequences of obesity should be considered. Such trials should focus on individuals with elevations (.1.0 mg/L) in CRP, because studies with low-risk persons are less likely to show an effect, resulted in misleading outcomes. If persons with lower CRP levels must be included, separate randomization of those with CRP .1.0 mg/L would justify separate examination of this subgroup, assuming adequate power in this stratum. In addition, if the potential independent effect of vitamin C is to be determined, it would be necessary to exclude persons who are taking other anti-inflammatory drugs (except low-dose aspirin for heart disease prevention) and to exclude users of multiple vitamins (something which has not been done in most large antioxidant trials), because multiple vitamins alone can raise plasma ascorbic acid levels substantially and make the control group insufficiently different from the active treatment group. Finally, it may be prudent to evaluate vitamin C alone, unpaired with vitamin E, as we found a weaker CRP-lowering effect with the combination than with vitamin C alone in our previous trial [56].

5. C - reactive protein concentrations in cerebral spinal fluid in gram-positive and gram-negative bacterial meningitis

Several reports have shown an ability of CRP to discriminate between patients with bacterial meningitis and patients with aseptic (viral) meningitis. Although a recent Meta-analysis suggested that a negative CRP test in either cerebrospinal fluid (CSF) or serum can be used with a very high probability to rule out bacterial meningitis, a more recent report suggested that serum concentrations are a better screening tool for this differential diagnosis.

The substantial increase in CSF CRP, as well as the trend of an increased CSF/blood ratio of CRP, suggests that infection with gram-negative bacteria enhances permeability of CRP through the blood-brain barrier. It is possible that these findings reflect the ability of the endotoxin lipopolysaccharide-s, present in gram-negative but not in gram-positive bacteria, to affect the permeability of the blood-brain barrier [57][58]. CSF nitric oxide (NO) may be involved in this mechanism because its concentration in CSF is higher in gram-negative meningitis. This possibility is supported by the higher potency of gram-negative bacteria to promote macrophage NO production [59], the enhanced production of NO in the CSF of septic meningitis [60], and the role of NO in permeability changes of the blood-brain barrier in LPS-induced experimental meningitis [61].

Another interesting potential explanation for the present observation is that lipopolysaccharide-s produced by gram-negative bacteria could induce local CRP synthesis in the central nervous system. CRP can be produced in neurons [62], and lipopolysaccharide-s can induce CRP in extrahepatic sites [63]. This may also explain the increase, albeit nonsignificant, in serum CRP in the gram-negative cases. There is currently no single test to diagnose the etiology of meningitis promptly and accurately. Given its high sensitivity and easy measurability, CRP may be a useful supplement for rapid diagnosis and categorization of bacterial meningitis.

Author details

Moneer Faraj and Nihaya Salem
Department of Neurosurgery, Hospital of Neurosciences, Baghdad, Iraq

6. References

[1] http://en.wikipedia.org/wiki/C-reactive_protein
[2] Tillett WS, Francis T (September 1930). "Serological reactions in pneumonia with a nonprotein somatic fraction of pneumococcus". *J. Exp. Med.* 52 (4): 561–71.
[3] Pepys, MB; Hirschfield, GM (June 2003). "C-reactive protein: a critical update" (PDF). *J Clin Invest* 111 (12): 1805–12. doi:10.1172/JCI18921. PMC 161431. PMID 12813013.

http://www.jci.org/articles/view/18921/files/pdf?disposition=attachment.
[4] http://en.wikipedia.org/wiki/C-reactive_protein
[5] Peter J. Kennelly; Murray, Robert F.; Victor W. Rodwell; Kathleen M. Botham (2009). *Harper's illustrated biochemistry*. McGraw-Hill Medical. ISBN 0-07-162591-7.
[6] Matthew R. Pincus; McPherson, Richard A.; Henry, John Bernard (2007). *Henry's clinical diagnosis and management by laboratory methods*. Saunders Elsevier. ISBN 1-4160-0287-1.
[7] John J. Ratey MD; Gary A. Noskin MEd MD; MD, Ralph Braun; Edward N. Hanley Jr MD; Iain B. McInnes; Shaun Ruddy MD (2008). *Kelley's Textbook of Rheumatology: 2-Volume Set, Expert Consult: Online and Print (Textbook of Rheumatology (Kelley's)(2 Vol))*. Philadelphia: Saunders. ISBN 1-4160-3285-1.
[8] http://www.jbc.org/content/279/47/48487
[9] http://www.genecards.org/cgi-bin/carddisp.pl?gene=CRP
[10] Thompson, D; Pepys, MB; Wood, SP (February 1999). "The physiological structure of human C-reactive protein and its complex with phosphocholine". Structure 7 (2): 169–77. doi:10.1016/S0969-2126(99)80023-9. PMID 10368284.
[11] Dhillon, B; Yan, H; Szmitko, PE; Verma, S (May 2005). "Adipokines: molecular links between obesity and atheroslcerosis". Am J Physiol Heart Circ Physiol 288 (5): H2031–41. doi:10.1152/ajpheart.01058.2004. PMID 15653761. http://ajpheart.physiology.org/content/288/5/H2031.full.pdf.
[12] http://www.genecards.org/cgi-bin/carddisp.pl?gene=CRP
[13] A C-reactive protein promoter polymorphism is associated with type 2 diabetes mellitus in Pima Indians. (PubMed id 12618085)[1, 4, 5] Wolford J.K....Hanson R.L. *(2003)*
[14] http://www.genecards.org/cgi-bin/carddisp.pl?gene=CRP
[15] A C-reactive protein promoter polymorphism is associated with type 2 diabetes mellitus in Pima Indians. (PubMed id 12618085)[1, 4, 5] Wolford J.K....Hanson R.L. *(2003)*
[16] Mantovani A, Garlanda C, Doni A, Bottazzi B (January 2008). "Pentraxins in innate immunity: from C-reactive protein to the long pentraxin PTX3". J. Clin. Immunol. 28 (1): 1–13. doi:10.1007/s10875-007-9126-7. PMID 17828584
[17] Clyne B, Olshaker JS (1999). "The C-reactive protein". J Emerg Med 17 (6): 1019–25. doi:10.1016/S0736-4679(99)00135-3. PMID 10595891
[18] NCBI Entrez Protein #CAA39671
[19] http://en.wikipedia.org/wiki/ELISA
[20] http://www.proz.com/kudoz/english_to_spanish/medical_general/1100998-immunoturbidimetric_method.html
[21] http://en.wikipedia.org/wiki/Immunodiffusion
[22] http://en.wikipedia.org/wiki/C-reactive_protein
[23] Pepys, MB; Hirschfield, GM (June 2003). "C-reactive protein: a critical update" (PDF). *J Clin Invest* 111 (12): 1805–12. doi:10.1172/JCI18921. PMC 161431. PMID 12813013. http://www.jci.org/articles/view/18921/files/pdf?disposition=attachment.
[24] Clyne B, Olshaker JS (1999). "The C-reactive protein". *J Emerg Med* 17 (6): 1019–25. doi:10.1016/S0736-4679(99)00135-3. PMID 10595891.

[25] http://labtestsonline.org/understanding/analytes/hscrp/tab/test .
[26] http://en.wikipedia.org/wiki/C-reactive_protein
[27] http://labtestsonline.org/understanding/analytes/hscrp/tab/test.
[28] http://www.ncbi.nlm.nih.gov/pmc/articles/PMC2832720/
[29] http://labtestsonline.org/understanding/analytes/hscrp/tab/test.
[30] http://en.wikipedia.org/wiki/C-reactive_protein
[31] http://boneandspine.com/definitions/c-reactive-protein/
[32] http://en.wikipedia.org/wiki/C-reactive_protein
[33] The New Iraqi Journal of Medicine 2009 ; 5 (3): http://www.scopemed.org/journal.php?jid=20
[34] The New Iraqi Journal of Medicine 2009 ; 5 (3): http://www.scopemed.org/journal.php?jid=20
[35] Munoz M. , Garcia – Vallejo JJ , Sempere JM , Romero R. , Ollala E , Sebastian C acute phase response in patients undergoing lumbar spinal surgery ; modulation by per operative treatment with Naproxen and Famotidine . Eur Spine J. 2004 Jul; 13(4):367-73.
[36] The New Iraqi Journal of Medicine 2009 ; 5 (3): http://www.scopemed.org/journal.php?jid=20
[37] Qrrego LM, Perez CM, Perez YM, Cheyre EJ, Mardones PR, Plasma C- reactive protein in elective orthopedic surgery Rev. Med Chil. 2005 Nov. 133 (11): 1341 – 8 .
[38] Sugimori K , Kawaguchi Y , Morita M , Kitajima I , Kimura T. High – sensitivity analysis of serum C- reactive protein in young patients with lumbar disc herniation .J Bone Joint surg. Br. 2003 Nov, 85 (8) : 1151-4
[39] Thelander U , Larsson S. Quantitation of C- reactive protein level and ESR after spinal surgery. Spine 1992 April 17 (4):400-4.
[40] http://chestjournal.chestpubs.org/content/108/5/1288.abstract
[41] http://www.jbc.org/content/279/47/48487
[42] Lusic I, Radonic V, Pavelin S, and Bilic I (2006) Is C-reactive protein a better predictor of recurrent carotid disease following carotid endarterectomy than established risk factors for atherosclerosis? Vasa 35: 221-225.
[43] Verma S, Devaraj S, and Jialal I (2006) Is C-reactive protein an innocent bystander or proatherogenic culprit? C-reactive protein promotes atherothrombosis. Circulation 113: 2135-2150.
[44] Li JJ, Fang CH, and Hui RT (2005) Is hypertension an inflammatory disease? Med Hypotheses 64: 236-240.
[45] Vainas T, Lubbers T, Stassen FR, Herngreen SB, van Dieijen-Visser MP, Bruggeman CA, Kitslaar PJ, and Schurink GW (2003) Serum C-reactive protein level is associated with abdominal aortic aneurysm size and may be produced by aneurysmal tissue. Circulation 107: 1103-1105.
[46] Tambyraja AL, Dawson R, Valenti D, Murie JA, and Chalmers RT (2007) Systemic inflammation and repair of abdominal aortic aneurysm. World J Surg 31: 1210-1214.

[47] Sung KC, Suh JY, Kim BS, Kang JH, Kim H, Lee MH, Park JR, and Kim SW (2003) High sensitivity C-reactive protein as an independent risk factor for essential hypertension. Am J Hypertens 16: 429-433.
[48] Kim JS, Kang TS, Kim JB, Seo HS, Park S, Kim C, Ko YG, Choi D, Jang Y, and Chung N (2007) Significant association of C-reactive protein with arterial stiffness in treated non-diabetic hypertensive patients. Atherosclerosis 192: 401-406.
[49] Vainas T, Lubbers T, Stassen FR, Herngreen SB, van Dieijen-Visser MP, Bruggeman CA, Kitslaar PJ, and Schurink GW (2003) Serum C-reactive protein level is associated with abdominal aortic aneurysm size and may be produced by aneurysmal tissue. Circulation 107: 1103-1105.
[50] Jabs WJ, Theissing E, Nitschke M, Bechtel JF, Duchrow M, Mohamed S, Jahrbeck B, Sievers HH, Steinhoff J, and Bartels C (2003) Local generation of C-reactive protein in diseased coronary artery venous bypass grafts and normal vascular tissue. Circulation 108: 1428-1431.
[51] Safar ME, Peronneau PA, Levenson JA, Toto-Moukouo JA, and Simon AC (1981) Pulsed Doppler: diameter, blood flow velocity, and volumic flow of the brachial artery in sustained essential hypertension. Circulation 63: 393-400.
[52] Shaw A and Xu Q (2003) Biomechanical stress-induced signaling in smooth muscle cells: an update. Curr Vasc Pharmacol 1: 41-58.
[53] http://jpet.aspetjournals.org/content/330/1/206.full
[54] http://www.creactiveprotein.net/c-reactive-protein.html
[55] http://www.healthy-heart-guide.com/crp-blood-test.html
[56] Vitamin C treatment reduces elevated C-reactive protein.(Gladys Block a, Christopher D. Jensen a, Tapashi B. Dalvi a, Edward P. Norkus b, Mark Hudes a, Patricia B. Crawford a, Nina Holland a, Ellen B. Fung c, Laurie Schumacher c, Paul Harmatz) Free Radical Biology & Medicine 46 (2009) 70–77
[57] http://www.clinchem.org/content/48/3/591.full
[58] Wispelwey B, Lesse AJ, Hansen EJ, Scheld WM. Haemophilus influenzae lipopolysaccharide-induced blood-brain barrier induced permeability during experimental meningitis in the rat. J Clin Invest 1988;82:1339-1346
[59] Jungi TW, *Valentin-Weigand P, Brcic M. Differential induction of NO synthesis by gram-positive and gram-negative bacteria and their components in bovine monocyte-derived macrophages.* Microb Pathog 1999;27:43-*53.*
CrossRefMedlineOrder article via InfotrieveWeb of Science
[60] Tsukahara H, Haruta T, Hata I, Mayumi M. Nitric oxide in septic and aseptic meningitis in children. Scand J Clin Invest 1998;58:71-80.
[61] Boje KMK. *Inhibition of nitric oxide synthase attenuates blood-brain barrier disruption during experimental meningitis.* Brain Res 1996;720:75-*83.*
CrossRefMedlineOrder article via InfotrieveWeb of Science
[62] Yasojima K, *Schwab C, McGeer EG, McGeer PL. Human neurons generate C-reactive protein and amyloid P: upregulation in Alzheimer's disease.* Brain Res 2000;887:80-*89.*

CrossRefMedlineOrder article via InfotrieveWeb of Science

[63] Introna M, Alles VV, Castellano M, Picardi G, De Gioia L, et al. Cloning of mouse ptx3, a new member of the pentraxin gene family expressed at extrahepatic sites. Blood 1996;87:1862-1872.

Chapter 6

Whole Blood RNA Analysis, Aging and Disease

Junko Takahashi, Akiko Takatsu, Masaki Misawa and Hitoshi Iwahashi

Additional information is available at the end of the chapter

http://dx.doi.org/10.5772/48226

1. Introduction

Microarray techniques allow to detect genome-wide perturbations during various treatments and to measure various responses by multitude of gene probes. Toxicogenomics, in which microarray techniques are specifically used in toxicology test, has been widely recognized as one of standard safety procedures for chemicals [1-3]. Gene expression microarrays have been used particularly for screening of genes involved in specific biological processes of interest, such as diseases or responses to environmental stimuli. Such experiments adopt the "healthy state" as a control, and identify highly expressed or suppressed genes. However, few studies deal with the features of gene expression and its variation at the "healthy state" to be influenced by species, age, sex, and individual variability. In measuring the state of disease and drug response, minimally invasive blood sampling, which allows for direct measurement of immune-responsive blood cells, excels other invasive biopsy techniques upon disease diagnostics and assessment of drug response, as well as health monitoring. Blood RNA contains an enormous amount of information on expression of messenger RNA and non coding functional RNA which remains without being translated into protein. Thus, blood RNA offers an opportunity to detect subtle change in physiological state. In this chapter, we discuss the potential of the RNA diagnosis using whole blood, showing a series of whole blood microarray experiments to evaluate variations of correlation among individuals and ages [4], dietary-induced hyperlipidemia, and other stresses using specific pathogen-free (SPF) miniature pigs.

2. The use of whole blood RNA analysis

Use of whole blood was intended on two accounts. First, RNA expression and degradation is susceptible to artificial manipulation such as cell separation and extraction. The whole blood manipulation avoids this risk, unlike dealing with extracted white blood cells. In addition, whole-blood RNA can be stabilized immediately by using RNA blood sampling tube such as PAXgene. This avoids the cell separation process after sampling and minimizes the possibility of RNA denaturation. Usually, peripheral blood mononuclear cells (PBMCs) separation employs the difference of specific gravity between other blood components, which should be followed immediately after the blood sampling. Such manipulation requires a skilled operator to reduce the influence of separation procedures on gene expression. Second, the whole blood is a heterogeneous population of lymphocytes (monocytes, T-cells, and B-cells), granulocytes (neutrophils, eosinophils, and basophils), and platelets. One can expect that representative subpopulations in white blood cells may vary depending on the health condition of an individual. When a great alteration occurs in some subpopulations, the whole blood may also depart from the normal state of its age, because whole blood is a heterogeneous mixture of such subpopulations. Therefore, identification of gene expression characteristics and age-related variation in subpopulations in whole blood are essential issues.

3. The advantage of using miniature pigs

Pigs are a useful model animals of humans because they have similar anatomy and digestive physiology to human [5-6]. In particular, miniature pigs are easier to breed and handle than other nonprimates, making them an optimal species for preclinical test [7]. Moreover, blood samples can be taken repeatedly and human medical devices such as endoscopes and MRI and CT scanners are also applicable. These advantages increasingly allow miniature pigs for laboratory animals, with recent progress in upgraded supply systems. In spite of some large-scale microarray studies on pigs, only a limited amount of fundamental data is available for pigs compared to other laboratory species [8-9]. In September 2003, the Swine Genome Sequencing Consortium (SGSC) was formed by industry, government, and academia, to promote pig genome sequencing under international coordination [10]. In November 2009, since the announcement of completed swine genome map by members of the SGSC, its research environment has been enhanced [11].

4. Gene expression profiles change related to aging

It is particularly important to identify gene expression characteristics and variation of heterogeneous population of cells with age in whole blood.

Fractions of lymphocytes, monocytes, neutrophils, eosinophils, and basophils in white blood cells showed insignificant differences with age as a result of ANOVA analysis. This study attempted to identify characteristics of age-related gene expression by taking into account of change in the number of expressed genes by age and similarities of gene expression intensity between individuals.

4.1. Characteristics of study subjects

Five males and five females of 12 week old Clawn miniature pigs were housed individually in cages of 1.5 m^2 at the SPF facility of the breeder (Japan Farm Co., Ltd, Kagoshima, Japan) for 18 weeks. Mean body weights of males and females at the beginning of the experiment were 7.0 kg and 6.9 kg respectively. During this period, all animals were fed with 450g/day standard dry feed (Kodakara73, Marubeni Nisshin Feed Co., Ltd., Tokyo Japan) with free access to water. Fetuses were taken out from their mothers on days 77 to the 84 days of the pregnancy by a Caesarean section. The unborn baby's sex was determined based on the shape of the vulva.

Sex	n	12 weeks	16 weeks	20 weeks	24 weeks	30 weeks	*P* †
Male	5	7.0 ± 0.6	10.7 ± 3.8	12.1 ± 2.6	15.0 ± 1.7	17.7 ± 1.7	< 0.001
Female	5	6.9 ± 0.5	7.9 ± 3.2	10.1 ± 2.6	13.5 ± 2.1	16.0 ± 2.6	< 0.001

Values are mean±SD. †*P* values were calculated using one-way factorial ANOVA.

Table 1. Subject body weight results
doi:10.1371/journal.pone.0019761.t001

All blood samples were collected from the superior vena cava at 12, 16, 20, 24, and 30 weeks of age. Blood (EDTA), plasma (EDTA) and serum samples for hematology and biochemical tests were collected 24 hours after fasting. Hematology and biochemical tests were conducted by Clinical Pathology Laboratory, Inc. (http://www.patho.co.jp/index.html) (Kagoshima, Japan) using standard clinical methods.

Body weight change and hematological variation during breeding period are shown Table 1 and Table 2, respectively. One-way ANOVA analysis for age-related variations in red blood cell count (RBC), hemoglobin concentration (HGB), and hematocrit value (HCT) showed significant differences for both males and females. However, the mean corpuscular volume (MCV), mean corpuscular hemoglobin (MCH), and mean corpuscular hemoglobin concentration (MCHC) remained unchanged. Differences in platelet count (PLT) and fibrinogen level (Fbg) were significant only for females. Any significant differences were not observed for both males and females for Prothrombin time (PT), activated partial thromboplastin time (ATPP), and the white blood cell count (WBC). Similarly to humans, the ratio of lymphocytes to white blood cells increased with maturation from 16 to 30 weeks of age. However, its difference was statistically insignificant according to ANOVA analysis. From 12 to 30 weeks of age, the ratios of granulocytes (neutrophils, eosinophils, and basophils), lymphocytes, and monocytes to white blood cells were unchanged, and differences were also insignificant.

4.2. Microarray gene expression profiles - Number of expressed genes

To characterize the age-related gene expression in whole blood from miniature pigs, RNA analysis was conducted on bloods sampled from fetal stage, 12, 20, and 30 weeks subjects. Each RNA sample was analyzed by an Agilent #G2519F#20109 Porcine Gene Expression Microarray (44K) consisting of 43603 oligonucleotide probes.

The change in the number of expressed genes to identify age-related characteristics was examined. Microarray gene expressions were divided into two groups; "absent" and "present", using flag indicators given by the scanner. Background level was determined from spot intensities outside the gene probing area. "Absent" was assigned to the spots whose intensities were less than the background level, while the rests were marked as "present." Then each gene was judged as either "expressed" or "unexpressed" based on the number of "present" events. We defined a certain gene as "expressed" when "present" exceeds 75% out of replicated events. A threshold of 75% was chosen by considering experimental deviation.

Hematological analysis	Sex	n	12 weeks	16 weeks	20 weeks	24 weeks	30 weeks	*P* †
RBC, 10^4/μL	Male	5	742.7 ± 72.6	858.0 ± 97.7	894.8 ± 55.8	919.0 ± 21.0	866.2 ± 24.5	< .05
	Female	5	727.0 ± 20.2	886.6 ± 62.2	921.2 ± 64.5	901.4 ± 46.1	838.4 ± 44.2	< .001
HGB, g/dL	Male	5	14.9 ± 1.6	16.4 ± 1.2	17.3 ± 0.6	18.3 ± 0.4	17.7 ± 0.3	< .001
	Female	5	14.9 ± 0.4	17.5 ± 0.8	18.0 ± 0.9	18.4 ± 1.1	17.5 ± 0.6	< .001
HCT, %	Male	5	50.9 ± 5.1	53.6 ± 2.7	54.7 ± 2.1	58.4 ± 2.8	55.3 ± 1.2	< .05
	Female	5	49.0 ± 1.8	56.1 ± 2.2	57.8 ± 4.2	57.9 ± 3.0	54.8 ± 2.8	< .01
MCV, fL	Male	5	65.8 ± 1.0	66.3 ± 2.5	67.3 ± 2.9	65.1 ± 1.4	65.8 ± 2.2	NS
MCH, Pg	Male	5	19.8 ± 0.5	20.0 ± 1.1	20.1 ± 0.9	20.5 ± 0.6	20.6 ± 0.8	NS
CHC, %	Male	5	30.1 ± 0.4	30.2 ± 1.0	29.9 ± 0.9	31.5 ± 0.9	31.2 ± 0.8	NS
PLT, 10^4/μl	Male	5	21.3 ± 0.4	31.6 ± 10.8	18.1 ± 4.4	25.0 ± 8.6	24.9 ± 5.1	NS
	Female	5	34.5 ± 2.0	24.8 ± 5.5	19.0 ± 5.0	24.8 ± 8.9	19.7 ± 5.7	< .05
PT, sec	Male	5	13.8 ± 3.2	15.5 ± 0.3	16.5 ± 0.9	15.9 ± 0.7	16.1 ± 0.6	NS
	Female	5	-	15.8 ± 1.1	16.1 ± 0.5	16.4 ± 0.5	16.0 ± 0.7	NS
APTT, sec	Male	5	< 20	< 20	< 20	< 20	< 20	
	Female	5	< 20	< 20	< 20	< 20	< 20	
Fbg, mg/dl	Male	5	171.3 ±36.9	185.8 ± 93.8	169.4 ± 39.4	158.6 ± 9.0	147.8 ± 34.2	NS
	Female	5	-	160.2 ± 19.4	145.2 ± 16.3	176.5 ± 20.1	123.3 ± 27.5	< .05
WBC, 10^2/μL	Male	5	62.0 ± 18.7	86.6 ±12.7	78.8 ± 24.7	79.6± 24.0	71.8 ± 13.2	NS
	Female	5	66.0 ± 23.4	74.0 ± 13.7	78.0 ± 18.7	72.4 ± 10.4	61.8 ± 11.3	NS
Lymphocyte, %	Male	5	34.8 ± 12.1	45.2 ± 7.4	44.6 ± 9.3	36.8 ± 6.9	33.6 ± 7.6	NS
Neutrophil, %	Male	5	55.0 ± 10.9	43.1 ± 10.3	44.8 ± 7.4	52.2 ± 7.0	56.2 ± 9.2	NS
Eosinophil, %	Male	5	3.8 ± 2.2	3.1 ± 1.4	3.0 ± 1.9	5.0 ± 2.7	4.6 ± 1.7	NS
Basophil, %	Male	5	0.3 ± 0.5	0.3 ± 0.4	0.2 ± 0.4	0.0 ± 0.0	0.2 ± 0.4	NS
Monocyte, %	Male	5	6.3 ± 1.0	8.0 ± 3.2	7.4 ± 1.5	6.0 ± 2.1	5.4 ± 1.3	NS

Biochemical variables for miniature pigs during the experiment are shown. Values are mean±SD. RBC, red blood cell count; HGB, hemoglobin concentration; HCT, hematocrit value; MCV, mean corpuscular volume; MCH, mean corpuscular hemoglobin ; MCHC, mean corpuscular hemoglobin concentration; PLT, blood platelet count; PT, prothrombin time; ATPP, activated partial thromboplastin time; Fbg, fibrinogen level; WBC, white blood cell count; and NS: not significant. †*P* values were calculated using one-way factorial ANOVA.

Table 2. Subject hematology results
doi:10.1371/journal.pone.0019761.t002

The number of expressed genes was less in fetal stage and infancy period but increased with age, reaching a steady state of gene expression after 20 weeks of age (Figure 1). Expressed genes for male and female were analyzed by one-way factorial ANOVA. Then Tukey-Kramer's method was applied only to significant groups. Differences between age groups (fetal stage, 12, 20, and 30 weeks of age) were significant for male, female, and mixed subjects of male and female. A Tukey-Kramer's multiple comparisons test revealed that differences between fetal stage and other age groups were statistically significant ($p<0.001$) for both male and female. Also, differences were significant ($P<0.05$) between 12 and 30 weeks females.

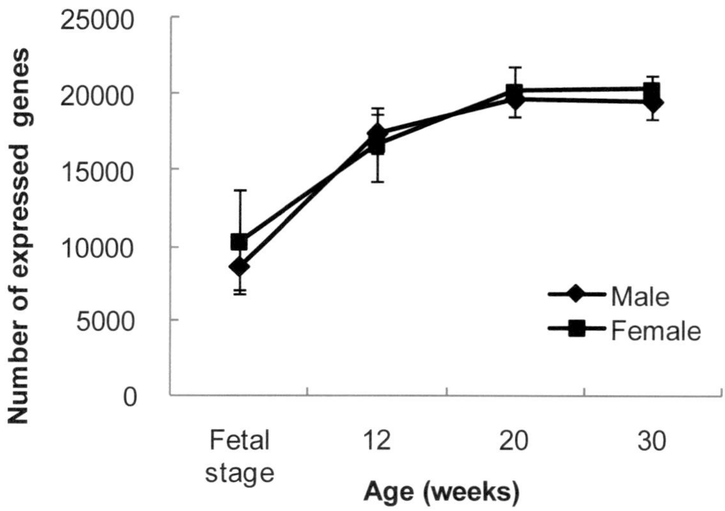

Figure 1. Number of genes expressed in whole blood of miniature pigs at different ages. In the graph, ◆ represents male and ■represents female. Values are means±SD.
doi:10.1371/journal.pone.0019761.g001

4.3. Microarray gene expression profiles – Correlation of gene expression

Variations in correlation coefficients among individuals of the same age and different age groups were evaluated. Pearson correlation coefficient was used for correlation analysis. Correlation coefficients for a total of 31 microarrays were obtained in normalized signals log-scale after excluding "absent" spots. A color-coded pairwise correlation matrix is shown in Figure 2. The color scale at the bottom indicates correlation strength.

The average correlation coefficient within the same age group is shown in Figure 3. Variations in gene expression were greater for younger subjects, but it diminished with age while generating resembling expression patterns. Correlation coefficient within 30 weeks age group was slightly smaller than that within 20 weeks age group. However, this difference is smaller than other distant age groups. Significant differences were observed between any age groups according to an ANOVA analysis using Fisher's Z-transform. The average correlation coefficient between different age groups is shown in Figure 4. Significant differences were observed except between "fatal stage vs. 20 weeks" and "fatal stage vs. 30 weeks", and between "12 weeks vs. 20 weeks" and "12 weeks vs. 30 weeks" according to an ANOVA analysis using Fisher's Z-transform ($P < 0.05$). These results suggest that the variation in gene expression intensity within the same age was great in fetal stage and infancy period, but converged with age.

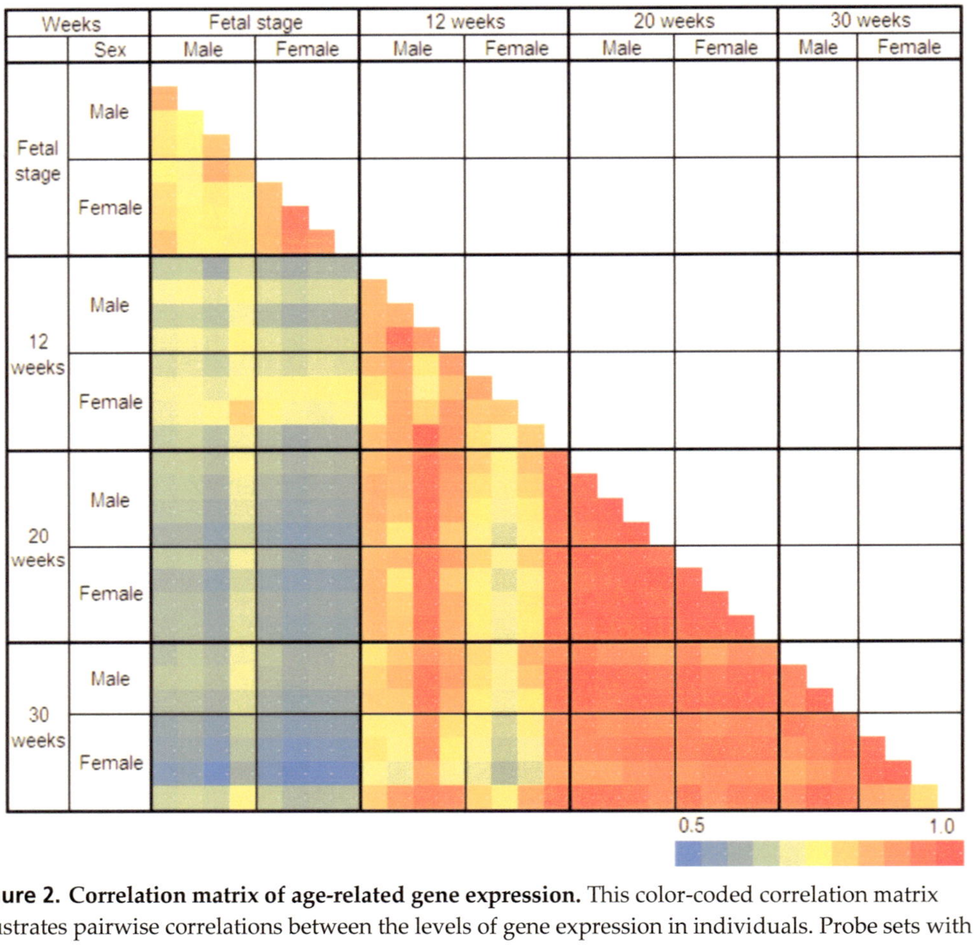

Figure 2. Correlation matrix of age-related gene expression. This color-coded correlation matrix illustrates pairwise correlations between the levels of gene expression in individuals. Probe sets with normalized signals (log-transformed and scaled) were used to calculate correlations between 31 arrays using Pearson correlation coefficient; signals flagged as "absent" were excluded. doi:10.1371/journal.pone.0019761.g002

4.4. Classification of genes depending on the status of age-related expression

All spots on the microarray were divided into 16 categories as shown Table 3 after assigning "1" for expressed genes and "0" for unexpressed genes. Here, definitions of "expressed" and "unexpressed" are described in "Materials and methods." Category 1 consists of a total of 6,763 genes expressed in the fetal stage, 12, 20, and 30 weeks of age. Category 2 consists of a total of 7,564 genes expressed at 12, 20, and 30 weeks of age. Category 4 consists of a total

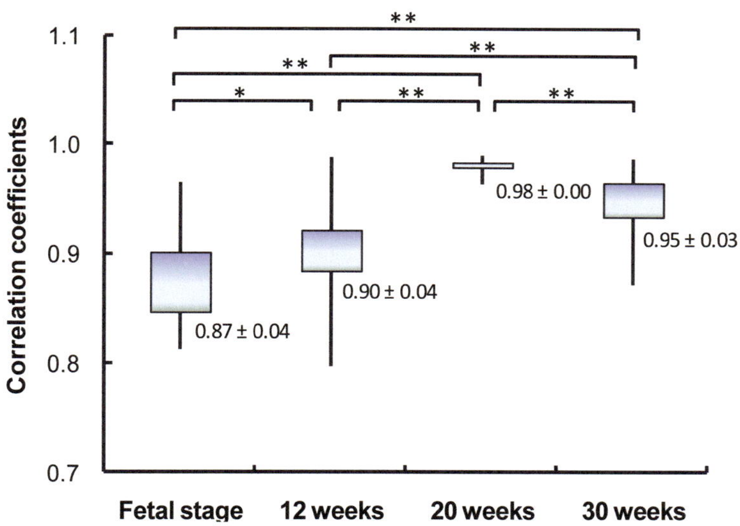

Figure 3. Age-related correlation coefficients within the same age groups. Correlation coefficients were calculated between individuals within the same age groups. The bottom and top of the boxes represent the 25th and 75th percentiles respectively. The lower and upper whiskers denote the minimum and maximum values of the data. Comparisons of the groups were made with the ANOVA test. * $p < 0.05$, ** $p < 0.01$.

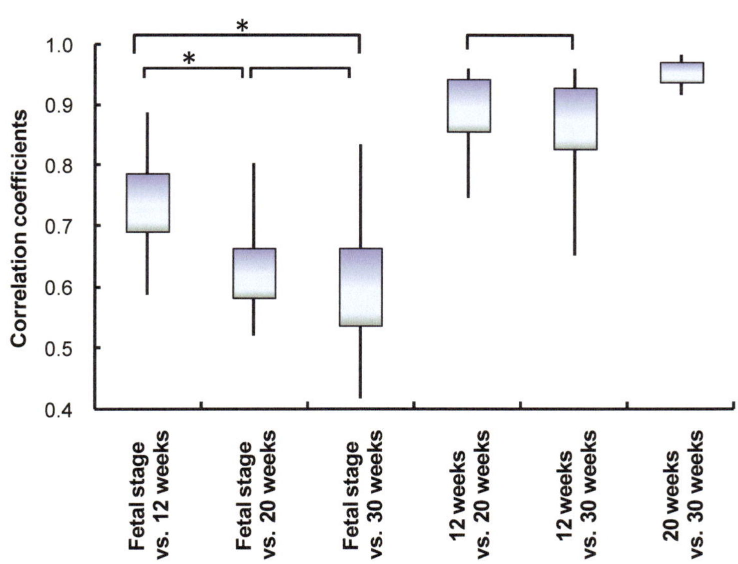

Figure 4. Age-related correlation coefficients between the different age groups. Correlation coefficients were calculated between the different age groups. The bottom and top of the boxes represent the 25th and 75th percentiles respectively. The lower and upper whiskers denote the minimum and maximum values of the data. Comparisons of the groups were made with the ANOVA test. * $p < 0.01$.

of 3,547 genes expressed after 20 weeks of age. Category 8 consists of a total of 827 genes expressed after 30 weeks of age. Sum of the genes expressed at certain age and those unexpressed (Categories 3, 5, 6, 7, 9, 10, 11, 12, 13, 14, and 15) was 1,051. Its fraction was 5.6% of 18,701 genes (Categories 1, 2, 4, and 8) expressing constantly once they appeared. Category 16 consists of genes unexpressed throughout the breeding period. Figure 5 shows the ratio of the genes belonging to each category.

Category	Fetal stage	12 weeks	20 weeks	30 weeks	Number of genes	Definition
1	1	1	1	1	6763	genes expressed from fetal stage to 30 weeks
2	0	1	1	1	7564	genes expressed from 12 to 30 weeks
3	1	0	1	1	49	
4	0	0	1	1	3547	genes expressed from 20 to 30 weeks
5	1	1	0	1	14	
6	0	1	0	1	80	
7	1	0	0	1	7	
8	0	0	0	1	827	genes expressed at 30 weeks
9	1	1	1	0	73	
10	0	1	1	0	124	
11	1	0	1	0	29	
12	0	0	1	0	428	genes expressed at 20 weeks
13	1	1	0	0	16	
14	0	1	0	0	147	genes expressed at 12 weeks
15	1	0	0	0	84	genes expressed in fetal stage
16	0	0	0	0	23851	genes not expressed from fetal stage to 30 weeks

Depending on the status of expression, all spots on the microarray can be divided into 16 categories. Here, "1" represents an expressed gene and "0" represents an unexpressed gene.

Table 3. Genes classified into 16 categories according to the status of age-related expression doi:10.1371/journal.pone.0019761.t005

To characterize gene expression in each category, TC Annotator List (Porcine version 14.0 3-11-10) was downloaded from the TIGR gene Indices. TC Annotator List includes the gene number and the GO terms. Out of 43,603 probes in the Agilent porcine microarray (#G2519F#20109), 6,019 genes bear GO annotation. Microarray cDNA probes were classified by GO terms of "biological processes". Out of all genes, fraction in Categories 1, 2, 4, 8, and 16 were 31%, 20%, 8%, 2%, and 38% respectively.

Then the difference in gene expression between all spots and those in 4 categories (Categories 1, 2, 4, and 8) was examined. GO groups dominantly expressed in Category 1 relates to mitosis (GO:0000070, GO:0000022, GO:0007052, and GO:0007100) and to immune

(GO:0043161, GO:0045059, GO:0019886), while those highly expressed in Category 2 related to cellular defense and regulation.

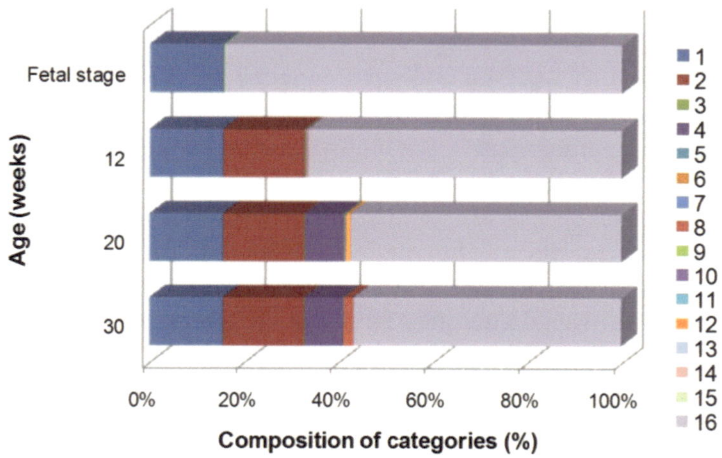

Figure 5. Ratios of categories for groups of the same age. The ratios of the genes in each category were calculated for groups in the fetal stage and at 12, 20, and 30 weeks of age. Categories are defined in Table 3.
doi:10.1371/journal.pone.0019761.g003

4.5. Age-related changes in gene expression levels for the immune system

Expression intensity of immunity gene was examined. Antigen processing and presentation (GO:0019882) and T cell selection (GO0045058) include the major histocompatibility complex (MHC) genes. By presenting antigens, MHC is involved in elimination of bacterial or viral pathogen, rejection of cancer cells, and rejective response on organ transplantation. Also MHC is indispensable in the immune system. Swine leukocyte antigens (SLA) are important immunogens for humoral responses and important mediators of the cellular immune responses through both direct and indirect presentation of peptides to T-cells [12]. SLA includes 6 of classical class I genes (SLA-1, SLA-2, SLA-3, SLA-6, SLA-7, and SLA-8) and 8 of classical class II genes (SLA-DMA, SLA-DMB, SLA-DOA, SLA-DOB1, SLA-DQA, SLA-DQB1, SLA-DRA, and SLA-DRB1) [13-14]. SLA class II lacks DPA1, DPB1, DRB3, DRB4, and DRB 5 in humans. On the Agilent porcine microarray, all of SLA genes except DOA are mounted on 28 spots. Among these, 11 SLA genes fell under Category 1, 1 fell under Category 2, and 1 fell under Category 8. Expression of SLA classical class I and class II genes are shown in Figure 6A and 6B, respectively. Both genes expressed in fatal stage, 12, 20, and 30 weeks in an increased manner by age.

The Agilent porcine microarray had 7 probes with 7 types of interferon and 7 probes for 4 types of interferon receptors. All of 7 interferon genes fell under Category 16. Normally these genes remain unexpressed but expressed upon necessity. In contrast, 1 type of interferon receptor gene fell under Category 1, 3 fell under Category 2, and were expressed until 12 weeks of age. Their signal intensities stayed at constant levels after 12 weeks (Figure 6C).

Toll-like receptors (TLRs) are the principal pattern recognition receptors. With this innate immunity, the first immune response is mediated into reserved foreign patterns on recognition. TLRs recognize reserved molecular patterns, start rapid response to protect the host upon infection, and produce signals, such as cytokines and co-stimulatory molecules to activate the adaptive immune system [15-16]. Regulation of the TLR signaling cascade is important for inflammatory responses, innate host defense, and adaptive immune responses [17-18]. Most mammalian species are estimated to have between 10 and 15 types of TLRs. The Agilent porcine microarray has 10 types of TLRs probes. Among these TLRs, 5 of TLR genes fell under Category 2 (expressed until 12 weeks of age), 1 under Category 8, and 4 under Category 16. Their signal intensities remained constant after 12 weeks of age (Figure 6D).

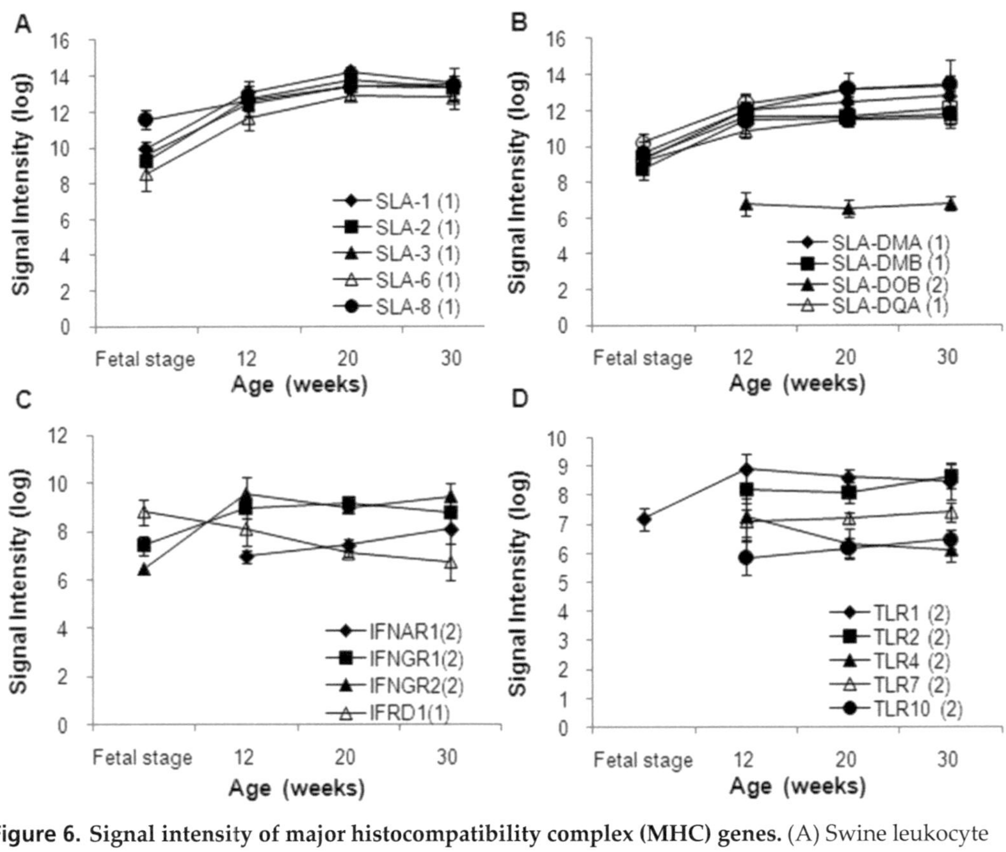

Figure 6. Signal intensity of major histocompatibility complex (MHC) genes. (A) Swine leukocyte antigens (SLA) classical class I genes. (B) Swine leukocyte antigens (SLA) classical class II genes. (C) Interferon receptor genes. (D) Toll-like receptor (TLR) genes. Signal intensities were normalized using quantile normalization and log-transformed after excluded signals flagged as "absent." The category numbers are shown in graph legends. Genes in Categories 1, 2, and 4 are shown in the graph. doi:10.1371/journal.pone.0019761.g005

5. Gene expression profiles change related to hyperlipidemia

To examine the usage of whole blood RNA analysis for the early diagnosis of the disease, we showed transitions in dietary induced hyperlipidemia gene expression profiles of whole blood RNA in miniature pigs.

Hyperlipidemia is well recognized as a risk factor for cardiovascular disease (CVD). As diet represents the most important determinant of hyperlipidemia, dietary animal models can be useful for the study of CVD progression [19]. High-fat, high-cholesterol, and high-sugar diets have been shown to induce hyperlipidemia, obesity, and insulin resistance in humans and rodents [20-22]. Dietary-induced hyperlipidemia pig models have also been established [23-29].

A high-fat and high-cholesterol diet (HFCD) as a typical dietary treatment were used for dietary-induced hyperlipidemia miniature pig models, by using specific pathogen-free (SPF) Clawn miniature pigs.

Eight 12-week-old, male Clawn miniature pigs were housed individually in cages of 1.5 m^2 at the breeder's specific pathogen-free (SPF) facility (Japan Farm Co., Ltd, Kagoshima, Japan) for 27 weeks. Body weights at the beginning of the experiment were 5.1 (2.6) kg (mean (standard deviation; SD)). During this period, 5 pigs were fed with 450 g/day standard dry feed (Kodakara73, Marubeni Nisshin Feed Co., Ltd., Tokyo Japan), and had unlimited access to water (control group). Five pigs were fed a high-fat, high-cholesterol diet containing 15% lard and 2% cholesterol (HFCD group).

Almost no changes were observed in fasting plasma triglyceride levels. Fasting plasma total cholesterol concentrations had increased in the HFCD group by week 5 of the feeding period ($P<0.001$) and were maintained between 350 and 1150 mg/dL from weeks 10–27. Fasting plasma high-density lipoprotein cholesterol (HDL-C) concentrations increased and showed significant differences ($P < 0.001$) from weeks 10–27. Fasting plasma low-density lipoprotein cholesterol (LDL-C) concentrations also increased and showed significant differences from weeks 5–27. Fasting plasma glucose concentrations remained unchanged.

5.1. Gene expression profiles of dietary-induced hyperlipidemia for whole blood RNA

RNA analyses were conducted on blood samples obtained at weeks 10, 19, and 27 of the feeding periods to characterize the dietary effects on gene expression profiles in whole blood and white blood cells of miniature pigs. Each RNA sample was analyzed by aporcine gene expression microarray consisting of 43603 oligonucleotide probes.

Variation in correlation coefficients among individuals on the same diet and between different diet groups was evaluated. Pearson correlation coefficients were used for the correlation analysis. Correlation coefficients for 23 microarrays in total were obtained for a normalized signals log-scale after excluding "absent" spots, definition of "absent" were described in Materials and Methods. A color-coded pairwise correlation matrix is displayed in Figure 7.

The correlation coefficients of whole blood expression profiles within the same diet groups were 0.97 (0.01) (mean (standard deviation; SD)), and 0.94 (0.05) for the control, HFCD whole blood at 10 weeks, 0.94 (0.03), and 0.93 (0.06) at 19 weeks, and 0.95 (0.02), and 0.95 (0.03) at 27 weeks, respectively. Using Fisher's Z-transformation to normalize the correlation distributions, no significant differences in correlation coefficients among dietary groups were observed at any period during the treatments. This indicates uniformity of dietary-induced hyperlipidemia for our protocols.

The whole blood correlation coefficients among the different diet groups were 0.95 (0.04) for control vs. HFCD at 10 weeks, 0.93 (0.03) at 19 weeks, and 0.95 (0.03) at 27 weeks, respectively.

5.2. Assigning known functions to gene expression - Gene ontology annotation

Up- and down-regulated genes were identified and classified these according to function using information from the Gene Ontology (GO) Database to understand the observed differences in whole blood gene expression profiles for the different dietary groups. Top-ranked genes with fold changes in expression greater than 2.0 ($p < 0.05$) and less than 0.5 ($p < 0.05$) were selected at 10, 19, and 27 weeks. As a result, the GO categories of many genes up-regulated at the end of the 19-week dietary period were related to nucleotide binding (GO: 0000166, GO: GO: 0005524, 0005525, GO: 0017076, GO: 0019001, GO: 00032553, GO: 00032555, GO: 0032561), and catabolic processes (GO: 0009057, GO: 0019941, GO: 0030163, GO: 0043632, GO: 0044257, GO: 0044265,). Many genes down-regulated after 27 weeks were in the GO categories related to biological adhesion (GO: 0007155, GO: 0022610).

5.3. Effect of white blood cells on whole blood gene expression profiles in dietary-induced hyperlipidemia

Microarray analyses were conducted from white blood cells at the end of the dietary period to evaluate the effect of white blood cells on whole blood gene expression profiles (Figure 8). The correlation coefficients of white blood cells expression profiles within the same dietary groups were 0.94 (0.05) and 0.95 (0.03) for the control and HFCD groups at 27 weeks. The white blood cells correlation coefficients was 0.94 (0.04) between control and HFCD. The average correlation coefficients between whole blood and white blood cells were 0.83 (0.04) and 0.79 (0.05) for control and HFCD. Using Fisher's Z-transformation to normalize the correlation distributions, no significant differences in correlation coefficients of white blood cells were observed between control and HFCD groups.

Up- and down-regulated genes were identified and classified these according to function using information from the Gene Ontology (GO) Database to understand the observed differences in white blood cells gene expression profiles for the different dietary groups, as the same as whole blood gene expression profiles. Top-ranked genes with fold changes in expression greater than 2.0 ($p < 0.05$) and less than 0.5 ($p < 0.05$) were selected at 27 weeks. As a result, many genes down-regulated related oxidation-reduction process (GO:0055114) and keg pathways of steroid biosynthesis.

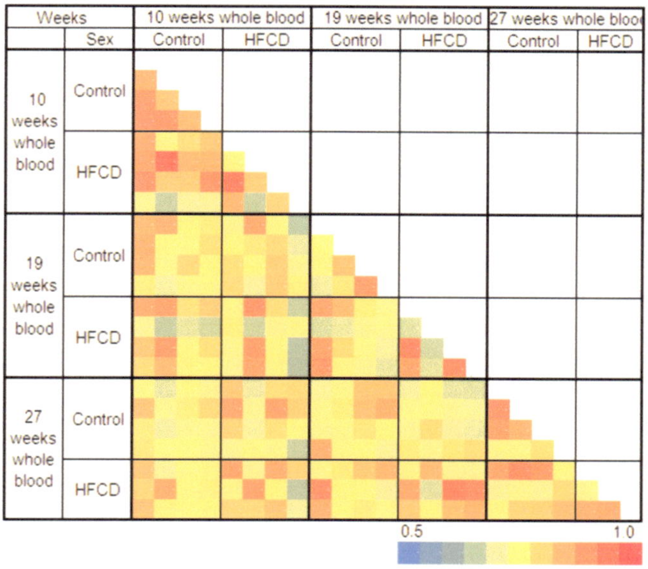

Figure 7. Correlation matrix of dietary-related gene expression profiles of whole blood. This color-coded correlation matrix illustrates pairwise correlations between the levels of gene expression in individuals. Probe sets with normalized signals (log-transformed and scaled) were used to calculate correlations between 23 arrays using Pearson correlation coefficient; signals flagged as "absent" were excluded. The color scale at the bottom indicates the strengths of the correlations.

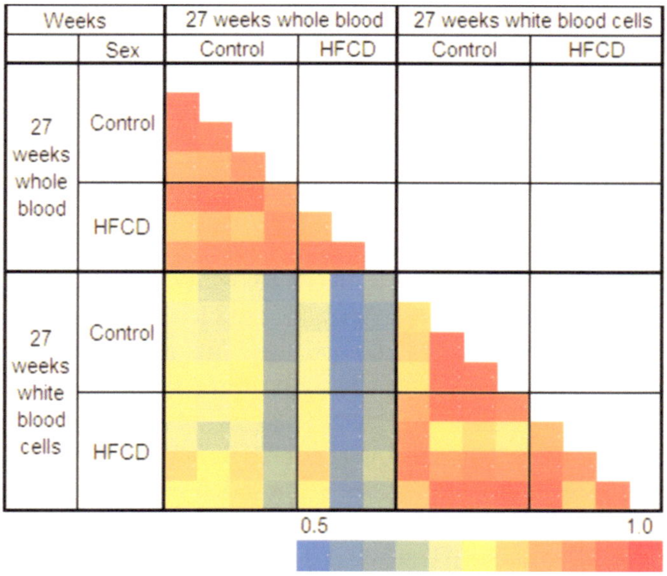

Figure 8. Correlation matrix of dietary-related gene expression profiles of whole blood and white blood cells. This color-coded correlation matrix illustrates pairwise correlations between the levels of gene expression in individual at feeding period at week 27. Probe sets with normalized signals (log-transformed and scaled) were used to calculate correlations between 15 arrays using Pearson correlation coefficient; signals flagged as "absent" were excluded. The color scale at the bottom indicates the strengths of the correlations.

6. Gene expression profiles change with other stresses

Furthermore, a possibility was shown that whole blood RNA analysis is applicable to evaluation of physiological state.

The degree of stress can be comparable according to the numbers of up-regulated and down-regulated genes, even if the stress is different in quality from the others.

Sodium azide was given orally to the miniature pigs over 20 weeks. There were no significant changes of hematological and biochemical properties for administrated dose of 300μg/kg, one hundredth of LD_{50}. On the other hand, gene expression profiles were obviously changed. Anesthesia group showed a slight degree, but the one week fasting group showed a significant difference. This can be clearly noticed when the contents of stress is classified by the function of up-regulated and down-regulated genes. Consequently, grade of the stress can be estimated according to the expression state of genes.

Stresses	P<0.05, Fold change>2		
	total	up regulation	down regulation
sodium azide 300μg/kg ; LD_{50} 1/100	893	339	554
blood removal (150ml) after 6 hours	1747	227	1520
Fasting a week	3136	1840	1296
anesthesia after 6 hours	160	87	73
non treatment (blood removal 20ml)	73	14	59

Table 4. Summery of gene expression condition of several types of stress
Number of genes

7. Effects of white blood cells on whole blood gene expression profiles

Whole blood contains a variety of cell types as red blood cells, granulocytes, lymphocytes, and platelets. Most of the nucleated cells in blood are white blood cells such as neutrophils, T-cells, B-cells, and monocytes. The number of white blood cells in humans is known to decrease steadily from infancy to adulthood, and its composition (i.e. lymphocytes, granulocytes) also changes with age [30]. In study of the gene expression profiles change related to aging, hematological data of the fetal stage was unavailable because the amount of collected blood was insufficient for the analysis. From 12 to 30 weeks of age, ANOVA analysis indicated no significant differences in the fractions of lymphocytes, neutrophils, eosinophils, basophils, and monocytes. In addition, these compositions were almost equal to those in human adults. The above result suggests that the gene expression profile change of age-related whole blood RNA is not due to the composition of white blood cell subpopulations.

The intraclass correlation between Staphylococcus enterotoxin B-stimulated and unstimulated blood from healthy subjects was significantly higher in leukocyte-derived samples the in whole blood, suggesting that the method of RNA isolation from whole blood can be a critical step in blood RNA assay [31]. Although PBMCs do not contain neutrophils, eosinophils, basophils, nor platelets, Min et al. reported highly correlated results (r^2 = 0.85) for 8,273 genes expressed between the whole blood RNA, by using the PAX gene Blood RNA system, and peripheral blood mononuclear cell (PBMC) RNA samples isolated from healthy volunteers by using a Ficoll-Paque gradient and TRI Reagent (SIGMA) [32]. Other workers conducted a large scale genome-wide expression analysis of white blood cells subpopulations. This study indicates that correlation coefficients for T-cells and monocytes among different healthy subjects were 0.98±0.01 and 0.97±0.01, respectively. However, for the same subjects (n=5), correlation coefficients between T-cells and monocytes was 0.88±0.01, indicating varied correlation between white blood cells subpopulations. In addition, gene expression analysis were showed a varying dependence on the isolation method such as PAXgene, Buffy coat, and lysis. The correlation coefficients between isolation methods were 0.89±0.04, 0.91±0.04, 0.96±0.06, for PAXgene vs. lysis, PAXgene vs. Buffy coat, and Buffy coat vs. lysis, respectively [33]. In order to ensure the reliability for to clinical use of whole blood RNA diagnosis, the development of standard method and measurement standards needs to be sought.

The Gene Ontology (GO) Database was used to categorize gene expression profiles functionally to conduct the effects of white blood cells on whole blood gene expression profiles in our study of hyperlipidemia. As a result, the GO term, related to white blood cell function (GO: 0006954, 0007166), had a high correlation coefficient. In contrast, GO terms related to the repair of damaged organs, including translation (GO: 0006412), positive regulation of growth rate (GO: 0040010), and growth (GO: 004007), showed low correlation coefficients. We, therefore, conclude that the difference in the gene expression profiles between the whole blood and white blood cells are not only caused by differences in experimental protocols, but also by differences in RNA origin [34].

8. Conclusion

Whole blood RNA is easy to handle compared to isolated white blood cell RNA and can be used for health and disease monitoring and animal control. In addition, whole blood is a heterogeneous mixture of subpopulation cells. Once a great change occurs in composition and expressing condition of subpopulations, their associated change will be reflected on whole blood RNA.

Whole blood microarray analyses were conducted to evaluate variations of correlation among individuals and ages using specific pathogen-free (SPF) Clawn miniature pigs. The characteristics of age-related gene expression by taking into account of change in the number of expressed genes by age and similarities of gene expression intensity between individuals were identified. As a result, the number of expressed genes was less in fetal stage and infancy period but increased with age, reaching a steady state of gene expression after 20 weeks of age. Variation in gene expression intensity within the same age was great in fetal stage and infancy period, but converged with age. The variation between 20 and 30 weeks of age was comparable to that among 30 weeks individuals. These results indicate that uniformity of laboratory animals is expected for miniature pigs after 20 weeks of age.

In dietary-induced hyperlipidemia study, feeding treatments commenced when the pigs were 12 weeks old, RNA analysis was conducted on whole blood sampled after 10, 19, and 27 weeks of the feeding period. Variation in whole blood gene expression intensity among individuals within the HFCD group was in the same range as that of the controls at any period, indicating uniformity of dietary-induced hyperlipidemia expression profiles in miniature pigs. Dietary-induced transitions of gene expression profiles for genes bearing GO terms were examined. Major changes included an induction of proteins involved in catabolic processes and protein metabolism after a 19-week dietary period, and a reduced expression of proteins involved in steroid metabolism and lipid biosynthesis after a 27-week dietary period.

In several kinds of stress study, the degree (extent) of stress can be comparable according to the gene number of up-regulate, or down-regulate, even if the stress is different in kind from the others.

A possibility was shown that whole blood RNA analysis is applicable to evaluation of physiological state. By considering variation in gene expression profiles of miniature pigs, whole blood RNA analyses can be used in practical applications. The blood RNA diagnostics under development may eventually be useful for monitoring human health.

Author details

Junko Takahashi* and Akiko Takatsu
National Metrology Institute of Japan, National Institute of Advanced Industrial Science and Technology, Tsukuba, Ibaraki, Japan

Masaki Misawa
Human Technology Research Institute, National Institute of Advanced Industrial Science and Technology, Tsukuba, Ibaraki, Japan

Hitoshi Iwahashi
Health Research Institute, National Institute of Advanced Industrial Science and Technology, Takamatsu, Kagawa, Japan
Faculty of Applied Biological Sciences, Gifu University, Gifu, Japan

9. References

[1] Williams-Devane CR, Wolf MA, Richard AM (2009) Toward a public toxicogenomics capability for supporting predictive toxicology: survey of current resources and chemical indexing of experiments in GEO and ArrayExpress. Toxicol Sci 109(2):358-371.

[2] Pennie W, Pettit SD, Lord PG (2004) Toxicogenomics in risk assessment: an overview of an HESI collaborative research program. Environ Health Perspect 112(4):417-419.

* Corresponding Author

[3] Tong W, Cao X, Harris S, Sun H, Fang H, et al. (2003) ArrayTrack--supporting toxicogenomic research at the U.S. Food and Drug Administration National Center for Toxicological Research. Environ Health Perspect 111(15):1819-182
[4] Takahashi J, Misawa M, Iwahashi I (2011) Oligonucleotide microarray analysis of age-related gene expression profiles in miniature pigs. PLoS ONE 6(5):e19761.
[5] Lunney JK (2000) Advances in Swine Biomedical Model Genomics. Int J Biol Sci 3(3):179–184.
[6] Simon GA, Maibach HI (2000) The Pig as an Experimental Animal Model of Percutaneous Permeation in Man: Qualitative and Quantitative Observations – An Overview. Skin Pharmacol Appl Skin Physiol 13(5):229-234.
[7] Vodicka P, Smetana K Jr, Dvoránková B, Emerick T, Xu YZ, et al. (2005) The miniature pig as an animal model in biomedical research. Ann N Y Acad Sci 1049:161-171.
[8] Hornshøj H, Conley LN, Hedegaard J, Sørensen P, Panitz F, et al. (2007) Microarray expression profiles of 20.000 genes across 23 healthy porcine tissues. PLoS One 21;2(11):e1203.
[9] Steibel JP, Wysocki M, Lunney JK, Ramos AM, Hu ZL, et al. (2009) Assessment of the swine protein-annotated oligonucleotide microarray. Anim Genet 40(6):883-893.
[10] Schook LB, Beever JE, Rogers J, Humphray S, Archibald A, et al. (2005) Swine Genome Sequencing Consortium (SGSC): a strategic roadmap for sequencing the pig genome. Comp Funct Genomics 6(4):251-255.
[11] Archibald AL, Bolund L, Churcher C, Fredholm M, Groenen MA, et al. (2010) Pig genome sequence--analysis and publication strategy. BMC Genomics 11:438
[12] Ierino FL, Gojo S, Banerjee PT, Giovino M, Xu Y, et al. (1999) Transfer of swine major histocompatibility complex class II genes into autologous bone marrow cells of baboons for the induction of tolerance across xenogeneic barriers. Transplantation 67(8):1119-1128.
[13] The Immuno Polymorphism Database (IPD) - major histocompatibility complex (MHC) Database. Swine (SLA) Sequences - Release 1.2.0 16/05/2008. http://www.ebi.ac.uk/ipd/mhc/sla/. Accessed November 1,2010.
[14] Ho CS, Lunney JK, Ando A, Rogel-Gaillard C, Lee JH, et al. (2009) Nomenclature for factors of the SLA system, update 2008. Tissue Antigens 73(4):307-315.
[15] Frei R, Steinle J, Birchler T, Loeliger S, Roduit C, et al. (2010) MHC class II molecules enhance Toll-like receptor mediated innate immune responses. PLoS One 5(1):e8808
[16] Takeda K, Kaisho T, Akira S (2003) Toll-like receptors. Annu Rev Immunol 21:335–376.
[17] Medzhitov R (2001) Toll-like receptors and innate immunity. Nat Rev Immunol 1:135–145.
[18] Akira S, Takeda K (2004) Toll-like receptor signalling. Nat Rev Immunol 4:499–511.
[19] Lissner L, Heitmann BL (1995) Dietary fat and obesity: evidence from epidemiology. Eur J Clin Nutr 49(2):79–90.
[20] Radonjic M, de Haan JR, van Erk MJ, van Dijk KW, van den Berg SAA, et al. (2009) Genome-wide mRNA expression analysis of hepatic adaptation to high-fat diets reveals switch from an inflammatory to steatotic transcriptional program. PLoS ONE 4(8):e6646.

[21] Russell JC, Proctor SD. (2006), Small animal models of cardiovascular disease: tools for the study of the roles of metabolic syndrome, dyslipidemia, and atherosclerosis. Cardiovasc Pathol 15(6):318-330.

[22] Oron-Herman M, Kamari Y, Grossman E, Yeger G, Peleg E, et al. (2008) Metabolic syndrome: comparison of the two commonly used animal models. Am J Hypertens 21(9):1018-1022.

[23] Kobari Y, Koto M, Tanigawa M. (1991) Regression of diet-induced atherosclerosis in Güttingen Miniature Swine. Lab Anim 25 (2):110-116.

[24] De Keyzer D, Karabina SA, Wei W, Geeraert B, Stengel D, et al. (2009) Increased PAFAH and oxidized lipids are associated with inflammation and atherosclerosis in hypercholesterolemic pigs. Arterioscler Thromb Vasc Biol 29(12):2041-2046.

[25] Orbe J, Rodriguez JA, Calvo A, Grau A, Belzunce MS, et al. (2001) Vitamins C and E attenuate plasminogen activator inhibitor-1 (PAI-1) expression in a hypercholesterolemic porcine model of angioplasty. Cardiovasc Res 49(2):484-492.

[26] de Smet BJ, Kuntz RE, van der Helm YJ, Pasterkamp G, Borst C, et al. (1997) Relationship between plaque mass and neointimal hyperplasia after stent placement in Yucatan micropigs. Radiology 203(2):484-488.

[27] Bowles DK, Heaps CL, Turk JR, Maddali KK, Price EM. (2004) Hypercholesterolemia inhibits L-type calcium current in coronary macro-, not microcirculation. J Appl Physiol 96(6):2240-2248.

[28] W Yin, D Liao, M Kusunoki, S Xi, K Tsutsumi, et al. (2004) NO-1886 decreases ectopic lipid deposition and protects cells in diet-induced diabetic swine pancreatic. J Endocrinol 180(3):399-408.

[29] Zhang C, Yin W, Liao D, Huang L, Tang C, et al. (2006) NO-1886 upregulates ATP binding cassette transporter A1 and inhibits diet-induced atherosclerosis in Chinese Bama minipigs. J Lipid Res 47(9):2055-2063.

[30] Hulstaert F, Hannet I, Deneys V, Munhyeshuli V, Reichert T, et al. (1994) Age-Related Changes in Human Blood Lymphocyte Subpopulations: II. Varying Kinetics of Percentage and Absolute Count Measurements. Clin Immunol Immunopathol 70(2):152-158.

[31] Feezor RJ, Baker HV, Mindrinos M, Hayden D, Tannahill CL, et al. (2004) Whole blood and leukocyte RNA isolation for gene expression analyses. Physiol Genomics 19:247–254.

[32] Min JL, Barrett A, Watts T, Pettersson FH, Lockstone HE, et al. (2010) Variability of gene expression profiles in human blood and lymphoblastoid cell lines. BMC Genomics 11:96

[33] Cobb JP, Mindrinos MN, Miller-Graziano C, Calvano SE, Baker HV, et.al. (2005) Application of genome-wide expression analysis to human health and disease. Proc Natl Acad Sci USA. 102(13):4801-4806.

[34] Takahashi J, Waki S, Matsumoto R, Odake J, Miyaji T, et al. (2012) Oligonucleotide microarray analysis of dietary-induced hyperlipidemia gene expression profiles in miniature pigs. PLoS ONE 7(5):e37581.

Chapter 7

Proliferation and Differentiation of Hematopoietic Cells and Preservation of Immune Functions

Osamu Hayashi

Additional information is available at the end of the chapter

http://dx.doi.org/10.5772/48322

1. Introduction

A limited number of pluripotent stem cells are mainly located in the bone marrow, and give rise to all blood cell 1ineages. Because of their relatively short lifespan, circulating cells must be continually replaced in living body throughout the life. The task performed by hematopoietic stem cells is shared in two main features, that is, the capacity of regeneration which prevents depletion of the cells and the ability of preservation of blood homeostasis. The mechanisms behind the critical choice between lineage-commitment and maintenance of the stem-cell pool involve a number of complex interactions between hematopoietic progenitor cells at different stages of maturation, stromal cells and their extracellular matrix, as well as a variety of stimulatory or inhibitory cytokines provided by the microenvironment.

Hematopoietic growth factors were first identified in the 1960s as soluble agents produced in spleen, uterus or lung, and found to maintain the formation of differentiated colonies from hematopoietic progenitor cells in semisolid culture systems. Hence they were named colony-stimulating factors, CSFs (Schneider and Dy, 1999). Most of these molecules have been purified and their genes have been sequenced. They are currently available in recombinant form and have been used with success in clinical trials.

Hematopoietic growth factors or CSFs can be divided into two categories, according to their target cell specificity (Figure 1). One group comprises the factors whose activity is relatively restricted to particular cell types, such as macrophage colony-stimulating factor (M-CSF) for macrophages, granulocyte colony-stimulating factor (G-CSF) for neutrophils, interleukin-5 (IL-5) for eosinophils and B cells, and thrombopoietin (Tpo) for megakaryocytes and erythropoietin (Epo) for the erythroid lineage. The second category of growth factors has a relatively wide spectrum of activities, such as IL-3 and granulocyte-macrophage colony-stimulating factor (GM-CSF). The factors target a heterogeneous population of cells, including both primitive and lineage-committed progenitors. Action of these two molecules can be modulated by a number of cytokines which are not essentially growth factors. Among these, IL-1, IL-6, IL-9, IL-1l and leukemia inhibitory factor (LIF) are involved. An interleukin 6 class cytokine or stem cell factor (SCF) plays a particularly important role in the amplification of early stem cell commitment. IL-7 is also noteworthy in this context, with respect to its crucial role in lymphopoiesis, as evidenced by the strong lymphopenia in IL7-deficient mice. Hematopoiesis can be also regulated negatively by a heterogeneous set of molecules, such as interferon, tumor necrosis factor-alpha (TNF-α), transforming growth factor beta (TGFβ) and compounds like prostaglandins, ferritin and lactoferrin.

The precise function of cytokines during constitutive hematopoiesis in a healthy organism is still unclear, although much evidence has been accumulated from the study using genetically modified mice. The purpose of hematopoiesis, however, is not only the maintenance of homeostasis, but also a rapid and controlled response to stress situations. The immune response induced by infection, the number of circulating white blood cells can be remarkably increased (Schneider and Dy, 1999). In the process, the cytokines generated by sensitized lymphocytes and activated cells of the immune system play a crucial role in the recruitment and the differentiation of hematopoietic cells.

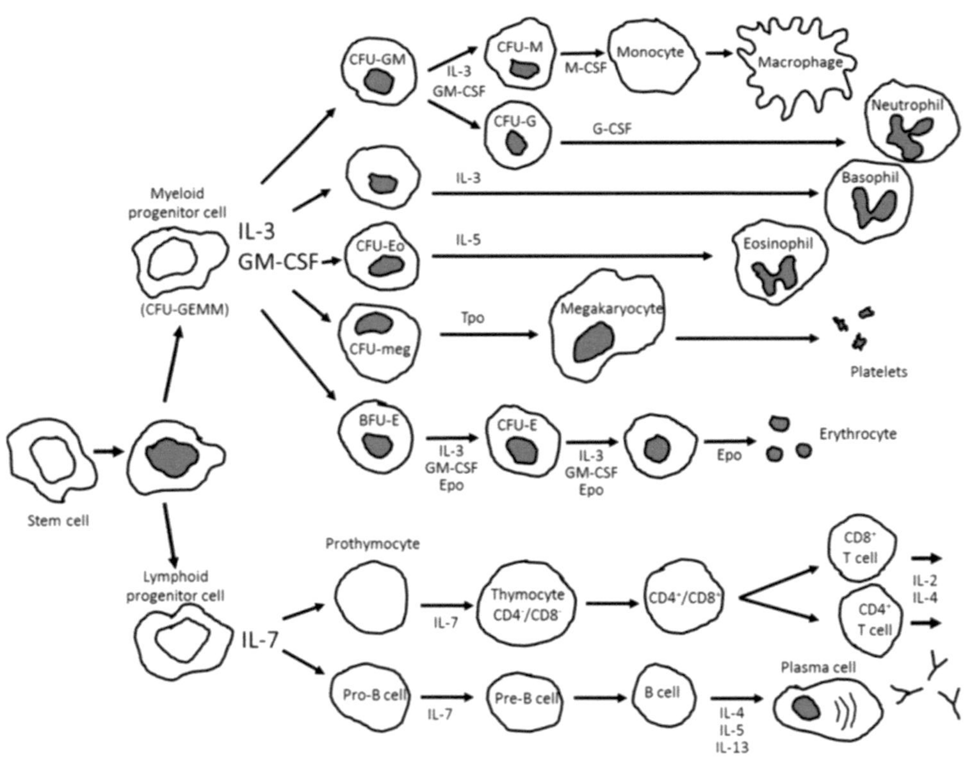

Figure 1. Simplified haematopoietic differentiation scheme and cytokines (modified from Elk and Dy, 1999)

In the chapter, we focus on relations and networks of cytokines, induced by ingesting *in-vivo* study of *Spirulina* and by *in-vitro* cultured cells, to differentiation of hematopoietic cells and preservation of immune functions, and discuss the possibility of their medicinal application for sustaining a healthy state.

2. *Spirulina*

Spirulina platensis is a helicoidal filamentous blue-green alga (cyanobacterium) and has a history of being used as food for over a thousand years, and has been commercially produced for more than 40 years as a food supplement (Ciferri, 1983; Gershwin and Belay, 2008). *Spirulina platensis* is prokaryote and belongs to the class Cyanophyceae, or Cyanobacteria. In its commercial use, the common name, *Spirulina*, refers to the cyanobacterium, *Arthrospira platensis*, and is a whole product of biological origin. In its taxonomic use, *Spirulina* is a name used to describe mainly two species of Cyanobacteria, *Arthrospira platensis* and *A. maxima*, which are commonly used as food, dietary supplement, and feed supplement (Vadiraja et al., 1998) . These and other *Arthrospira* species forming helical trichomes were once combined and classified into a single genus, *Spirulina* (Geitler, 1932). Before Geitler, on the basis of the presence of septa or division in the trichomes, the two genera were placed separately, that is, the *Spirulina* species being without septa and the *Arthrospira* species with septa. Recent morphological, physiological, and biochemical studies have shown that these two genera are distinctively different and that the edible forms commonly referred to as *Spirulina platensis* have little in common with other much smaller species. This distinction has been also based on results from the complete sequence of the 16S ribosomal RNA gene and the internal transcribed spacer (ITS) between the 16S and 23S rRNA genes determined for two *Arthrospira* strains and one *Spirulina* strain (Nelissen et al., 1992) showing that the two *Arthrospira* strains formed a close cluster distant from the *Spirulina* strain.

Blue green algae *Spirulina platensis* (*Arthrospira platensis*) is gaining more and more attention as a nutraceutical and source of potential pharmaceuticals. *Spirulina* is known to have nutritional advantages of high-quality protein contents and other components such as vitamins; minerals, and essential fatty acids, including γ-linolenic acid, and β-carotene (Belay et al., 1993) , and has been approved its safety in the report from United Nations International Development Organization, UNIDO (Chamorro-Cevallos, 1980). Moreover, sulfated polysaccharides, called calcium-spirulan (Ca-Sp) and isolated from a hot-water extract of *Spirulina*, exhibit immunomodulatory activity and inhibit metastasis of melanoma cells to the lungs (Mishima et al., 1998) , and can also inhibit virus entry (Hayashi et al., 1996). Immolina, a high-molecular-weight polysaccharide fraction of *Spirulina*, promotes chemokine expression in human monocytic THP-1 cells (Grzanna et al., 2006). *Spirulina* contains phycocyanin (CPC; C-phycocyanin), a blue, 270-kDa photosynthetic pigment protein, which accounts for approximately 15% of the dry weight of *Spirulina* (Ciferri, 1983).

Recently, more attention has been given to the study of the therapeutic effects of *Spirulina*. In addition to its effectiveness in reducing hyperlipidemia, diabetes, and high blood pressure in humans and animals, anti-viral and anti-cancer effects of orally administered *S. platensis* involving immune functions have also been reported (Belay, 2002).

3. Structure of phycocyanin

The biological and pharmacological properties of *Spirulina* were attributed mainly to C-phycocyanin (CPC). CPC is a major light-harvesting or photosynthetic pigment protein present in the antenna rods of *Spirulina platensis*. *S. platensis* also contains allophycocyanin (APC) as a minor component present at the core of the antenna rods. CPC and APC including phycoerythrin (PE) are the principal classes of phycobiliproteins which form supramolecular complexes known as phycobilisomes assemblies in cyanobacteria (Figure. 2a). In phycobiliproteins, a linear tetrapyrrole (bilin) as the chromophore is covalently attached to the apoprotein by thioether bonds to cysteine residues. CPC molecule is composed of two kinds of subunits, α- and β-subunits to form trimeric aggregation $\alpha3\beta3$ (Figures. 2b and 2c). Padyana et al. (2001) solved the crystal structure of CPC by molecular replacement technique (Figures. 2d and 2e). The α- and β-subunit polypeptides exhibit high affinity for one another and associate into (αβ)-monomers, which in turn aggregate into $(\alpha\beta)_3$-trimers and $(\alpha\beta)_6$-hexamers (Figure. 2f).

The medicinal and pharmacological properties of CPC have been reported earlier (Romay et al., 1998). Recent studies have demonstrated the antioxidant (Vadiraja et al., 1998; Wu and Annie Ho, 2008), anti-inflammatory (Reddy et al., 2000), and hepatoprotective properties (Vadiraja et al., 1998), in addition to anticancer, anti-allergic, immune-enhancing (Hayashi et al., 2008), blood-vessel-relaxing and blood-lipid-lowering effects of CPC (Gershwin and Belay, 2008).

a.

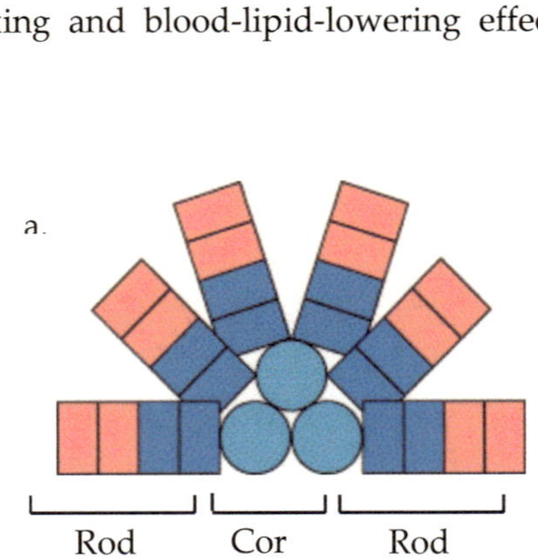

b.

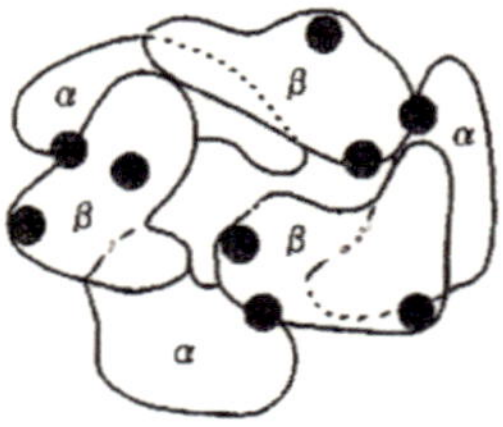

c.

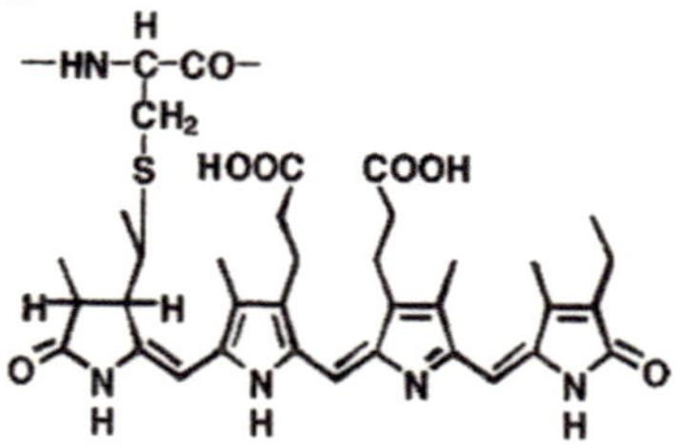

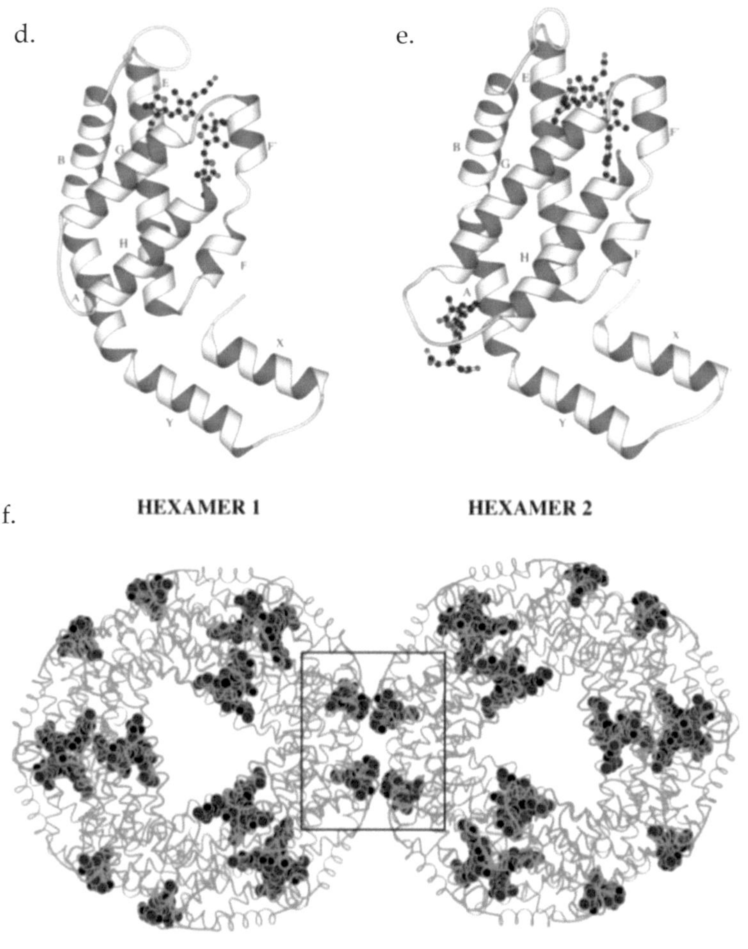

A phycobilisome (a) has six antenna rods with a three-cylinder core of allophycocyanin, APC (circles), two of the core cylinders lie on the thylakoid membrane, while the third one does not. Each rod has four hexameric disk-like structures, two of phycoerythrin, PE (red), and two of phycocyanin, CPC (blue) (MacColl, 2004). CPC consists of α- and β-subunit polypeptides to form trimeric aggregation $\alpha_3\beta_3$ and nine phycocyanobilin moieties as a chromophore shown in closed circles (b). c shows chemical structure of phycocyanobilin (Li et al., 2006). d and e show ribbon representation of CPC α-subunit and CPC β-subunit, respectively, with chromophores shown in ball and stick representation (Padyana et al., 2001). f shows coil representation of the two $(\alpha\beta)_6$-hexamers in the crystal asymmetric unit, and the box drawn at the center highlights the close proximity of phycocyanobilins at the position 155 on each β-subunit in the region between the adjacent hexamers (Padyana et al., 2001).

Figure 2. Schematic representation of one type of phycobilisome (a), and various representations of C-phycocyanin (b - f).

Preparation of phycocyanin solution in the experiments Phycocyanin was extracted from spray-dried *Spirulina platensis* with 50 mM sodium-phosphate buffer (pH 6.0). The crude extract was partially purified by DE-52 ion-exchange chromatography. The eluate was dialyzed against distilled water and lyophilized. Phycocyanin contents of the resultant powder were over 80%, and the recovery from the crude extract was approximately 6%. The phycocyanin powder was dissolved in distilled water to a concentration of 0.05%, centrifuged in a refrigerated machine for 10 min at 1,500 g, and the supernatant was sterilized by filtration through a 0.20-μm-pore filter (Hayashi et al., 2006).

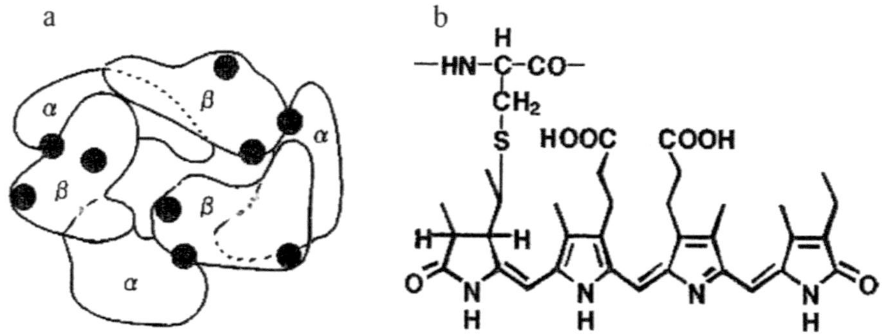

a. CPC molecule composed of two kinds of subunits(α- and β-subunits) to form $\alpha_3\beta_3$ and nine phycocyanobilin moieties as a chromophore (closed circles). b. Chemical structure of phycocyanobilin. Phycocyanobilin was covalently bound to polypeptide chain of CPC by ways of thioetherlinkage to cysteine residues, one on the α-chain and two on the β-chain (Li et al., 2006).

Figure 3. Structure of CPC $(\alpha\beta)_3$-trimer and phycocyanobilin

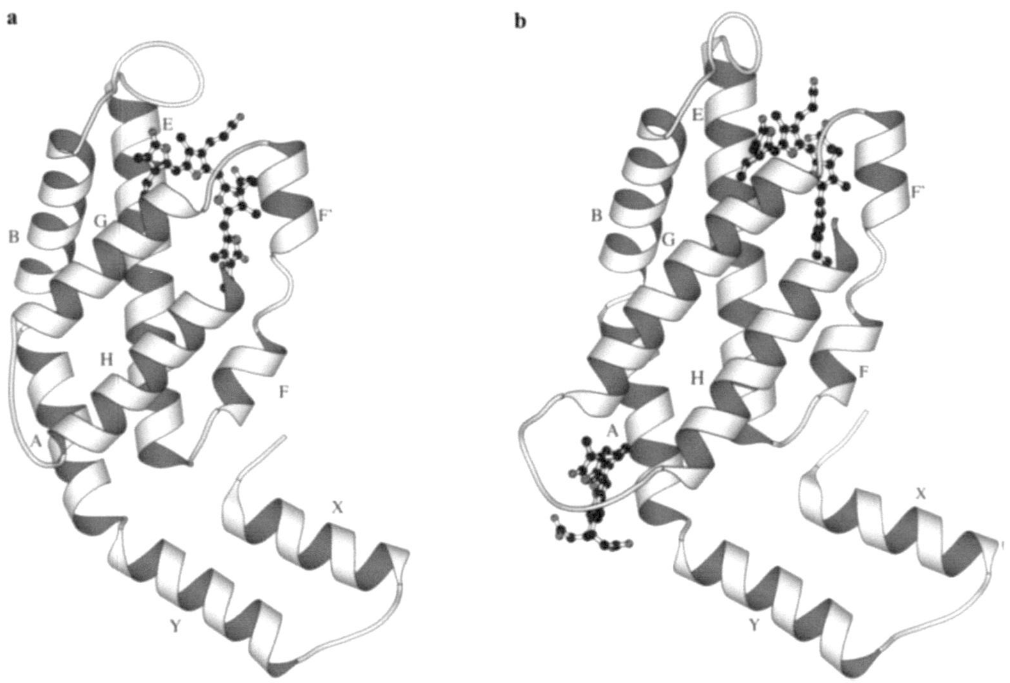

Figure 4. Ribbon representation of (a) CPC α-subunit (b) CPC β-subunit. Chromophores are shown in ball and stick representation (Padyana et al., 2001).

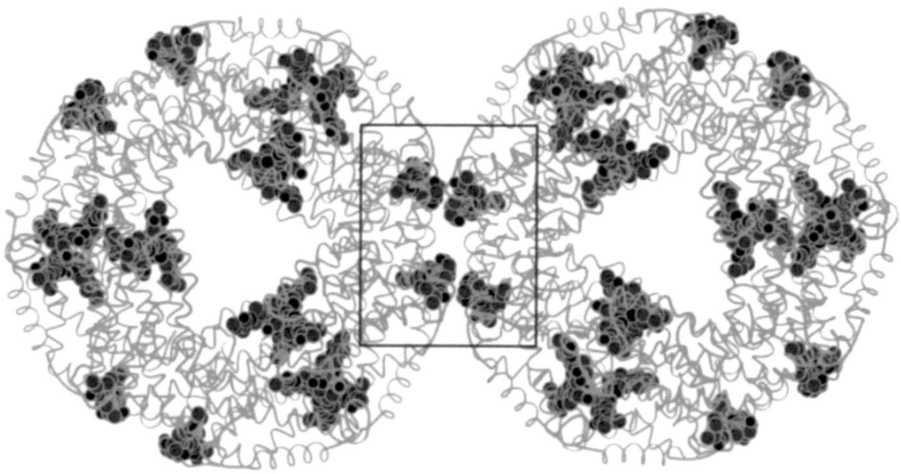

The figure illustrates the arrangement of chromophores at various locations within the hexamers. The box drawn at the center highlights the close proximity of phycocyanobilins at the position 155 on each β-subunit in the region between the adjacent hexamers (Padyana et al., 2001).

Figure 5. Coil representation of the two hexamers in the crystal asymmetric unit, a view through the approximate central axis of hexamers.

4. Enhancement of proliferation and differentiation of bone marrow cells stimulated with *Spirulina* and its extracts

Immunomodulation properties of *Spirulina* have been widely studied in chickens, prawns and fish, other animals, and humans. Generally, *Spirulina* and its extracts, such as hot-water extracts and phycocyanin, tended to enhance immune functions including mucosal or innate immunity through macrophage and secretions of the related cytokines (Belay, 2002; Hirahashi et al., 2002; Nemoto-Kawamura et al., 2004). Mao et al. (Mao et al., 2000) demonstrated that *Spirulina* stimulated the secretion of IL-1ß and IFN-γ in human peripheral blood mononuclear cells (PBMC) examined to nearly 2.0 and 3.3 times basal levels, respectively, and suggested that *Spirulina* helped balance the production of Th1 and Th2 cytokine stimulation. Phycocyanin, a characteristic photosynthesis pigment protein and an antioxidant in *Spirulina*, has been known to promote the growth of a human myeloid cell line, RPMI 8226 (Shinohara et al., 1988). Liu et al. (2000) reported that phycocyanin inhibited growth of human leukemia K562 cells and enhanced the arrest of the cell growth at G1 phase, suggesting enhancement of differentiation of the cells.

We have reported that *Spirulina* and its extracts enhanced immune responses in mice, mainly through increased production of interleukin-1 (IL-1) in macrophages (Hayashi et al., 1994; Hayashi et al., 1998). In the mice which ingested phycocyanin for 6 weeks, a marked increase of OVA antigen-specific IgA, as well as total IgA level was observed in the Peyer's patches, mesenteric lymph nodes and intestinal mucosa, as well as in the spleen cells

(Nemoto-Kawamura et al., 2004). These findings suggest that *Spirulina* or its components such as phycocyanin, affects immune functions by promoting immune competent-cell proliferation or differentiation in lymphoid organs.

We first investigated the effects of *Spirulina* and its extracts on proliferation of hematopoietic cells of mice and induction of colony-forming activity.

Colony-formation of bone marrow cells in *in-vitro* study

Spirulina extracts such as a hot-water extract (SpHW), phycocyanin (Phyc), and cell-wall fraction (SpCW) recovered from *Spirulina* treated with 0.1 % sodium dodecyl sulfate to remove cytoplasmic material were used in this study. Culture supernatants of spleen (SP), Peyer's patch (PP), and peritoneal-exudated (PE) cells cultured with 20 μg/mL of the *Spirulina* extracts significantly enhanced proliferation of bone marrow cells (Figure 3). Each of the *Spirulina* extracts, SpHW, Phyc, and SpCW, itself, also directly enhanced proliferation of bone marrow cells in the concentration of 100 μg/mL of culture medium. In addition to that, colony- and cluster-formations of the bone marrow cells supplemented with culture supernatants of the spleen cells stimulated with *Spirulina* extracts, 50–400 μg/mL, were measured by soft agar method. The supernatants of cells cultured with Phyc and SpCW significantly increased the colony- and cluster-formations of the bone marrow cells in comparison to that of control or of the smallest concentration of each extract (Figure 4a). Culture supernatants of PE cells, which consisted of macrophages and lymphocytes in a ratio of about 50 % each and a small ratio of mast cells and neutrophils, also enhanced colony- and cluster-formations (Figure 4b). The numbers of these colonies, however, were almost the same as that by each other culture supernatant. Furthermore, Both granulocyte macrophage-colony stimulating factor (GM-CSF) and interleukin 3 (IL-3) contents in the culture supernatant or the serum as colony-forming activities were measured by commercially supplied ELISA assay kits. High amounts of GM-CSF or IL-3 were detected in the culture supernatants of the spleen and peritoneal-exudates cells stimulated with the *Spirulina* extracts, especially those with SpCW (Table 1). The amounts of IL-3 in the culture supernatants of the cells stimulated with SpHW and Phyc were relatively high, although colony formation by the supernatant was not so high. Culture supernatant of the cells stimulated with SpCW contained high amounts of GM-CSF but not of IL-3.

stimulated with	Colonies/well		GM-CSF pg/mL of CS		IL-3 pg/mL of CS	
	SP	PE	SP	PE	SP	PE
Control	0.5 ± 0.7	2.0 ± 2.3	<4	<4	47.3 ± 4.0	<3
SpHW	2.8 ± 2.6	33.0 ± 7.1	<4	7.1	76.7 ± 8.0	10.7
Phycocyanin	14.0 ± 5.9	37.3 ± 9.3	9.2 ± 0.7	4.3	94.7 ± 10.8	11.0
SpCW	28.2 ± 5.5	32.2 ±4.6	1,206 ± 333	104.7	481.7 ± 144.4	<3

Table 1. GM-CSF and IL-3 contents in the culture supernatants (SC) of the spleen (SP)and the peritoneal-exudates (PE) cells stimulated with *Spirulina* extracts (values are mean ± SD, N = 3)

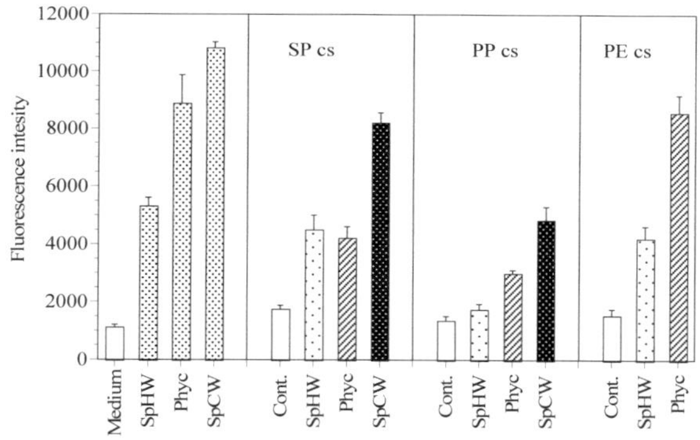

Figure 6. Bone marrow-cell proliferation by *Spirulina* extracts, SpHW, Phy, and SpCW, and by culture supernatant (CS) of lymphoid organ, spleen (SP) and Peyer's patch (PP), and peritoneal-exudates (PE) cells stimulated with the *Spirulina* extracts (Hayashi et al., 2006) (values are mean ± SD, n = 6)

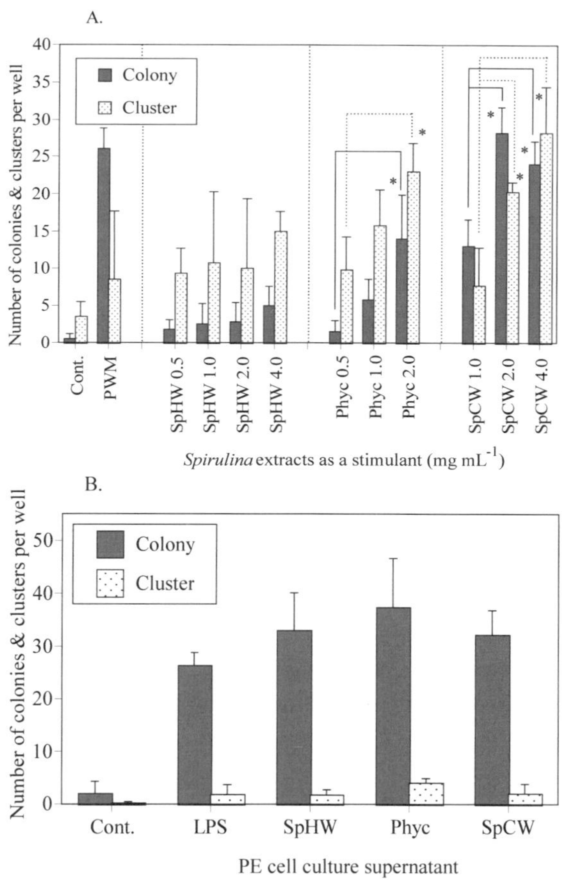

Figure 7. Bone marrow-cell colony and cluster formation in soft agar assay with the culture supernatant of the spleen cells (a) and peritoneal-exudates cells (b) stimulated with Spirulina extracts. Spleen cells were stimulated with 0.5, 1.0, 2.0 and 4.0 mg Spirulina extract/mL. Peritoneal-exudates cells were stimulated with 2.0 mg Spirulina extract /mL (Hayashi et al., 2006) (values are mean ± SD, n = 3).

Colony-formation activity in the mice fed *Spirulina* in *in-vivo* study

As a preliminary experiment for *in-vivo* study, we measured next colony forming activity in the mice fed with the *Spirulina* extracts, SpHW, Phyc and SpCW, for 5 consecutive days or in the mice treated with an intra-peritoneal single injection of the extracts.

The sera from the mice which ingested Phyc or SpCW (1 mg/0.2 mL) for 5 consecutive days with feeding catheter enhanced colony formation of bone marrow cells (Figure 5). The serum from Phyc-feeding group significantly increased it in comparison to controls in which normal serum was added. All of the sera obtained from the mice which were treated with intra-peritoneal single injection of the *Spirulina* extracts (10 mg/0.5 mL) also showed significantly high colony formation in comparison to control of normal serum, although levels of the activities of the sera were almost the same each other (data were not shown). Colony-stimulating factors, GM-CSF and IL-3, in the sera from the mice which were either fed or intra-peritoneally injected with the extracts, however, were under detection limit (<4 and 3 pg/mL serum, respectively). Concentration of GM-CSF in the LPS serum obtained by *i.p.* injection was 50.1 pg/mL.

For longer-period experiment in *in-vivo* study, colony- and cluster-formation in the bone marrow cells with culture supernatants of the spleen (SP), Peyer's patch (PP), and peritoneal-exudated (PE) cells from the mice, which ingested the *Spirulina* extracts, SpHW, Phyc, and SpCW, for 5 weeks were then measured to confirm the former results. Culture supernatants of each lymphoid-organ, SP, PP, and PE cells from the groups were prepared under stimulation with or without phycocyanin. Colony formation by the culture supernatant of SP cells from the mice of SpHW group, as well as by that of PE cells from Phyc or SpCW group, under stimulation with phycocyanin, was significantly higher than that by each culture supernatant of cells from control group, and thus colony-forming activity was also significantly induced in the blood, spleen, and Peyer's patch cells in the mice which ingested *Spirulina* extracts for 5 weeks although neither significant amount of GM-CSF nor IL-3 was detected in the blood (data not shown). On the other hand, ratios of neutrophils in the SpHW-ingesting group and of lymphocytes in the SpCW-ingesting group were significantly higher than in controls, while ratios of lymphocytes, neutrophils, and monocytes in the peripheral blood of control group were in the normal range. A significant increase in ratio of lymphocytes was also observed in bone marrow cells in Phyc-ingesting group, although the number of cells was small. In addition, increased ratio of reticulocytes was observed in the bone marrow of the mice fed with SpHW.

In the mice ingested 0.05% phycocyanin solution for 6 weeks, a marked increase in the antigen-specific IgA antibody level as well as the total IgA antibody level was observed in the intestinal mucosa, the Peyer's patches and mesenteric lymph nodes, which comprise a major part of the gut-associated lymphoid tissues (GALT), whereas neither IgG1 nor IgE was affected in the spleen cells (Nemoto-Kawamura et al., 2004). Phycocyanin ingestion for 8 weeks, on the other hand, suppressed the production of antigen-specific IgG1 and IgE antibody in the serum. Further, we investigated the effect of *Spirulina* on salivary IgA antibody level of the subjects who customarily ingested the *Spirulina* tablets as health food in various period of usage in their daily life, and measured correlation between the salivary IgA level and the amount of *Spirulina* ingested (Ishii et al., 1999). Total S-IgA level of the group ingesting *Spirulina* for more than one year was significantly increased ($p < 0.01$) in comparison to the group ingesting *Spirulina* for less than half a year, and statistically significant correlation between S-IgA levels in the saliva and total amount of *Spirulina* ingested by the subjects was observed (correlation coefficient $R = 0.288$, $n = 72$, $p < 0.05$).

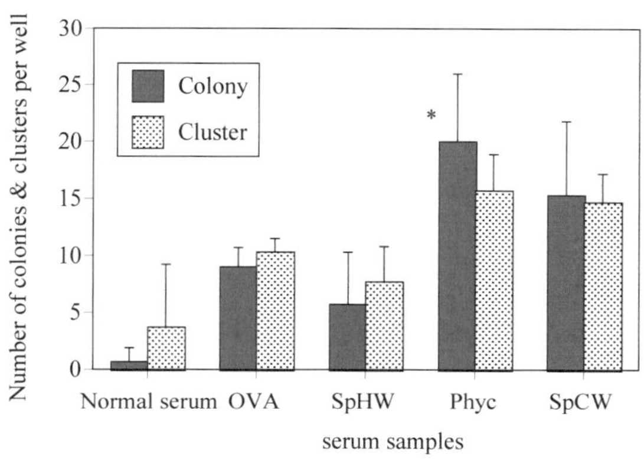

Figure 8. Bone marrow-cell colony and cluster formation in soft agar assay with the serum from the mice fed with *Spirulina* extracts for 5 consecutive days (Hayashi et al., 2006) (values are mean ± SD, n = 3). *; p<0.05 compared to Normal

It is known that multi-potent colony-stimulating factors such as G- and GM-CSF and IL-3, which are produced by a variety of cells including monocytes and lymphocytes can support proliferation of immature hematopoietic cells (Ihle, 1992). Liu et al. (2000) reported that phycocyanin from *Spirulina platensis* inhibited growth of human leukemia K562 cells in a dose-dependent manner, arresting them at the G1 phase with increased level of c-*myc* expression, suggesting that phycocyanin may enhance differentiation of the leukemia cells. Seya et al. (Hirahashi et al., 2002; Akao et al., 2009) reported that hot-water extract of *Spirulina* when taken orally in adult human enhances NK activation through the MyD88 pathway via Toll-like receptor (TLR) 2 and TLR4 on myeloid dendritic cells. From these findings, it appeared that *Spirulina*, including its components such as phycocyanin can affect enhancing proliferation or differentiation of immune competent-cells including bone marrow cell, which may cause normally sustaining or enhancing immune functions. Colony-stimulating activity other than IL-3 or GM-CSF, for example arginase and G-CSF, in the serum may contribute to the cell differentiation, although this is still not clear.

Zhang et al. (Zhang, 1994) found that C-phycocyanin and polysaccharide isolated from *Spirulina* increased leukocyte and bone marrow nucleated cell counts as well as colony formation of colony forming unit-granulocyte and macrophage (CFU-GM) in the gamma-ray irradiated mice, and also found that C-phycocyanin possessed high erythropoietin activity. Some institution facilities have reported the potential radiation protection effects of *Spirulina* against radiation-induced membrane damage and cellular dysfunction by reactive oxygen species in mice and against reduced levels of the leukocytes in the blood and nucleated cells in the bone marrow in dog (Zhang et al., 2001; Verma et al., 2006). Doctors in Belarus reported that ingestion of 5 g of *Spirulina* a day resulted in the reduction of Cesium-137 in urine by 50%, in children subjected to low level of radiation over a long period of time (Loseva and Dardynskaya, 1993). Rahadiya and Patel in India (Rabadiya and Patel, 2010) also reported radiation-effect-reducing activity of *Spirulina* in their review. Anti-oxidant and anti-inflammatory effects as well as proliferation and differentiation activity of *Spirulina* possibly contribute to the radiation protection effects.

5. Effect of phycocyanin on differentiation of human myeloid leukemia cell lines

A study of aerosolized GM-CSF demonstrated tolerance and possible efficacy in patients with malignant metastases to the lungs, possibly through upregulation of antigen-specific cytotoxic T-cells (Rao et al., 2003). It is known that various food compounds and the metabolites involving phycocyanin can influence the processes in cellular differentiation, apoptosis, and proliferative potential, and there is considerable evidence that vitamins and micronutrients are able to regulate gene expression of cancer cells, resulting in influence on the carcinogenic process (Sacha et al., 2005). All-trans-retinoic acid and vitamin D3 are known as one of the physiologic agents which can modulate the proliferation and differentiation of hematopoietic cells (Collins, 2002). The vitamin plus interferon-γ (IFNγ) treatment and enrichment with polyunsaturated fatty acids such as arachidonic acid, eicosapentaenoic acid or docosahexaenoic acid also significantly enhanced immunoregulatory effects, or enhanced the expression of monocytic surface antigens CD11b and CD14 on human premonocytic U937 cells (Obermeier et al., 1995). In this section, we investigated the effects of phycocyanin on differentiation and morphological and cytochemical changes of human myeloid leukemia cell lines, U937 and HL-60 cells, generally used for the studies of cell differentiation.

A human hematopoietic cell line, U-937, was derived from a patient with generalized histiocytic lymphoma. The histiocytic origin of the cell line was shown by its capacity of lysozyme production and the strong esterase activity (naphtol AS-D acetate esterase inhibited by NaF) of the cells (Sundstrom and Nillson, 1976). The cell line was morphologically identical to that of the tumor cells in the pleural effusion, and is known to be functionally differentiated to phagocytic macrophage by cytokines from lymphocytes (Koren et al, 1979).

A continuous human myeloid cell line, HL-60, was derived from the peripheral blood leukocytes of a patient with acute promyelocytic leukemia and established. The predominant cell type is a neutrophilic promyelocyte with prominent nuclear/cytoplasmic asynchrony (Gallangher et al., 1979). HL-60 cells lack specific markers for lymphoid cells, but express surface receptors for Fc fragment and complement (C3), which have been associated with differentiated granulocytes. They exhibit phagocytic activity and responsiveness to a chemotactic stimulus commensurate with the proportion of mature cells.

Preparation of Conditioned Medium (CM) of peripheral blood mononuclear cells cultured with phycocyanin

Human peripheral blood mononuclear cells (PBMCs) from 7 healthy volunteers were separated by density centrifugation (800 g, 30 mins) using a Lymphoprep™ (Density 1.077 g/mL, NYCOMED) under approving by the Institutional Review Board of our University. Cells from each subject were suspended in RPMI-FBS medium and adjusted to 1×10^6 cells/mL and were cultured with and without 2 mg/mL of phycocyanin (Phyc) using 24-well cultured plates. The conditioned mediums (CMs), both with and without Phyc (Phyco-CM and Cont-CM, respectively), were harvested on the 7th day and filtered through an 0.45 μmφ filter to remove cell debris.

Cell growth of U937 as well as HL-60 cells supplemented with Phyco-CM resulted in significant inhibition during the 7-day culture in comparison with those of control without supplementation, while supplementation with 2 mg/mL Phyc itself had no effect on growth in these cells. Both U937 and HL-60 cells stimulated with Phyc and Phyco-CM were more than 80% viable, as were those cells stimulated with phorbol-12-myristate-13-acetate (PMA) 0.02 μg/mL as a positive control of differentiation.

Morphology and flow cytometric assay of cell surface antigens on U937 and HL-60 Cells

U937 cells cultured in the medium supplemented with Phyco-CM morphologically changed into the cells with large cytoplasm with vacuoles, non-condensed nuclear chromatin, and a persistence of nucleolus that resembled to those stimulated with PMA as a positive control (Figure 6a) while control U937 cells, without stimulation, were promonocyte-like with variable nuclear shapes and regular indentations and comprised moderate cytoplasm containing numerous small eosinophilic granules and a few vacuoles. Cont-CM or conditioned medium of lymphocytes cultured without phycocyanin, only partially changed U937 cells into monocytic cells comprising moderate cytoplasm with large indented nucleus (Figure 6a). U937 cells stimulated with Phyco-CM and Cont-CM consisted of monocytes/macrophages in the ratio of 57% and 21%, respectively, and each ratio was significantly higher than that of control (1.4%) without stimulation. Stimulation by Phyc changed U937 cells partially to promonocytes with indents on the nuclei. The ratio of monocytes/macrophages was only 3.4 %.

Control HL-60 cells, without stimulation, was predominantly promyelocytes with azurophilic granules, large round nuclei, and prominent nucleoli. Morphological classification of the cells, especially those stimulated with Phyco-CM, was relatively difficult because various features of promyelocytes coexisted. The Phyco-CM-stimulated HL-60 cells showed a morphologically matured monocytic cell lineage (about 15.4%), that is, with decreased nuclear/cytoplasmic ratio and a paler cytoplasm with vacuoles (Figure 6b). The cells (about 80%) other than monocytic cells consisted of granulocytes, including promyelocytes and myelocytes, with large nuclei, less prominent cytoplasmic granules and a marked decrease or complete disappearance of nucleoli. Almost of all HL-60 cells stimulated with Phyc and Cont-CM were promyelocyte-like, while all-*trans* retinoic acid (ATRA) induced cells to differentiate into granulocytes (Figure 6b).

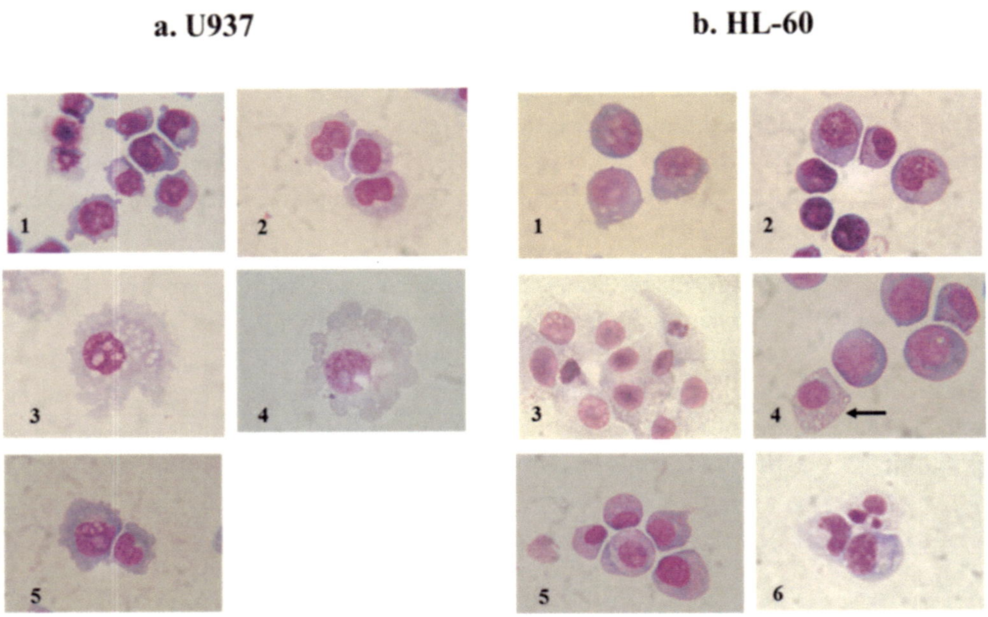

Cell morphology was measured under light microscopy. U937 cells (a) and HL-60 cells (b), 0.5 x 10^6 cells/mL of medium, were cultured for 3 days with RPMI-FBS (Cont.)
(1); with Phyc (2); with PMA (3); with Phyco-CM (4); with Cont-CM (5); with ATRA (6) (Ishii et al., 2009).
(Original magnification x 1000)

Figure 9. Morphology of U937 and HL-60 cells stimulated with Phyco-CM and others.

Flow cytometric assay was carried out using a Flow Cytometer (FCM; EPICS® ALTRA™, Beckman Coulter, Inc., Fullerton, CA). The expression of cell surface antigens, CD14, CD11b, CD66b and CD15, on U937 and HL-60 cells stimulated with various CMs, as described above, were determined by direct immunofluorescence method using appropriate fluorescent labeled monoclonal antibodies. Typical patterns of FCM analysis for CD14 antigen in both U937 and HL-60 cells stimulated with Phyco-CM were shown in Figure 7.

Ratio of CD14-antigen positive cells in U937 cells stimulated with Phyco-CM, 53%, was significantly high in comparison with those of Cont-CM and Cont without stimulation, 30% and 15%, respectively, while ratio of CD14-positive cells in HL-60 cells was originally low but was significantly increased by Phyc and Phyco-CM stimulations, about 20% (Figure 8a). Ratio of FcγR positive cells in U937 cells was originally high and those of the cells stimulated with Phyco-CM and Cont-CM were almost the same as Cont without stimulation, 65%. In HL-60, on the other hand, Phyco-CM increased FcγR positive cells significantly, 41%, compared with Cont and Cont-CM, 24% and 20%, respectively (Figure 8b). Further, a final concentration of 0.01 mg/mL of Phyc significantly increased the population of CD11b-antigen positive cells in U937 cells compared with Cont and Cont-CM (Figure 9a). Although the fluorescence intensity of anti-CD14 antibody per cell in U937 cells stimulated with Phyc was marginally higher than that of Cont (Figure 7a), the ratio of CD14-antigen positive cells was low (Figure 8a) and morphologically comprised 3.4% of monocytes/macrophages. This suggests that phycocyanin stimulates U937 cells to some extent to differentiate or express some CD antigens such as CD11b and CD14. CD11b as well as CD66b is specific in monocytes and granulocytes. Expression of CD11b is known to be up-regulated during granulocytic and monocytic differentiation, and is used as a marker of differentiation of myelomonocytic lineage (Lubbert et al., 1991). It has been also recognized that morphological changes of differentiating U937 cells are accompanied by cellular adherence and are paralleled by an expression of the β_2 integrins, CD11a, CD11c, CD18, and particularly CD11b (Hass et al., 1989). CD11b glycoprotein represents the α-subunit of a heterodimeric association with the common β-subunit CD18 in β_2 integrin, an adhesion molecule. Their extracellular domains with the CD11b/CD18 (CR3/Mac-1) β_2 integrin contribute to adhesion to adjacent cells, for example, the regulation of leukocyte-endothelial cell interactions (Ebnet et al., 2004). In the study using stably-transfected U937 cells with a vector containing the β_2 integrin gene in antisense orientation, Otte et al. (2011) suggested that induced adherence predominantly mediated by a functional CD11b/CD18 integrin contributed to cell cycle regulation and apoptosis during monocytic maturation. Concerning apoptotic cell death, photodynamic therapy (PDT) for tumors which is based on the tumor-selective accumulation of protoporphyrin IX (PpIX), as a photosensitizer after addition of 5-aminolevulinic acid (ALA) followed by irradiation with visible light has been demonstrated by some investigators, and it was reported that ALA-based photodynamic action (PDA) induced apoptotic cell death in U937 cells through a mitochondrial pathway and that ferrochelatase inhibitors might enhanced the effect of PDT for tumors (Amo et al., 2009). Furthermore pulsating electromagnetic field (PEMF) can affect cancer cells proliferation and death (Kaszuba-Zwoinska et al., 2010). They reported that U937 cells exposed to a pulsating magnetic field 50Hz, 45±5 mT three times for each 3 h with 24 h intervals induced cells death in higher cell density and conversely prevented puromycin-induced cell death. We could take advantage of the halfway differentiated U937 cells induced by phycocyanin as a cell culture model of cell differentiation and apoptotic cell death to investigate the molecular mechanism of these various tumoricidal treatments.

Both Phyc and Phyco-CM significantly increased the ratio of CD11b-antigen positive cells in U937 cells, about 30%, in comparison with those of Cont and Cont-CM, 12% and 22%, respectively, while in HL-60 neither CD11b nor CD66b cells showed significant increases in ratio when stimulated with Phyco-CM (16%, 22%) or Cont-CM (10%, 18%) cells. In contrast, the ratio of CD15-antigen positive cells in the U937 cells was low regardless of stimulation (Figure 9a). CD15-antigen is generally characteristic of granulocytes and monocytes. The ratio of CD15-antigen positive cells in the HL-60 cells showed insignificant changes when stimulated with Phyc, Phyco-CM and other CMs (Figure 9b).

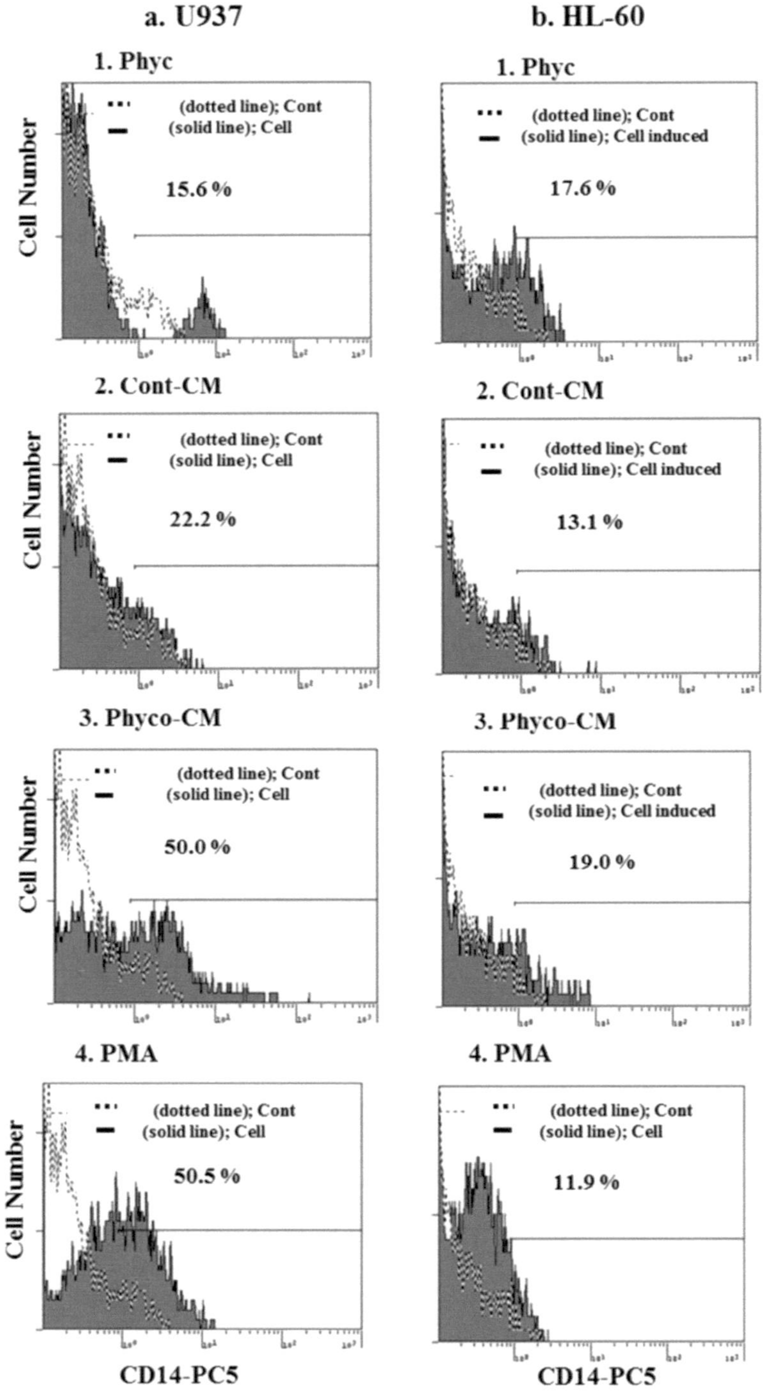

Patterns of U937 and HL-60 cells (0.5 x 10^6 cells/mL of medium) stimulated with Phyc (1), Cont-CM (2), Phyco-CM (3) and PMA (4) were shown in solid lines and that of Cont was shown in dotted lines (Ishii et al., 2009).

Figure 10. Typical patterns of CD14-positive cells in U937 and HL-60 cells.

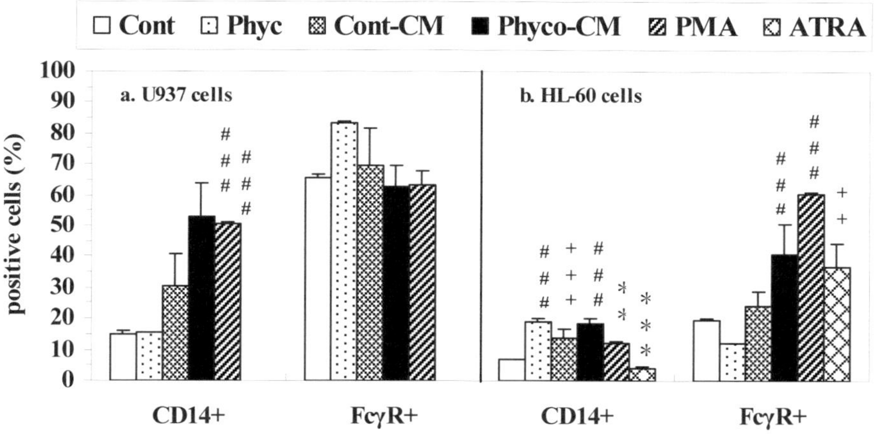

Data analysis was based on examination of 5000 cells/sample.
++; p < 0.01, +++; p < 0.001 to each Cont, **; p < 0.01, ***; p < 0.001 to each Cont-CM, ###; p < 0.001 to each Cont and Cont-CM. Each value shows mean ± SD, n=3~7 (Ishii et al., 2009)

Figure 11. Percentage of CD14 and FcγR positive cells in U937 and HL-60 cells stimulated with Phyco-CM and other stimulants.

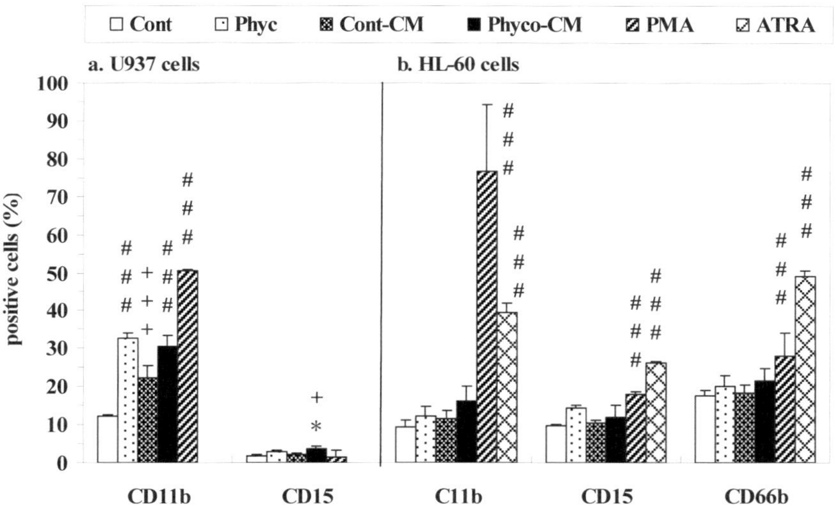

Data analysis was based on examination of 5000 cells/sample. Each value shows mean ± SD, n= 3 (Ishii et al., 2009)

Figure 12. Percentage of CD11b-, CD15- and CD66b-antigen positive cells in U937 and HL-60 cells stimulated with Phyco-CM and other stimulants.

Phagocytic activity and TNF-α production, cytochemical analysis

Differentiation of both HL-60 and U937 cells was also assessed by cytochemical analysis with specific and non-specific esterase (SE/NSE) double staining method and Nitro-blue tetrazolium (NBT) reducing activity which is characteristic of phagocytic cells (Table 2).

Although U937 cells were originally NSE positive, the Phyco-CM stimulated cells showed equally high ratio, while most HL-60 cells were SE positive under all stimulants. Phyco-CM stimulation significantly increased the ratio of NBT-positive cells in both U937 and HL-60 cells, while that of Cont-CM was almost the same as Cont. In addition to that, phagocytic activity in U937 cells stimulated with Phyco-CM was significantly higher than that of the cells stimulated with Cont-CM. In HL-60 cells, both Phyco-CM and Cont-CM increased phagocytic activity, as compared with Cont. Increased levels of TNF-α in both U937 and HL-60cells stimulated with Phyco-CM, were relatively high in comparison with Cont-CM but not significant, and were not synergistically increased by supplementation with LPS (1000 ng/mL) in the culture. Level of TNF-α in the cells stimulated with Phyc was under the detection limit.

Stimulators	Phagocytic activity (%)	TNF-α (pg/mL)	NBT reducing activity (%)
U937			
Cont	18 ± 5.2	ND	1.3 ± 0.3
Phyc	23 ± 5.1	< 15.6	5.0 ± 3.0
Cont-CM	32 ± 5.5 $^{++}$	46 ± 31	1.3 ± 0.8
Phyco-CM	81 ± 13 $^{+++, ***}$	66 ± 15	7.5 ± 4.1**
PMA	96 ± 4.6 $^{+++, ***}$	968 ± 150 ***	5.2 ± 2.9
HL-60			
Cont	17 ± 6.2	ND	0.7 ± 0.3
Phyc	16 ± 3.8	< 15.6	2.0 ± 1.0
Cont-CM	35 ± 12 $^{++}$	32 ± 29	2.1 ± 0.7
Phyco-CM	36 ± 13 $^{++}$	71 ± 18	5.3 ± 1.9$^{+++, **}$
PMA	84 ± 13 $^{+++}$	585 ± 39	1.7 ± 0.8
ATRA	72 ± 5.2 $^{+++}$	ND	10.8 ± 3.3 $^{+++, ***}$

Phagocytic activity was determined by ingestion of opsonin-treated latex beads. NBT reducing activity was measured as percentage of the positive cells, which contained intracellular blue-black formazan deposits. Positive cells out of 200 cells were counted under light microscopy. ++; $p < 0.01$, +++; $p < 0.001$ compared to Cont, **; $p < 0.01$, ***; $p < 0.001$ compared to Cont-CM, < ; under detection limit (15.6 pg/mL), ND; not detected (values are mean ± SD, n=3)

Table 2. Cytochemical analysis of U937 and HL-60 cells stimulated with Phyco-CM

Phyco-CM and Phyc quite significantly increased the population of CD14-antigen positive cells in HL-60 cells, although the level was lower than that in U937 cells (Figure 8). In addition to that, Phyco-CM increased also the NBT reducing activity of HL-60 cells. Tamagawa et al. (1998) reported that NBT reducing activity was used as a marker of HL-60 cell differentiation into granulocytes and monocytes. Fontana et al. (1981) suggested that HL-60 cells were able to commit themselves to the development of two different program of hematopoietic differentiation, that is, either myeloid or macrophage depending on cytokine or stimulant. In fact, both monocytic and granulocytic cells coexisted in HL-60 cells stimulated with Phyc and Phyco-CM as the result of differentiation in two types of directions. However, NSE and SE ratios in HL-60 cells did not necessarily correspond to morphological observation. Normally NSE has been thought to be specific for monocyte/macrophage activity (Tanaka et al., 1983), and Chiao et al. (1981) reported that conditioned medium of normal human peripheral blood lymphocytes induced HL-60 cells into macrophage and monocyte-like cell lines, but most HL-60 cells stimulated with Phyco-CM in the present study were SE positive, and only about 15% of monocytic matured cells were found in the cells after Phyco-CM stimulation. It appeared that the effects of Phyco-CM on HL-60 cells may insufficiently induce to matured cells.

CD14 antigen has been reported to be a receptor for the complex of LPS and LPS-binding protein (LBP). It is known that LPS and Gram negative bacteria as triggers (Beutler, 2000; Lu et al., 2008) can cause TNF-α release in human monocytes through TLR4 (Tudhope et al., 2008). The U937 cells stimulated with Phyco-CM, that showed high ratio of CD14-positive cells, are expected to express TLR4 in addition to CD4 because expression of TLR4 needs CD14 and LBP in response to the binding of LPS with LBP. Phyco-CM induced TNF-α production in the culture supernatants of U937 and HL-60 cells. A high molecular weight polysaccharide, Immulina, from *Spirulina* was a potent activator of nuclear factor-kappaB (NF-κB) and induced both IL-1β and TNF-α mRNAs in THP-1 human monocytes (Pugh et al., 2001), and expression of TLR2 and CD14 probably contributed to the NF-κB activation and immune enhancing activity of the Immulina in mice (Balachandran et al., 2006). The levels of TNF-α, however, were not further increased with LPS stimulation (1000 ng/mL) in the U937 cells stimulated with phyco-CM. Phagocytic activity in the stimulated U937 cells was significantly higher than that of the cells stimulated with Cont-CM, and there was no stimulatory effect in the existence of LPS. Phyc alone did not induce TNF-α in U937 and HL-60 cells.

6. Age-related changes in intestine intraepitherial lymphocyte subsets and their functional preservation by *Spirulina* in mice

Age-related immune dysfunction has been reviewed by many researchers (Solana et al., 2006). The complex age-related changes in the immune system, collectively termed "immunosenescence," have been demonstrated in diverse species, including humans, and have been recognized as contributing to morbidity and mortality due to greater incidence of infectious diseases, autoimmune diseases, and cancer. The concept of age-related immunosenescence is in agreement with numerous data such as the change of cytokine balances, the decrease of interleukin (IL)-2 contrary to the increase of IL-6, and nutritional imbalance or malnutrition (Miquel, 2001; De la Fuente, 2002). It was reported that antigen-specific secretory immunoglobulin A titer in the intestinal lumen declined in senescent animals (Koga et al., 2000). Some studies have also reported that reduced bioavailability of key conditionally essential nutrients might limit immune response in aging (Cunningham-Rundles, 2004) and that well-nourished elderly people appear to have less significant or minimal changes in immune response (Krause et al., 1999).

It is generally accepted that the development of age-associated alterations occurs earlier in the mucosal immune system than in the systemic immune compartment (Schmucker et al., 2003). The mucosal immune system of the intestinal epithelia contains a functionally specialized T-cell population known as intraepithelial lymphocytes (IELs). Because of their unique location in the mucosal epithelium, IELs are recognized as a first-line mucosal barrier against infectious diseases and food-borne allergens (Hayday et al., 2001).

We have reported that ingestion of phycocyanin enhanced the antigen-specific immunoglobulin A response in the intestinal mucosa of mice (Nemoto-Kawamura et al., 2004). In this section, we investigated age-related changes in intestine IEL subsets in mice by flow cytometric (FCM) analysis and their functional preservation after the animals were fed *Spirulina*.

Characterization of IELs of adult and aged mice

IELs possess phenotypic features distinct from those of lamina propria lymphocytes in intestine. Lamina propria lymphocytes consist of predominantly activated T cells and are mainly $CD4^+$ and $CD8^+$ single-positive T cells in proportions of about 70% and 30%, respectively. The phenotype of lamina propria lymphocytes, in general, is similar to that of the cells in the peripheral lymphoid tissues and in the circulating blood, that is, over 95% of the cells possess a surface phenotype of T-cell receptor $\alpha\beta^+$ ($TCR\alpha\beta^+$), whereas less than 5% possess $TCR\gamma\delta^+$. These cells are known to be matured in the thymus (Lydyard and Grossi, 1998). IELs, on the other hand, possess $TCR\gamma\delta^+$ in a greater percentage (30–60%) and $TCR\alpha\beta^+$ in a percentage of 40–70%, which might be related to their state of activation (Ewijk et al., 1999). In adult mice bred in a conventional environment, about half of the IELs have a phenotype of surface CD antigen similar to that of most peripheral T lymphocytes, that is, Thy-1^+, $TCR\alpha\beta^+$, and either $CD4^+$ or $CD8^+$, which are made up of heterodimers of $CD8\alpha$ and β chains ($CD8\alpha\beta^+$). These cells were matured in a thymus-dependent manner (Kaminogawa and Nanno, 2004). Another major IEL population possesses the surface phenotype $TCR\alpha\beta^+$ or $TCR\gamma\delta^+$, which expresses CD8 homodimeric α chains ($CD8\alpha\alpha^+$) but does not express CD4 or CD8 heterodimeric molecules (Rocha et al., 1994). These cells are known to be of extrathymic origin. Small percentages of the $TCR\alpha\beta^+$ and $TCR\gamma\delta^+$ but no TCR cells are $CD8^-$ $CD4^-$. $TCR\alpha\beta^+$ IELs co-expressing both CD4 and CD8 molecules are rare but bear high levels of $TCR\alpha\beta$ and $CD8\alpha\alpha$ (Lefrancois, 1991). Our preliminary experiment showed that the number of $CD45^+$ (leukocyte-common antigen-positive) cells as IELs was significantly lower in aged mice than in adult mice. Either the proportion or the number of $CD8^+$ cells in addition to $CD45^+$ cells of aged mice was significantly lower than that of adult mice, corresponding to the previous article by Komuro et al (1990). The proportion and number of $CD4^+CD8^+$ double-positive cells in the aged mice, on the other hand, were higher than those in adult mice. It has been reported that $CD4^+CD8^+$ T cells bearing $TCR\alpha\beta$ in the epithelium, which were derived from thymus-dependent populations, expanded with aging at a local site of the intestine under the influence of intestinal microflora, contributing to the first line of defensive barrier in the epithelium (Takimoto et al., 1992).

Overall, increased or decreased levels of these surface antigen-positive cells observed in the aged mice tended to be restored by the ingestion of SpHW for 5 weeks in the aged-SP group. In fact, significant decreases of $CD45^+CD8^+$ cells and increases of $CD8^-CD4^-$ and

$CD45^+TCR\alpha\beta^+$ cells were observed in the aged mice, whereas neither an increase nor a decrease was observed in the aged-SP group fed with SpHW—that is, the levels were similar to those in adult mice. In particular, the proportions of $CD45^+CD8^+$ cells and $CD45^+TCR\gamma\delta^+$ cells in the aged-SP group significantly increased in comparison to the aged group. $CD8^+$ T cells expressing $\alpha\beta$TCR ($\alpha\beta$T cells) are engaged in antigen-specific cell cytotoxicity mediated by major histocompatibility complex (MHC) molecules, whereas T cells expressing $\gamma\delta$TCR ($\gamma\delta$T cells) often manifest preliminary target cell killing without MHC restriction (Cruse and Lewis, 1995). $\gamma\delta$T cells have also been shown to be associated with regulation of the generation and differentiation of IELs (Komano et al., 1995). These results suggest that ingestion of SpHW in the aged-SP group may contribute to the functional preservation of the intestinal epithelium as a first line of mucosal barrier against infectious agents through retaining the numbers of certain IELs.

Decreased levels of RBCs, especially the level of hematocrit, Ht, in the aged group, were also restored after ingestion of SpHW in the aged-SP group. Significant decreases in WBCs in the aged-SP group, in contrast to the increase in the aged group, may be ascribed to the anti-inflammatory activity of *Spirulina* (Vila et al., 2008) and/or to the restoration of immunological function by ingesting *Spirulina*. Some reports indicated that phycocyanin and the polysaccharide isolated from *Spirulina* increased bone marrow nucleated cell and erythrocyte counts in the gamma-ray irradiated mice or dog (Zhang, 1994; Zhang et al., 2001; Verma et al., 2006). Many studies have demonstrated that *Spirulina* including phycocyanin possesses antioxidant activity, as well as an anti-inflammatory activity (Romay et al., 1998; Remirez et al., 2002), which scavenges peroxyl radicals, and also acts as an inhibitor of cyclooxygenase, like nonsteroidal anti-inflammatory drugs. In addition, a down-regulation of pro-inflammatory cytokines, such as TNF-α and -γ, was observed in the aged animals on the *Spirulina*-enriched diet (Vila et al., 2008). Overexpression of MHC class I-related chain A in the intestine of experimental transgenic mice resulted in a clonal expansion of $CD4^+CD8\alpha\alpha^+$ IELs and attenuated acute colitis in an experimental model of inflammatory bowel disease induced by dextran sodium sulfate administration (Park et al., 2003). $CD8\alpha\alpha^+$ IELs developed along an extrathymic pathway may work as anti-inflammatory regulator T cells to sustain the mucosal intranet formed by intestinal epithelial cells and IELs and to diminish the expansion of enterotoxigenic *Escherichia coli* (Kim et al., 2001). Although ingesting SpHW did not significantly increase the level of $CD4^+CD8^+$ IELs in the present study, these facts, in addition to our present results, suggest that ingestion of *Spirulina* appears to be effective for protecting immune functions or improving immune systems vulnerable to age, thereby reducing the risk of infectious and autoimmune diseases. However, additional detailed study is needed.

7. Conclusions

Spirulina and its extracts enhanced proliferation of hematopoietic cells and colony formation of bone marrow cell, as a marker for cell differentiation activity, in *in-vitro* and *in-vivo* study using mice. Phycocyanin, a light-harvesting pigment of *Spirulina*, also induced cell differentiation of human leukemia cell lines, U937 and HL-60 cells, into monocyte/macrophage and granulocyte, respectively, to some extent directly and indirectly through enhancing cytokine production in human peripheral blood lymphocytes stimulated with phycocyanin. These distinguished activities of *Spirulina* as well as other certain functional foods can be preferably emphasized to be used, especially for elderly people. Recent intervention study showed that 6- and 12-week supplementation of *Spirulina* increased mean hemoglobin level and indoleamine 2,3-dioxygenase activity, as a sign of immune function, in the elderly subjects, suggesting that *Spirulina* may ameliorate anemia and immunosenescence in elderly people (Selmi et al., 2011). Pentón-Rol et al. (2011) demonstrated that phycocyanin triggered preventing or downgrading experimental autoimmune encephalitis (EAE) expression in rats, and that ingestion of phycocyanin induced a regulatory T cell (Treg) response in peripheral blood mononuclear cells from the patients with multiple sclerosis (MS). The authors suggested that phycocyanin may act as a neuroprotector and thereby may restore the functional damage in neurodegenerative disorders of the central nervous system (CNS). Another animal model in rats showed that *Spirulina* promoted stem cell genesis and protected against LPS-induced declines in neural stem cell proliferation, and that cytokines did appear capable of regulating several phases of the neurogenesis process, supporting their hypothesis that a diet enriched with *Spirulina* may help protect the stem/progenitor cells from insults (Bachstetter et al., 2010). These studies including reports summarized in this chapter show that *Spirulina* is useful in providing complementary nutrients for modulating or maintaining the immune system and that is also may have potential therapeutic benefits for improvement of immune dysfunctions caused by, for example, radiation, chemotherapy using anti-cancer and anti-infectious drugs, and certain microorganisms such as human immunodeficiency virus (HIV) itself, other than ageing. Further research along these lines is needed to validate these evidences.

Author details

Osamu Hayashi
Kagawa Nutrition University, Japan

8. References

Akao, Y, Ebihara, T, Masuda, H, Saeki, Y, Akazawa, T, Hazeki, K, Hazeki, O, Matsumoto, M, and Seya, T (2009). "Enhancement of antitumor natural killer cell activation by orally administered *Spirulina* extract in mice", *Cancer Sci*, 100, 1494-1501.

Amo, T, Kawanishi, N, Uchida, M, Fujita, H, Oyanagi, E, Utsumi, T, Ogino, T, Inoue, K, Shuin, T, Utsumi, K, and Sasaki, J (2009). "Mechanism of cell death by 5-aminolevulinic acid-based photodynamic action and its enhancement by ferrochelatase inhibitors in human histiocytic lymphoma cell line U937", *Cell Biochem Funct*, 27, 503-515.

Bachstetter, AD, Jernberg, J, Schlunk, A, Vila, JL, Hudson, C, Cole, MJ, Shytle, RD, Tan, J, Sanberg, PR, Sanberg, CD, Borlongan, C, Kaneko, Y, Tajiri, N, Gemma, C, and Bickford, PC (2010). "Spirulina promotes stem cell genesis and protects against LPS induced declines in neural stem cell proliferation", *PLoS One*, 5, e10496.

Balachandran, P, Pugh, ND, Ma, G, and Pasco, DS (2006). "Toll-like receptor 2-dependent activation of monocytes by Spirulina polysaccharide and its immune enhancing action in mice", *Int Immunopharmacol*, 6, 1808-1814.

Belay, A (2002). "The potential application of *Spirulina* (*Arthorspira*) as a nutritional and therapeutic supplement in health management", *J Am Nutraceutical Association*, 5, 27- 48.

Belay, A, Ota, Y, Miyakawa, K, and Shimamatsu, H (1993). "Current knowledge on potential health benefits of *Spirulina*", *J Appl Phycol*, 5, 235-241.

Beutler, B (2000). "TLR4: central component of the sole mammalian LPS sensor", *Current Opinion in Immunology*, 12, 20-26.

Chamorro-Cevallos, G (1980). "Toxicological research on the alga *Spirulina*", *Report: United Nations International Development Organization (UNIDO)* UF/MEX/78/048, Vienna.

Chiao, JW, Freitag, WF, Steinmetz, JC, and Andreeff, M (1981). "Changes of cellular markers during differentiation of HL-60 promyelocytes to macrophages as induced by T lymphocyte conditioned medium", *Leukemia Research*, 5, 477-489.

Ciferri, O (1983). "*Spirulina*, the edible microorganisms", *Microbiol Res*, 47, 551-578.

Collins, S (2002). "The role of retinoids and retinoic acid receptors in normal hematopoiesis", *Leukemia*, 16, 1896-1905.

Cruse, JM, and Lewis, RE (1995). Illustrated Dictionary of Immunology. Florida: CRC Press, Inc.

Cunningham-Rundles, S (2004). "The effect of aging on mucosal host defense", *J Nutr Health Aging*, 8, 20-25.

De la Fuente, M (2002). "Effects of antioxidants on immune system ageing", *European Journal of Clinical Nutrition*, 56, 55-58.

Ebnet, K, Suzuki, A, Ohno, S, and Vestweber, D (2004). "Junctional adhesion molecules (JAMs): more molecules with dual functions?", *J Cell Sci*, 117, 19-29.

Ewijk, Wv, Hayday, A, Merkenschlager, M, Robey, E, Bevan, MJ, and Zamoyska, R (1999). "7. The thymus and the developement of T lymphocytes", CA Janeway, P Travers, M Walport, & JD Capra (Ed.), In Immunobiology - The immune system in health and disease 4th edition (pp 227-260). New York: Grand Publishing.

Fontana, JA, Colbert, DA, and Deisseroth, AB (1981). "Identification of a population of bipotent stem cells in the HL60 human promyelocytic leukemia cell line", *Proc Natl Acad Sci USA*, 78, 3863-3866.

Geitler, L (1932). "Rabenhorst's Kryptogamenflora von Deutschland, Ostereiich nd de Scheweiz". Leipzig: Akad Verlag, pp.

Gershwin, ME, and Belay, A (2008). "*Spirulina* in Human and Health". Boca Raton, FL: CRC Press Taylor & Francis Group, 312 pp.

Grzanna, R, Polotsky, A, Phan, PV, Pugh, N, Pasco, D, and Frondoza, CG (2006). "Immolina, a high-molecular-weight polysaccharide fraction of *Spirulina*, enhances chemokine expression in human monocytic THP-1 cells", *J Altern Complement Med*, 12, 429-435.

Hass, R, Bartels, H, Topley, N, Hadam, M, Köhler, L, Goppelt-Strübe, M, and Resch, K (1989). "TPA-induced differentiation and adhesion of U937 cells: changes in ultrastructure, cytoskeletal organization and expression of cell surface antigens", *Eur J Cell Biol*, 48, 282-293.

Hayashi, O, Hirahashi, T, Katoh, T, Miyajjima, H, Hirano, T, and Okuwaki, Y (1998). "Class specific influence of dietary *Spirulina platensis* on antibody production in mice", *J Nutr Sci Vitaminol*, 44, 841-851.

Hayashi, O, Ishii, K, and Kato, Y (2008). "*Spirulina* and Antibody Production", M Gershwin, & A Belay (Ed.), In *Spirulina* in Human Nutrition and Health (pp 205-226). Boca Raton, FL: CRC Press Taylor & Francis Group.

Hayashi, O, Katoh, T, and Okuwaki, Y (1994). "Enhancement of antibody production in mice by dietary *Spirulina* platensis", *J. Nutr. Sci. Vitaminol.*, 40, 431-441.

Hayashi, O, Ono, S, Ishii, K, Shi, Y, Hirahashi, T, and Katoh, T (2006). "Enhancement of proliferation and differentiation in bone marrow hematopoietic cells by *Spirulina* (*Arthrospira*) *platensis* in mice", *Journal of Applied Phycology*, 18, 47-56.

Hayashi, T, Hayashi, K, Maeda, M, and Kojima, I (1996). "Calcium spirulan, an inhibitor of enveloped virus replication, from a blue-green alga Spirulina platensis", *J Nat Prod*, 59, 83-87.

Hayday, A, Theodoridis, E, Ramsburg, E, and Shires, J (2001). "Intraepithelial lymphocytes: exploring the Third Way in immunology", *Nat. Immun.*, 2, 997.

Hirahashi, T, Matsumoto, M, Hazeki, K, Saeki, Y, Ui, M, and Seya, T (2002). "Activation of the human innate immune system by *Spirulina*: augmentaion of interferon production and NK cytotoxicity by oral administration of hot water extract of *Spirulina platensis.*", *International Immunopharmacology*, 2, 423 - 734.

Ihle, JN (1992). "Interleukin-3 and hematopoiesis", *Chem. Immunol.*, 51, 65 - 106.

Ishii, K, Katoh, T, Okuwaki, Y, and Hayashi, O (1999). "Influence of dietary Spirulina platensis on IgA level in human saliva", *Joshi Eiyo Daigaku Kiyou*, 30, 27-33 (in Japanese).

Ishii, K, Shi, Y, Katoh, T, and Hayashi, O (2009). "Effect of Phycocyanin, one of the extracts of Spirulina, on differentiation of U937 and HL-60 human myeliod leukemia cell lines", *J Phys Fit Nutr Immunol*, 19, 222-232.

Kaminogawa, S, and Nanno, M (2004). "Modulation of Immune Functions by Foods", *Evid Based Complement Alternat Med*, 1, 241-250.

Kaszuba-Zwoinska, J, Wojcik, K, Bereta, M, Ziomber, A, Pierzchalski, P, Rokita, E, Marcinkiewicz, J, Zaraska, W, and Thor, P (2010). "Pulsating electromagnetic field stimulation prevents cell death of puromycin treated U937 cell line", *J Physiol Pharmacol*, 61, 201-205.

Kim, J, Takahashi, I, Kai, Y, and Kiyono, H (2001). "Influence of enterotoxin on mucosal intranet: selective inhibition of extrathymic T cell development in intestinal intraepithelial lymphocytes by oral exposure to heat-labile toxin", *Eur J Immunol*, 31, 2960-2969.

Koga, T, McGhee, JR, Kato, H, Kato, R, Kiyono, H, and Fujihashi, K (2000). "Evidence for early aging in the mucosal immune system", *Journal of Immunology*, 165, 5352-5359.

Komano, H, Fujiura, Y, Kawaguchi, M, Matsumoto, S, Hashimoto, Y, Obana, S, Mombaerts, P, Tonegawa, S, Yamamoto, H, Itohara, S, and et al. (1995). "Homeostatic regulation of intestinal epithelia by intraepithelial gamma delta T cells", *Proceedings of the National Academy of Sciences of the United States of America*, 92, 6147-6151.

Komuro, T, Sano, K, Asano, Y, and Tada, T (1990). "Analysis of aged-related degeneracy of T-cell repertoir: Localized functional failure in CD8+ T cells", *Scandinavian journal of immunology*, 32, 545-553.

Krause, D, Mastro, AM, Handte, G, Smiciklas-Wright, H, Miles, MP, and Ahluwalia, D (1999). "Immune function did not decline with aging in aooarently healthy, well-nourished women", *Mech Ageing Dev*, 112, 43-57.

Lefrancois, L (1991). "Phenotypic complexity of intraepithelial lymphocytes of small intestine", *Journal of Immunology*, 147, 1746.

Li, B, Gao, MH, Zhang, XC, and Chu, XM (2006). "Molecular immune mechanism of C-phycocyanin from *Spirulina platensis* induces apoptosis in HeLa cells in vitro", *Biotechnol Appl Biochem*, 43, 155-164.

Loseva, LP, and Dardynskaya, IV (1993) *Spirulina* natural sorbent of radionucleides. In the 6th International Congress of Applied Algology. Czech Republic.

Lu, YC, Yeh, WC, and Ohashi, PS (2008). "LPS/TLR4 signal transduction pathway", *Cytokine*, 42, 145-151.

Lubbert, M, Herrmann, F, and Koeffler, HP (1991). "Expression and regulation of myeloid-specific genes in normal and leukemic myeloid cells", *Blood*, 77, 909-924.

Lydyard, P, and Grossi, C (1998). "3. Lymphoid system", I Roitt, J Brostoff, & D Male (Ed.), In Immunology 5th edition (pp 31-41). London: Mosby International Ltd.

MacColl, R (2004). "Allophycocyanin and energy transfer", *Biochim Biophys Acta*, 1657, 73-81.

Mao, TK, Van De Water, J, and Gershwin, ME (2000). "Effect of *Spirulina* on the secretion of cytokines from peripheral blood mononuclear cells", *Journal of Medicinal Food*, 3 (3), 135-140.

Miquel, J (2001). "Nutrition and ageing", *Public Health Nutrition*, 4 (6A), 1385-1388.

Mishima, T, Murata, J, Toyoshima, M, Fujii, H, Nakajima, M, Hayashi, T, Kato, T, and Saiki, I (1998). "Inhibition of tumor invasion and metastasis by calcium spirulan (Ca-SP), a novel sulfated polysaccharide derived from a blue-green alga, Spirulina platensis", *Clin Exp Metastasis*, 16, 541-550.

Nelissen, B, Wilmotte, A, De Baere, R, Haes, F, Van De Peer, Y, and Neefs, J (1992). "Phylogenetic study of cyanobacteria on the basis of 16S ribosomal RNA sequences", *Belg J Bot*, 125, 210-213.

Nemoto-Kawamura, C, Hirahashi, T, Nagai, T, Yamada, H, Katoh, T, and Hayashi, O (2004). "Phycocyanin enhances secretory IgA antibody responses and suppresses allergic IgE antibody response in mice immunized with antigen-entrapped biodegradable microparticles", *J Nutr Sci Vitaminol*, 50, 129 -136.

Obermeier, H, Hrboticky, N, and Sellmayer, A (1995). "Differential effects of polyunsaturated fatty acids on cell growth and differentiation of premonocytic U937 cells", *Biochim Biophys Acta*, 1266, 179-185.

Otte, A, Mandel, K, Reinstrom, G, and Hass, R (2011). "Abolished adherence alters signaling pathways in phorbol ester-induced human U937 cells", *Cell Commun Signal*, 9, 20.

Padyana, AK, Bhat, VB, Madyastha, KM, Rajashankar, K, and Ramakumar, S (2001). "Crystal Structure of a Light-Harvesting Protein C-Phycocyanin from *Spirulina platensis*", *Biochemical and Biophysical Research Communications*, 282, 893-898.

Park, EJ, Takahashi, I, Ikeda, J, Kawahara, K, Okamoto, T, Kweon, MN, Fukuyama, S, Groh, V, Spies, T, Obata, Y, Miyazaki, J, and Kiyono, H (2003). "Clonal expansion of double-positive intraepithelial lymphocytes by MHC class I-related chain A expressed in mouse small intestinal epithelium", *Journal of Immunology*, 171, 4131-4139.

Pentón-Rol, G, Martínez-Sánchez, G, Cervantes-Llanos, M, Lagumersindez-Denis, N, Felino Acosta-Medina, E, Falcón-Cama, V, Alonso-Ramírez, R, Valenzuela-Silva, C, Rodríguez-Jiménez, E, Llópiz-Arzuaga, A, Marín-Prida, J, López-Saura, PA, Guillén-Nieto, GE, and Pentón-Arias, E (2011). "C-Phycocyanin ameliorates experimental autoimmune encephalomyelitis and induces regulatory T cells", *International Immunopharmacology* 11, 29-38.

Pugh, N, Ross, SA, ElSohly, HN, ElSohly, MA, and Pasco, DS (2001). "Isolation of three high molecular weight polysaccharide preparations with potent immunostimulatory activity from *Spirulina platensis*, *Aphanizomenon flosaquae* and *Chlorella pyrenoidosa*", *Planta Med*, 67, 737-742.

Rabadiya, B, and Patel, P (2010). "*Spirulina*: Potential clinical therapeutic application", *Journal of Pharmacy Research*, 3, 1726-1732.

Rao, RD, Anderson, PM, Arndt, CA, Wettstein, PJ, and Markovic, SN (2003). "Aerosolized granulocyte macrophage colony-stimulating factor (GM-CSF) therapy in metastatic cancer", *Am J Clin Oncol*, 26, 493 - 498.

Reddy, CM, Bhat, VB, Kiranmai, G, Reddy, MN, Reddanna, P, and Madyastha, KM (2000). "Selective inhibition of cyclooxygenase-2 by C-phycocyanin, a biliprotein from *Spirulina platensis*", *Biochem Biophys Res Commun*, 277, 599-603.

Remirez, D, Ledon, N, and Gonzalez, R (2002). "Role of histamine in inhibitory effects of phycocyanin in experimental models of allergic inflammatory response", *Mediators of Inflammation*, 11, 81-85.

Rocha, B, Vassalli, P, and Guy-Grand, D (1994). "Thymic and extrathymic origins of gut intraepithelial lymphocyte populations in mice", *J Exp Med*, 180, 681-686.

Romay, C, Armesto, J, Remirez, D, Gonzalez, R, Ledon, N, and Garcia, I (1998). "Antioxidant and anti-inflammatory properties of c-phycocyanin from blue-green algae", *Inflammation Research*, 47, 36-41.

Sacha, T, Zawada, M, Hartwich, J, Lach, Z, Polus, A, Szostek, M, Zdzi Owska, E, Libura, M, Bodzioch, M, Dembińska-Kieć, A, Skotnicki, A, Góralczyk, R, Wertz, K, Riss, G, Moele, C, Langmann, T, and Schmitz, G (2005). "The effect of beta-carotene and its derivatives on cytotoxicity, differentiation, proliferative potential and apoptosis on the three human acute leukemia cell lines: U-937, HL-60 and TF-1", *Biochim Biophys Acta*, 1740, 206-214.

Schmucker, DL, Owen, RL, Outenreath, R, and Thoreux, K (2003). "Basis for the age-related decline in intestinal mucosal immunity", *Clin Dev Immunol*, 10, 167-172.

Schneider, E, and Dy, M (1999). "Cytokines and haematopoiesis", J Theze (Ed.), In The Cytokine Network and Immune Functions (pp 146-161). New York: Oxford University Press.

Selmi, C, Leung, PS, Fischer, L, German, B, Yang, CY, Kenny, TP, Cysewski, GR, and Gershwin, ME (2011). "The effects of Spirulina on anemia and immune function in senior citizens", *Cell Mol Immunol*, 8, 248-254.

Shinohara, K, Okura, Y, Koyano, T, Murakami, H, and Omura, H (1988). "Algal phycocyanins promote growth of human cells in culture", *In Vitro Cellular and Developmental Biology*, 2, 1057 - 1060.

Solana, R, Pawelec, G, and Tarazona, R (2006). "Aging and innate immunity", *Immunity*, 24, 491-494.

Takimoto, H, Nakamura, T, Takeuchi, M, Sumi, Y, Tanaka, T, Nomoto, K, and Yoshikai, Y (1992). "Age-associated increase in number of $CD4^{+}CD8^{+}$ intestinal intraepithelial lymphocytes in rats", *Eur J Immunol*, 22, 159-164.

Tamagawa, K, Fukushima, S, Kobori, M, Shinmoto, H, and Tsushida, T (1998). "Proanthocyanidins from barley bran potentiate retinoic acid-induced granulocytic and sodium butyrate-induced monocytic differentiation of HL60 cells", *Bioscience, Biotechnology, and Biochemistry*, 62, 1483-1487.

Tanaka, H, Abe, E, Miyaura, C, Shiina, Y, and Suda, T (1983). "1 alpha, 25-dihydroxyvitamin D_3 induces differentiation of human promyelocytic leukemia cells (HL-60) into monocyte-macrophages, but not into granulocytes", *Biochem Biophys Res Commun*, 117, 86-92.

Tudhope, SJ, Finney-Hayward, TK, Nicholson, AG, Mayer, RJ, Barnette, MS, Barnes, PJ, and Donnelly, LE (2008). "Different mitogen-activated protein kinase-dependent cytokine responses in cells of the monocyte lineage", *The Journal of Pharmacology and Experimental Therapeutics*, 324, 306-312.

Vadiraja, BB, Gaikwad, NW, and Madyastha, KM (1998). "Hepatoprotective effect of C-phycocyanin: protection for carbon tetrachloride and R-(+)-pulegone-mediated hepatotoxicty in rats", *Biochem Biophys Res Commun*, 249, 428-431.

Verma, S, Samarth, R, and Panwar, M (2006). "Evaluation of Radioprotective Effects of *Spirulina* in Swiss Albino Mice", *Asian J Exp Sci*, 20, 121-126.

Vila, J, Gemma, C, Bachstetter, A, Wang, Y, Stromberg, I, and Bickford, PC (2008). "*Spirulina*, aging, and neurobiology", ME Gershwin, & A Belay (Ed.), In *Spirulina* in Human Nutrition and Health (pp 271-291). Boca Raton, FL: CRC Press Taylor & Francis Group.

Wu, L-c, and Annie Ho, J-a (2008). "Antioxidative and hepatoprotective effects of *Spirulina*", ME Gershwin, & A Belay (Ed.), In *Spiruilina* in Human Nutrition and Health (pp 119-151). Boca Raton, FL: CRC Oress Taylor & Francis Group.

Zhang, C-W (1994). "Effect of polysaccharide and phycocyanin from *Spirulina* on peripheral blood and hematopoietic system of bone marrow in mice", *Proceeding of 2nd Asia Pacific Conference on Algal Biotechnology, China*, 58.

Zhang, H-Q, Lin, A-P, Sun, Y, and Deng, Y-M (2001). "Chemo and radio-protective effects of polysaccharide of *Spirulina platensis* in hemopoeitic system of mice and dogs", *Acta Pharmacol Sin* 22, 1121-1124.

Chapter 8

Spontaneous Alternation Behavior in Human Neutrophils

Karen A. Selz

Additional information is available at the end of the chapter

http://dx.doi.org/10.5772/47851

1. Introduction

SAB: Spontaneous alternation behavior (SAB) generally refers to the tendency of animals, even single-celled organisms, to alternate their non-reinforced (Dember & Richman, 1989) choices of T- or Y-maze arms on subsequent trials, following an initial trial or turn. First described over 80 years ago (Tolman, 1925), the phenomenon has been ascribed to the operation of a variety of mechanisms including Hullian reactive inhibition (Solomon, 1948), stimulus satiation (Glanzer, 1953), action decrement (Walker, 1958), curiosity (Dember and Earl, 1957), habituation to novelty (Carlton, 1969), foraging strategies (Estes and Schoeffler, 1955) and spatial working memory (Sarter, et al., 1988). Studies have suggested that the primary cue for alternation among invertebrates to be is the body turn. Vertebrates rely primarily on directional and odor cues. The fitness benefits associated with stimulus seeking and behavioral exploration, foraging, remain the most compelling explanation of why SAB is found ubiquitously and reliably (Richman, et al.1986). Although the underlying mechanism of SAB is open to study, there is general agreement that the ability to alternate choices requires that the organism remember its previous choice (Hughes, 2004).

Because SAB implicates future behavior which is statistically dependent on prior behavior and accompanied by memorially-dependant loss of degrees of freedom, SAB has been used to suggest the presence of a functional short-term memory. A left or right turn in a T- or Y-maze is a statistical function of the presence and direction of the previous turn, when such a prior turn exists.

While theories of memory are many and not the focus of this chapter, SAB is generally suggested to be recent memory dependent in animals complex enough to possess the structures postulated to underlie recent memory, and to be dependent on a more basic sensory/membrane/receptor depletion time-limited memorial mechanism in simple organisms and cell systems that have also demonstrated SAB. Recent memory decays, some suggest exponentially in time (Eukaszewska and Deawichowska, 1982; Lalonde, 2002). This "decay" or, alternative, "interference" assumptions are explicit in many theories of short-term memory (e.g., Thorndike, 1914; Oberauer and Lewandowsky, 2008), so that the SAB effect would be expected to also diminish in the mean with the extension of the long leg of the T.

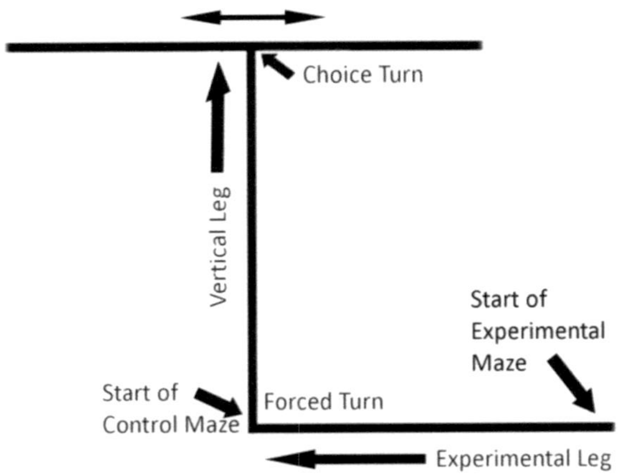

Figure 1. A general layout for T-mazes.

In fact, when the length of the vertical leg is treated as an experimental variable, using distance as a proxy for time, SAB consistently decreases as vertical leg length increases (Hughes, 1989). Similarly, with two-trial SAB, increasing the intertrial interval, and so the time between successive choice opportunities, has been shown to reduce alternation frequencies (Dember and Richman, 1989). This inverse relationship follows from a memory-based view of SAB, has been used to suggest that the longer the distance between successive turns, the greater the probability that the organism will "forget" the direction of its previous turn and choice will return to a statistically equiprobable condition (Hughes, 1989). No particular mechanism of "memory" is implied in this context. That is, any mechanism that causes current actions to be influenced by previous actions could potentially lead to SAB in general and to the loss of SAB with increased distance/time between the forced and choice turns.

PMN: Human polymorphonuclear leucocytes, PMN, are highly motile cells averaging 12 to 15 μm in diameter, exhibiting prominent, lobular nuclei. They emerge from bone marrow stem cells and are the most populous of the white blood cell category. PMNs are essential for host defense participating in both acute and chronic inflammatory processes. Other related properties include the regulation of immune responses, angiogenesis, and in physical interactions with neoplasms. Making this wide variety of functions possible is their dynamically adaptive behavior exemplified by the range of intrinsic patterns of motility. Following my recent work demonstrating phase transition scenarios in PMN morphodynamics (Selz, 2011), I developed a new method to assess the autonomous behavior of these human PMNs and whether single constituent cells exhibit SAB.

Recall that whereas the natural physiological environment for autonomous motion in human neutrophils contains the PMN's endogenous tropic peptide attractant, the classical "spontaneous alteration", SAB design of these studies requires that the observed behavior, the cell's spontaneous motion, be unperturbed. The necessary absence of these chemoattractants, leads to a multitude of required trials for the acquisition of a single data point. It was for this reason that I recorded hundreds of PMNs, increasing the number of trials until n>50 left/right decisions at the T-intersections in each of the three types of mazes will have been observed.

2. Methods and procedures

Three similar T-mazes were developed; 1) a control T-maze, 2) a forced-turn T-maze, and 3) a long-leg forced turn T-maze. As SAB is the tendency of an organism to alternate successively turning left and then right in a maze, the control maze is the one in which the first turn is the only turn. Cells in control mazes are expected to turn to the right or left with roughly equal probability. However, in the second, forced turn maze, in which the cell must always make a right turn before reaching the experimental left versus right choice point of the T, the statistical expectation is that more cells will turn left at the T. In the third maze, the SAB effect can decay in the mean with the extension of the long leg of the T.

The mazes were constructed on standard glass slides, inside a 12mm diameter, 25μm deep well. The specifications are indicated in the figures 2. Figure 3 is an electron micrograph of a set of the nano-structured mazes on a finished slide. Tolerances were ± 5%. Sidewall angles of mazes were 88-90^0. Surface variation (roughness) was in the neighborhood of 10nm.

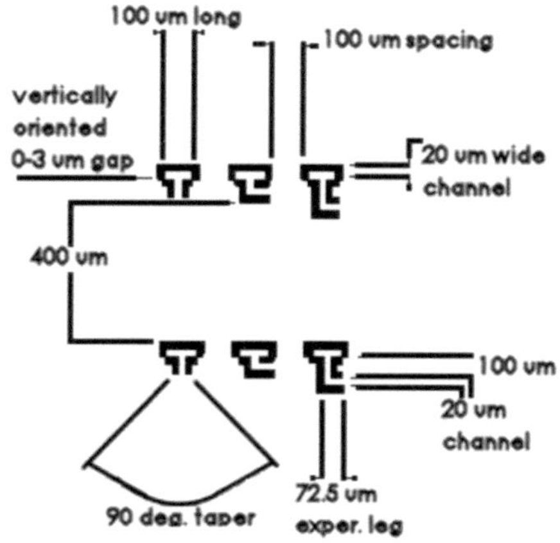

Figure 2. A rough schematic of the mazes on each slide.

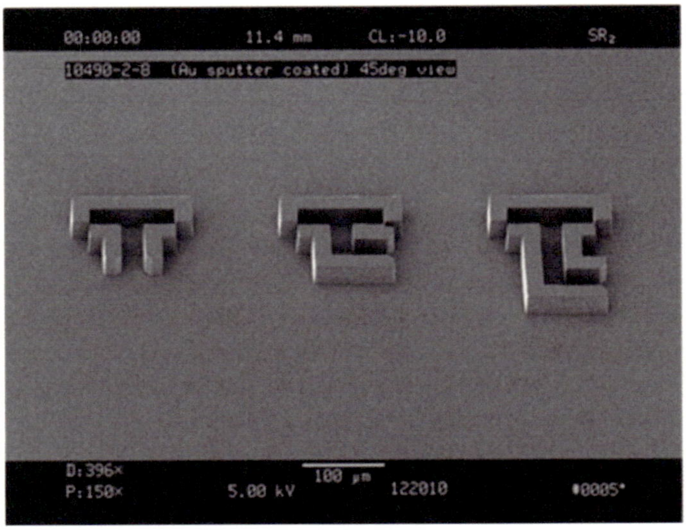

Figure 3. An EM image of one set of mazes on a slide. Note the taper at the entrance of each maze and the flow-through gap at the terminal ends of the mazes (0um at the base to 3um at the top of the maze walls). These allow the passage of medium, but not the entry or exit of PMN.

After gentle sedimentation, PMNs (along with some other white cells and platelets) were removed from the buffy coat by micropipette and, along with associated plasma. The 5.7 μm gap of standard slides and coverslips is smaller than the average diameter of PMNs, leading to some mechanical compression of the cells and contributing to their activation, as well as allowing the cell to move along the slide substrate and cover slip simultaneously (Malawista and deBoisfleury Chevance, 1997). The slides used in this study do not suffer from these deficits. All samples were drawn from 5 healthy, adult volunteers (3F, 2M, ages 25-47). All slides were pre-filled with Lactated Ringer's solution, that is isotonic with blood. This was done to avoid cells being deposited into the maze ends, as well as to avoid trapped air in the mazes, and to dilute the PMN sample.

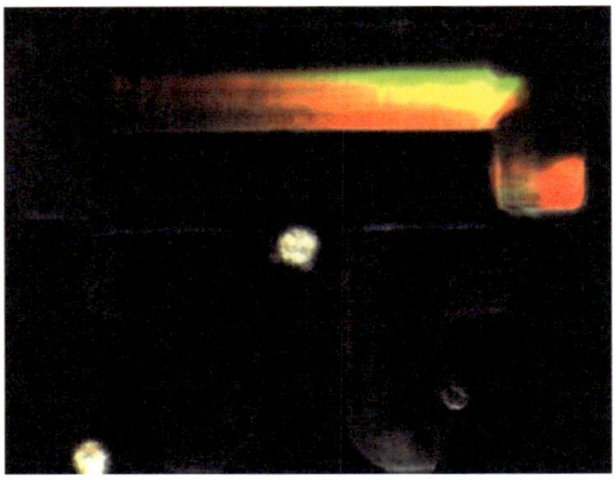

Figure 4. Shows a typical trial, in which a PMN (with evident lobular nuclei) translocates up the vertical leg of a control T-maze while another lingers outside the maze.

As implied by the word "spontaneous," SAB studies require that the cell's motion be observed without manipulating exogenous agents. Lactated Ringer's solution provided a uniform, "undoped" medium base. Without the activating influence of chemoattractants or physical activators (e.g. heat, pressure, sheer), many trials were required for the acquisition of each data point. In total, 102 PMN navigated the control maze past the decision point, 57 navigated the forced-turn maze, and 82 PMN completed the long-legged forced-turn T-maze.

PMN autonomous motions were observed through an Olympus BX41 microscope with a mixed CytoViva dark field and fluorescent optical illumination system. This incorporates a high-aperture, cardioid annular condenser (www.scitech.com.au) unique to this system and which makes possible visualization of objects below 90nm in diameter in real time, including cellular samples in an unfixed, living, active state (Samoylov, et al., 2005; Vainrub, et al. 2006). Because PMNs were treated gently, avoiding perturbations of column separation and elution, it became possible to reliably study a PMN continuously for extended times without the onset of granular clumping, membrane blebbing and other signs of impending apoptosis (Lodish, 2005). Whenever a PMN moved to the left or right beyond the choice point of a maze, its choice was recorded.

3. Results

Left-Right choices in the control maze were not significantly different from equiprobability (Left=49.02%; Right=50.98%; $\chi^2_{(1)}$=0.039, ϱ=0.843). However, in the forced-turn T-maze, 63.16% of the cells that had been forced to turn Right previously, turned Left at the decision point ($\chi^2_{(1)}$=3.947, ϱ=0.0469) . Contrary to initial expectation of the disappearance of the SAB effect with the increased length of the vertical leg of the maze, this effect persisted and even appeared to be strengthened in the long-legged forced-turn maze, in which 67.07% ($\chi^2_{(1)}$= 9.561, ϱ=0.0021) of completing cells turned Left at the decision point, long after a forced Right turn.

4. Conclusions

This is the first demonstration that SAB is present in PMN, a constituent cell of the human body. While SAB has been shown in human spermatozoa (Brugger, et. al., 2002), sperm cells are required to function in the world exterior to the body, while PMN are not.

The apparent strengthening of SAB in the long-legged forced-turn T-maze compared to the standard forced-turn maze, may be partially attributable to the higher n in the former and natural variation in data, but observation of hundreds of PMN in the maze environments suggests it might also result from a sort of practice effect of "frustrated" turn attempts in the channel, in a dose-response like paradigm. Length of time/distance spent in foiled attempts to turn may then serve as an order parameter. The persistence of SAB in this condition may also suggest multiple time scale, memory-like mechanisms operating in PMN.

There are, in fact, established physiological mechanisms and behavior that are consistent with this speculation and with my qualitative microscopic. PMNs are known to oscillate on multiple temporal and spatial scales, from 7sec, 70sec, and 260sec membrane potential fluctuations (Jäger, et al., 1988) and 25sec calcium flux oscillations, to the ~8sec G-F-actin oscillations (Marks and Maxfield, 1990), to 21.6sec and 230sec glycolytic cycles that produce NAD(P)H oscillations (Jäger, et al., 1988), and 10sec and 20sec pericellular proteolysis fluctuations (Marks and Maxfield, 1990), among many others. The time series in my recent study of PMN morphodynamics demonstrated scaling, board band power spectra with multiple resonances, suggesting a constellation of motility times (Selz, 2011). While there is debate over the specific fitness value(s) and mechanism(s) underlying SAB, it is clearly a phylogentically highly conserved behavior (Richman, et al.1986), and so, is assumed to be valuable. It follows that multiple mechanistically diverse time scales of function could be recruited to its service. This suggests the possibility of decentralized control in a highly interconnected, living dynamical system through local feedback. The necessary and sufficient conditions for a stable macro-system composed of multiple smaller systems operating on a variety of temporal and spatial scales are known in non-biological contexts (Ramakrishna and Viswanadham, 1982). Work is currently underway, adapting these constraints to a PMN model.

Because, with the prior forced turn, systems statistically deviate from equiprobability in a later choice circumstance, SAB represents a reduction in population behavioral entropy, and a situation in which a reduction in the behavior degrees of freedom and reduced statistical behavioral entropy is favored evolutionarily. This finding is contrary to some findings of increased entropic states being associated with greater biological health and/or function (e.g. Mandell, 1987; Paulus et al., 1980).

Author details

Karen A. Selz
Franklin-Fetzer Laboratory, Cielo Institute, Asheville, NC, USA

5. References

Brugger, P, Macas, E., and Ihlemann, J. (2002) Do sperm remember? *Behavl Brain Res.*, 136(1), 325-8.

Carlton PL. (1969). Brain-acetylcholine and inhibition. In: Tapp JT, editor. *Reinforcement and behavior*. New York: Academic Press,p. 286–327.

Dember WN, Earl RW.(1957). Analysis of exploratory, manipulatory and curiosity behaviors.*Psychol Rev*, 64:91–6.

Dember, W. N., & Richman, C. L. (Eds.) (1989). *Spontaneous alternation behavior*. New York: Springer.

Estes WK, Schoeffler MS. (1955). Analysis of variables influencing alternation after forced trials. J Comp *PhysiolPsychol*, 48:357–62.

Eukaszewska, I., Deawichowska, (1982). How long do rats remember the spatial arrangement of visual stimuli? *ActaNeurobiol.Exp*, 42, 127-133.;

Glanzer M. (1953). Stimulus satiation: an explanation of spontaneous alternation and related phenomena. *Psychol Rev*, 60:257–68.

Hughes, R. N. (1989). Phylogenetic comparisons. In W. N. Dember & C. L. Richman (Eds.), *Spontaneous alternation behavior* (pp. 38-57). NewYork: Springer.

Hughes, R. N. (2004). The value of spontaneous alternation behavior (SAB) as a test of retention in pharmacological investigations of memory. *Neuroscience & Biobehavioral Reviews*, 28, 497-505.

Jäger U, Gruler H, Bültmann B (1988) Morphological changes and membrane potential of human granulocytes under influence of chemotactic peptide and/or echo-virus type 9. *Klin Wochenschr* 66: 434.

Lalonde, R. (2002). The neurobiological basis of spontaneous alternation, *Neurosci&Biobehav Rev*, 26(1), 91-104.;

Lodish HF (2005) *Molecular and Cell Biology*. W.H. Freeman, New York.

Malawista SE, deBoisfleury Chevance A (1997) Random locomotion and chemotaxis of human blood polymorphonuclear leukocytes (PMN) in the presence of EDTA: PMN in close quarters require neither leukocyte integrins nor external divalent cations. *PNAS* 94:11577-82.

Mandell AJ (1987) Dynamical complexity and pathological order in the cardiac monitoring problem *Physica D* 27 235-42.

Marks PW, Maxfield FR (1990) Local and global changes in cytosolic free calcium in neutrophils during chemotaxis and phagocytosis. J Cell Biol 110:43.

Oberauer K, Lewandowsky S (2008) Forgetting in immediate serial recall: decay, temporal distinctiveness, or interference? *Psychology review*, 115(3), 544-576.

Paulus MP, Geyer MA, Gold LH, Mandell AJ (1990) Application of entropy measures derived from the ergodic theory of dynamical systems to rat locomotor behavior. *Proc.Natl.Acad.Sci.* 87: 723-727.

Ramakrishna A, Viswanadham N (1982) Decentralized Control of Interconnected Dynamical Systems. *IEEE Transactions on Automatic Control*, 27(1), 159-164.

Richman, R., et al.(1986). Spontaneous alternation behavior in animals: A review. *Current Psychology*, 5(4), 358-91.

Samoylov AM, Samoylova TI, Pustovyy OM, Samoylov AA, Toivio-Kinnucan MA, et al. (2005) Novel metal clusters isolated from blood are lethal to cancer cells. *Cells Tissues Organs* 179:115-124.

Sarter M, Bodewitz G, Stephens DN. (1988). Attenuation of scopolamine induced impairment of spontaneous alternation behaviour by antagonist but not inverse agonist and agonist beta-carbolines. *Psychopharmacology*, 94:491–5.

Selz KA, (2011).A Third Measure-Metastable State in the Dynamics of Spontaneous Shape Change in Healthy Human's White Cells.*PLoSComputBiol* 7(4): e1001117. doi:10.1371.

Solomon RL. (1948). The influence of work on behavior. *Psychol Bull*;45:1–40.502; R.N. Hughes (2004)*Neuroscience and Biobehavioral Reviews* 28, 497–505

Thorndike EL, *The Psychology of Learning*, N. Y., Teachers College, 1914

Tolman EC. (1925). Purpose and cognition: the determiners of animal learning. *Psychol Rev*, 32:285–97.

Vainrub A, Pustovyy O, Vodyanoy V (2006) Resolution of 90 nm (lambda/5) in an optical transmission microscope with an annular condenser. *Optics Lett* 31, 2855-2857

Walker EL. (1958). Action decrement and its relation to learning. *Psychol Rev*, 65:129–42.

Chapter 9

RBC-ATP Theory of Regulation for Tissue Oxygenation-ATP Concentration Model

Terry E. Moschandreou

Additional information is available at the end of the chapter

http://dx.doi.org/10.5772/48580

1. Introduction

It is known that red blood cells release ATP when blood oxygen tension decreases. ATP has an effect on microvascular endothelial cells to form a retrospective conducted vasodilation to the upstream arteriole. Local metabolic control of coronary blood flow due to vasodilation in microvascular units where myocardial oxygen extraction is relatively high occurs due to ATP.[5] Arterioles dilate or constrict in response to changing intravascular pressure.[6]

"It is well known that myogenic responses, flow-dependent vasodilation, local metabolic effects, and propagation all contribute to blood flow regulation. Primarily responsible for carrying oxygen in blood, red blood cells (RBCs) may also act as oxygen sensors and thus play a role in the communication of metabolic demand" [3,7]. The mechanisms for release of ATP from the RBC in response to lowered oxygen saturation have been studied. [8]. Jagger et al. [9] measured the ATP release at low O2 levels in the presence and absence of CO to demonstrate that the release of ATP from RBCs may be connected to the change of the hemoglobin molecule from its relaxed state to its deoxygenated state. Upon release, ATP binds to P2Y purinergic receptors on the luminal surface of the endothelium, starting the conducted response [10].An in vitro microfluidic experimental study to investigate the dynamics of shear-induced ATP release from human RBCs with millisecond resolution was conducted by Wan et al. [11].Conclusively it was shown that there is a sizable delay time between the onset of increased shear stress and the release of ATP. "It was seen that this response time decreases with shear stress, but does not depend significantly on membrane rigidity. It was shown that even though the RBCs deform significantly in short constrictions (duration of increased stress <3 ms), no measurable ATP is released."[11]

INTECH
open science | open minds

ATP is short for adenosine triposphate, which is a "currency" of biological energy. There exists an adenosine group with 3 phosphate groups attached to it. Hydrolizing this bond detaches one of the phosphate groups and produces ADP, which is adenosine di-phospahte plus a phosphate group and energy. Through chemical reaction if you pop off a phosphate group of ATP, energy will be generated for general heat or one can couple this reaction with other reactions that require energy. This chemical reaction of ATP to ADP involves going from stored energy to used energy. ADP can be recharged back to ATP by processes in the mitochondria.

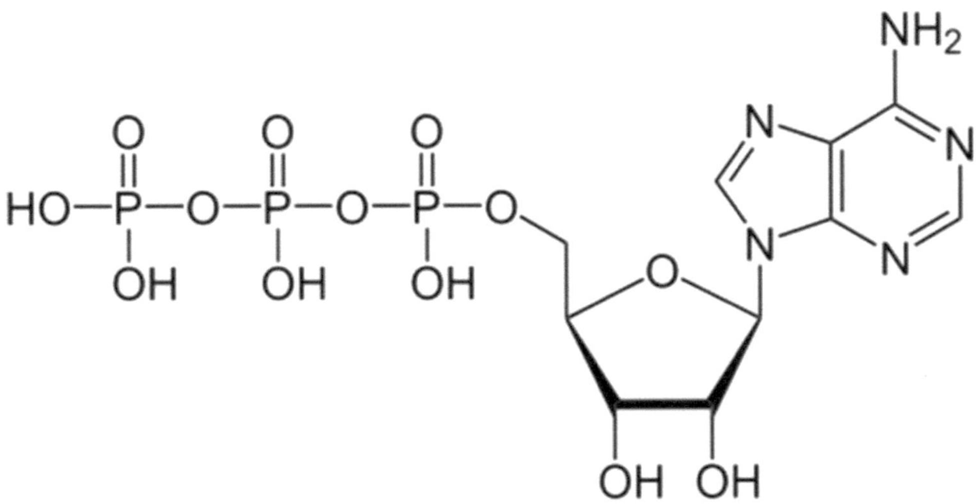

Figure 1. Adenosine Triphosphate[12]

The same part(adenine) that makes up DNA is that which makes up these energy currency molecules known as ATP molecules. Adenine makes part of adenosine which makes part of ATP. The other part of ATP is known as ribose from RNA, which is a five carbon sugar. ATP drives biological reactions. In terms of electrons when one pops off the phosphate group the electrons enter a lower energy state between phosphate and oxygen atoms which generates energy.

RBC's have no nucleus or mitochondria. As a result RBC's obtain their energy using glycolysis to produce ATP. There are both advantages and disadvantages to this. An advantage is due to the biconcave disk shape which optimizes the cell for the exchange of oxygen with its surroundings and optimizes space for the hemoglobin. The RBC's are deformable and flexible so that they can move through the tiny capillaries where oxygen is released. The disadvantage is that because of the absence of nuclei and organelles, mature RBC's do not contain DNA and cannot synthesize any RNA, and cannot divide or repair themselves. The Mitochondria enables cells to produce 15 times more ATP than usual. Lack of mitochondria means that the cells use none of the oxygen they transport. Instead they produce the energy carrier ATP by means of fermentation, via glycolysis of glucose and by lactic acid production.

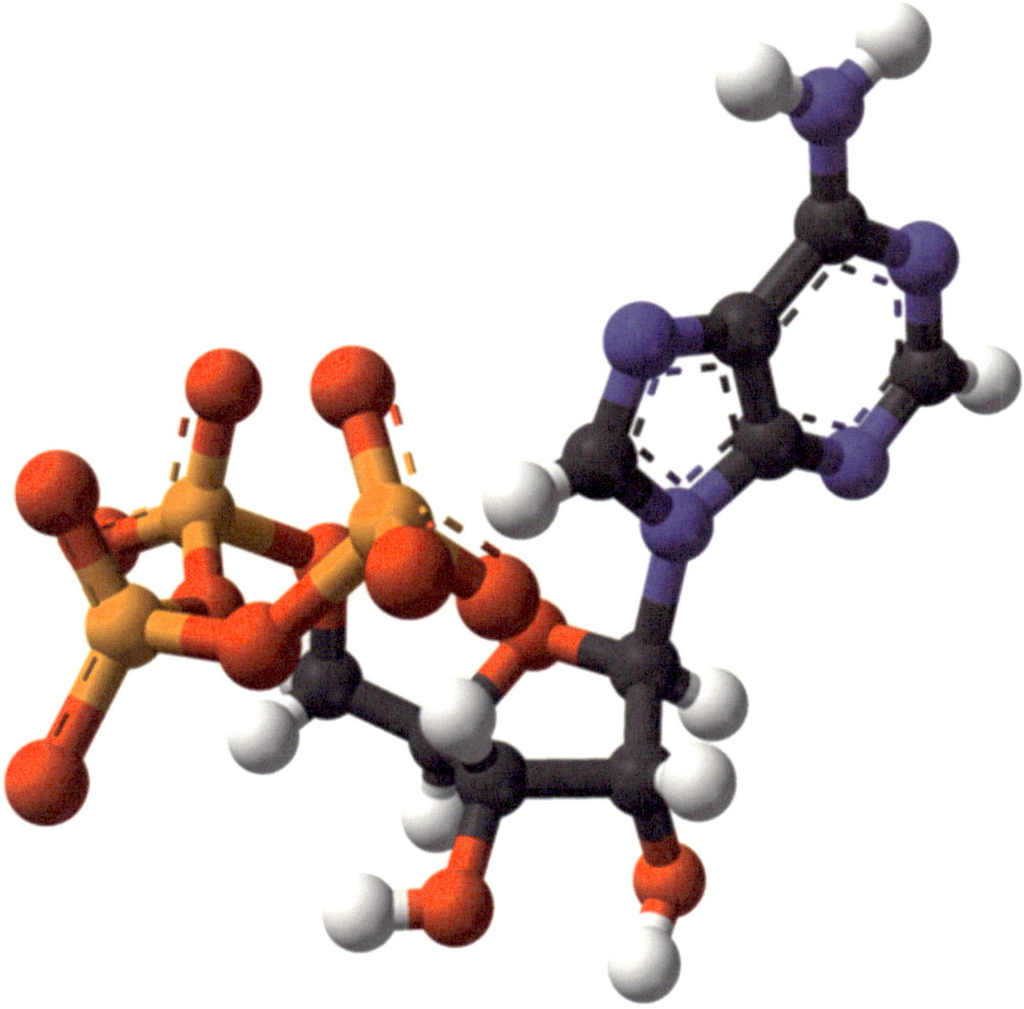

Figure 2. Ball and Stick Model of ATP based x-ray diffraction data[13]

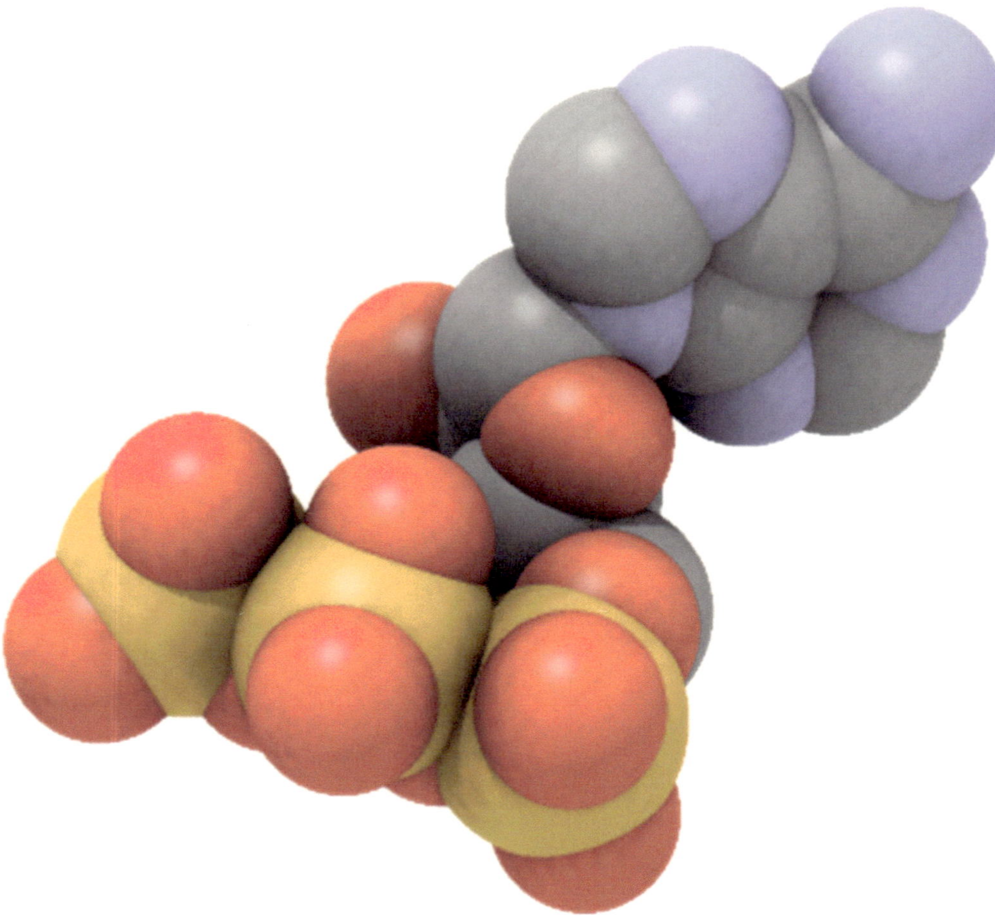

Figure 3. Space-Fill Representation of ATP[14]

2. Structural features erythrocyte and the erythrocyte membrane

Lacking organelles as nucleus, mitochondria, or ribosomes, the red cell does not synthesize new proteins, carrying out the oxidative reactions associated with mitochondria, or undergo mitosis.

The RBC consists of a membrane surrounding a solution of protein and electrolytes. About 95% of the protein is the oxygen-transport protein, hemoglobin. The remainder of the protein includes enzymes required for energy production and for maintenance of hemoglobin.

3. Shape of RBC

In immobile state, the normal human RBC is shaped as a biconcave disc. The disc shape is important to erythrocyte function. The ratio of surface to volume is optimized so that oxygen transfer is possible. Also the biconcave disc is more deformable than a sphere and undergoes the change in shape necessary for optimal movement in microvasculature.

The four possible forces to maintain the shape described are (1) elastic forces within the membrane, (2) surface tension, (3) electrical forces on the membrane surface, and (4) osmotic or hydrostatic pressures. The maintenance of RBC shape is dependent on the structure of the cell as well as in the external environment. If these are changed, the cell may become spherical.

When RBC's are suspended in hypotonic solutions andosmotic swelling occurs. This can make the cell spherical. These changes are associated with an increase in volume while the cell surface area remains the same or changes only slightly. When spherical shape is attained, the cell diameter decreases, and this shows the elastic properties of the membrane.

Discocyte-echinocyte transformation takes place when ATP is depleted, when intracellular calcium is increased, when the cell is exposed to plasma, anionic detergents, high pH, lysolecithin or fatty acids.

4. Dimensions of RBC

Photomicrographs are used to measure the dimensions of RBC's. Average values for the mean cellular volume in normal subjects are from approximately 85 to 91 fl. Ninety-five percent of normal red cells are between about 60 and 120 fl in volume. Various results have yielded an average normal value for red cell diameter of 7.2 to 7.4 microns.

5. Present objective

In this work we model the time delay of release of ATP as supporting work shows by Wan et al. [11] for shear-induced ATP release from red blood cells. A release rate which is a function of time and introduces a delay mechanism is introduced to show how the concentration of ATP is thus affected.

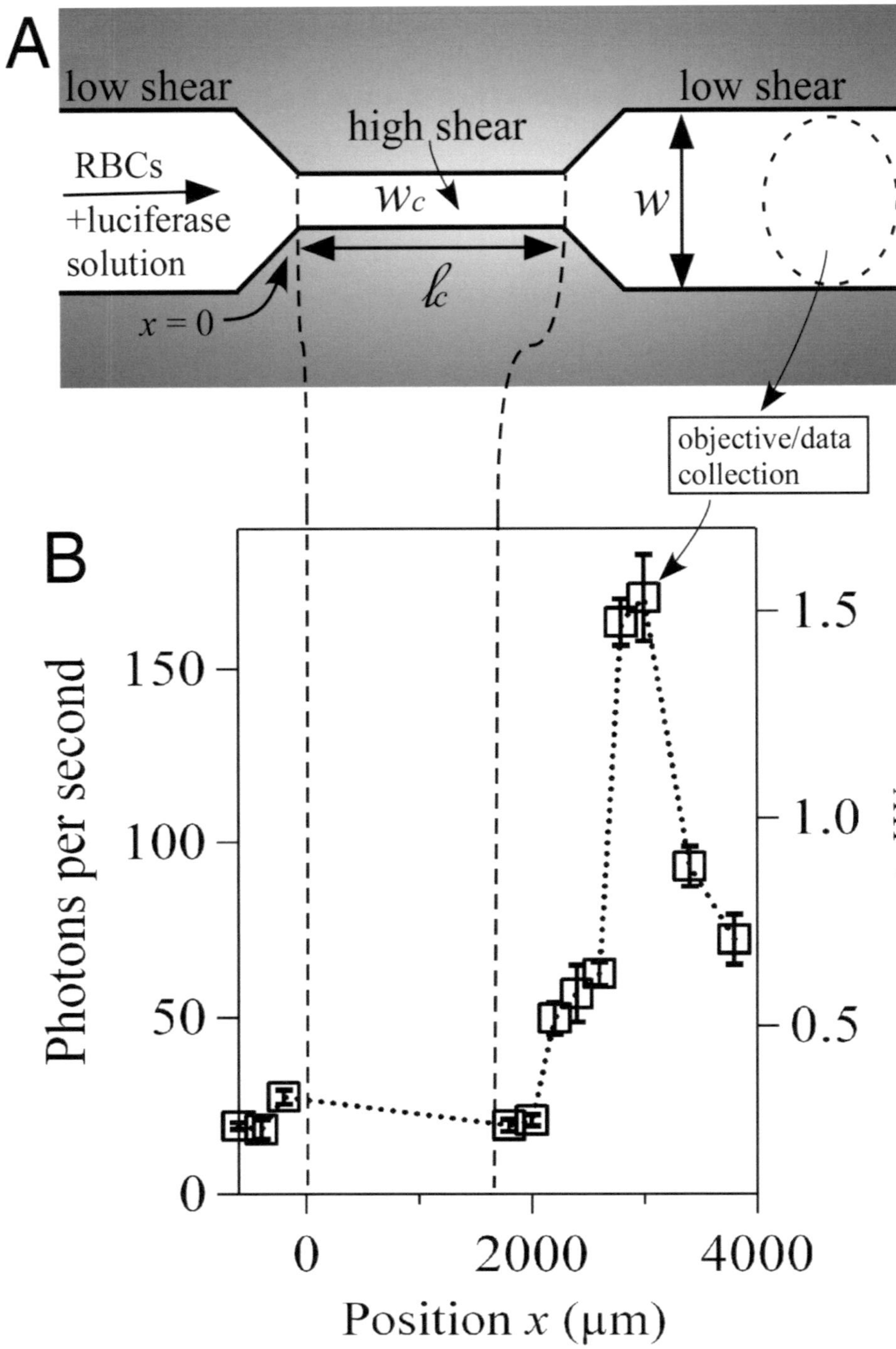
A
low shear
high shear
low shear
RBCs
+luciferase
solution
w_c
w
ℓ_c
$x = 0$
objective/data
collection
B
Photons per second
150
100
50
0
0
2000
4000
Position x (μm)
C_{ATP}(μM)
1.5
1.0
0.5

Figure 4. [11]

6. Method of solution

By conservation of mass, the decline in oxygen flux must equal the rate of oxygen consumption, giving the following equation for the change in oxygen saturation, S(x), with distance, x, along each arteriole:

$$\frac{d}{dx}\left[Qc_o H_D S(x)\right] = -q \tag{1}$$

where Q is volume flow rate in an individual vessel, c_o is the carrying capacity of RBCs at 100% saturation. H_D is the discharge hematocrit, and $q = \pi M_0 (r_{1,j}^2 - r_j^2)$ [3].

The release rate of ATP from an RBC, R[S(x)], is defined by a decreasing linear function of oxyhemoglobin saturation based on experimental data. ATP release from human erythrocytes in response to normoxia and hypoxia was observed in in vitro experiments.[3].

A linear fit of experimental values defines the ATP release function of saturation :

$$R\left[S(x)\right] = R_0\left[1 - R_1 S(x)\right] \tag{2}$$

In general,the rate of change in plasma ATP concentration, C(x,t), is given by the difference between the rates of ATP release and degradation:

$$\frac{\partial}{\partial t}[\pi R^2 \cdot (1 - H_T)C] + \frac{\partial}{\partial x}[(1 - H_D)QC(x)] = \pi R^2 H_T R[S(x,t)] - 2k_d \pi RC(x,t) \tag{3}$$

where H_T is tube hematocrit, R is radius of vessel and k_d is a concentration rate constant.([3])

We assume that there is no convection in the vessel and there is no x-dependence. Equation (3) simplifies to the following equation:

$$\frac{dC}{dt} = \frac{H_T}{1 - H_T} R(S(t)) - \frac{2}{R}\frac{k_d}{1 - H_T} C$$

In this chapter a model is developed which predicts tissue ATP concentrations as a variation of time and depth into the tissue due to changing oxygen tensions.

The ATP concentration within plasma as a variation of time due to changes in oxygen tension at the tissue surface is related to the release and degradation of ATP, by the following equation:

$$\frac{dC}{dt} = \eta \cdot R_{ATP}(t) - \delta C \tag{4}$$

where δ is some constant of degradation. $\delta = \frac{2}{R}\frac{k_d}{1-H_T}$ [Related to the RBC fraction], R is the release of ATP from the RBC and C is ATP concentration.

In this model the ATP concentration maximizes at some constant value, depending on the oxygen saturation. This model can be used to predict the plasma ATP concentration based on different oxygen saturations.

7. Discussion

From Equation (4), with varying degradation constant, related to the RBC fraction, and release rate , $R_{ATP}(t) = H(t-3)$ where H is the Heaviside function as a function of t, we show results in Figure 5 for concentration of ATP, (μM), versus time (ms). The value in the shifted Heaviside function corresponds to the experimental results of Wan et al [11] for time t< 3 ms. This is the time interval where there is no ATP release and can be confirmed in Figure 4 where there is no ATP release before and throughout the stenosis of the microfluidic device. In fact there is ATP release in the low shear expansion on the right of the microfluidic device. This can be seen in the increase in concentration of ATP released by RBC as shown in Figure 4. The parameter η represents the rate of increase of ATP release and for large η, the concentration of ATP increases rather steeply, wheras for smaller η the concentration of ATP increases less steeply as can be seen in Figure 6 for varying values of degradation constant. Also our model is consistent with the experimental results of Wan et al.[11] in that the greatest increase in ATP occurs approximately 29 ms after the onset of increased shear stress.

(See Figure 6 for $\delta = 0.1$ at time t=30ms.) It is noteworthy to see that these results for shear-induced ATP release can also be extended to ATP release due to a decrease in saturation.

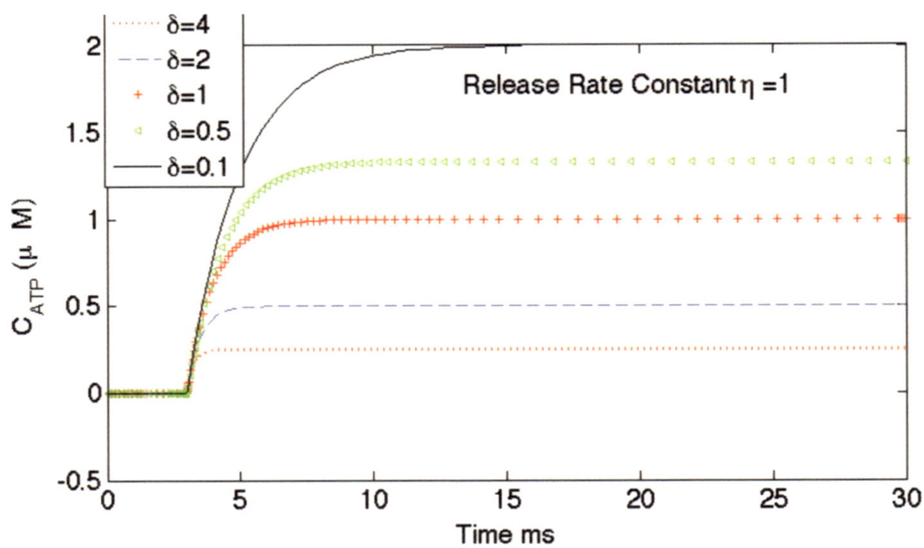

Figure 5.

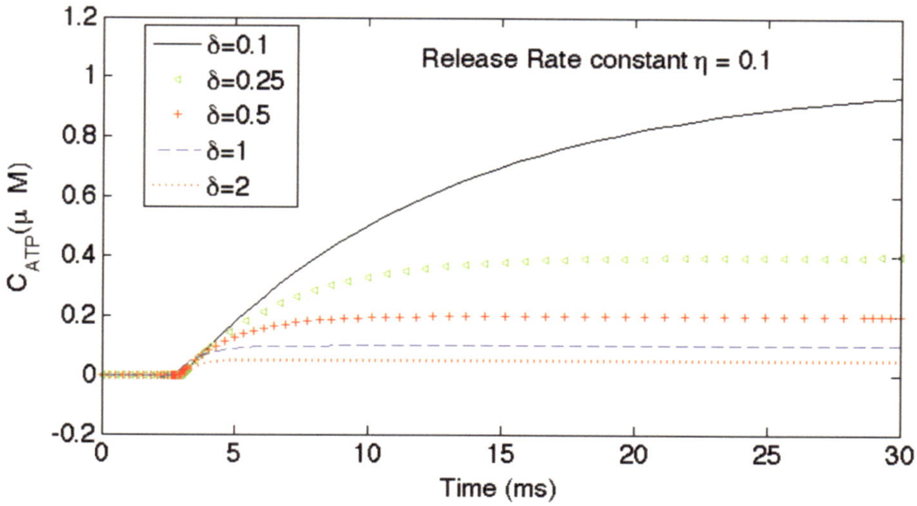

Figure 6.

8. Summary and conclusion

In this work we have outlined the importance of ATP as a signaling molecule in the microcirculation and have discussed the biochemical aspects of ATP and ADP as well as introduce a model for ATP release as used in microfluidic devices where RBC's are subject to compression and deform thus resulting in ATP release.

It is shown by Wan et al. [11] that even though the RBCs deform significantly in short constrictions (duration of increased stress <3 ms), no measurable ATP is released. This critical timescale is in proportion with a characteristic membrane relaxation time determined from observations of the cell deformation by using high-speed video[11]. "The results suggest a model wherein the retraction of the spectrin-actin cytoskeleton network triggers the mechano-sensitive ATP release and a shear-dependent membrane viscositycontrols the rate of release".[11]

It is noteworthy to see that these results for shear-induced ATP release can also be extended to ATP release due to a decrease in saturation.[3]

Author details

Terry E. Moschandreou
Department of Medical Biophysics, University of Western Ontario,
London Ontario, Canada

9. References

[1] Segal S.S. (2005) Regulation of blood flow in the microcirculation, Microcirculation 12(1): 33-45.

[2] M.L.EllsworthM.L.,Ellis C.G., Goldman D., Stephenson A.H., Dietrich H.H., Sprague R.S.(2009)Erythrocytes: oxygen sensors and modulators of vascular tone. Physiology (Bethesda)24: 107-16.

[3] ArcieroJ.C.,Carlson B.E., Secomb T.W.(2008) Theoretical model of metabolic blood flow regulation: roles of ATP release by red blood cells and conducted responses, Am. J. Physiol. Heart Circ. Physiol. 295(4): H1562-71.

[4] Bergfeld GR, Forrester T. (1992) Release of ATP from human erythrocytes in response to a brief period of hypoxia and hypercapnia. Cardiovas Res 26: 40-47.

[5] Farias Martin. III, Gorman Mark W., Savage Margaret V. and Feigl. Eric O. (2005) Plasma ATP during exercise: possible role in regulation of coronary blood flow AJP – Heart April 1, vol. 288 no.4: H1586-H1590.

[6] Johnson PC. (1980)The myogenic response.In:Handbook of Physiology.The Cardiovascular System.Vascular Smooth Muscle. Bethesda, MD: Am.Physiol. Soc., sect. 2, vol. II: p. 409 – 442.

[7] Ellsworth ML.(2000)The red blood cell as an oxygen sensor: what is the evidence? Acta Physiol Scand 168: 551–559.

[8] Buehler PW, Alayash AI.(2004)Oxygen sensing in the circulation: "cross talk"between red blood cells and the vasculature.Antioxid Redox Signal6:1000 –1010.

[9] Jagger JE, Bateman RM, Ellsworth ML, Ellis CG.(2001)Role of erythrocyte in regulating local O_2 delivery mediated by hemoglobin oxygenation. Am J Physiol Heart CircPhysiol280: H2833–H2839.

[10] Gorman MW, Ogimoto K, Savage MV, Jacobson KA, Feigl EO(2003)Nucleotide coronary vasodilation in guinea pig hearts.Am J Physiol HeartCircPhysiol285: H1040 – H1047.

[11] Wan Jiandi, Ristenpart William D., and Stone Howard A. (2008) Dynamics of shear-induced ATP release from red blood cells. PNAS: 1-7.

Section 2

Measurement of RBC Deformability and Microfluidics Technology for Cell Separation

Chapter 10

Measurement Techniques for Red Blood Cell Deformability: Recent Advances

Youngchan Kim, Kyoohyun Kim and YongKeun Park

Additional information is available at the end of the chapter

http://dx.doi.org/10.5772/50698

1. Introduction

Human red blood cells (RBCs) or erythrocytes have remarkable deformability. Upon external forces, RBCs undergo large mechanical deformation without rupture, and they restore to original shapes when released. The deformability of RBCs plays crucially important roles in the main function of RBCs - oxygen transport through blood circulation. RBCs must withstand large deformations during repeated passages through the microvasculature and the fenestrated walls of the splenic sinusoids (Waugh and Evans, 1979). RBC deformability can be significantly altered by various pathophysiological conditions, and the alterations in RBC deformability in turn influence pathophysiology, since RBC deformability is an important determinant of blood viscosity and thus blood circulation. Hence, measuring the deformability of RBCs holds the key to understanding RBC related diseases. For the past years, various experimental techniques have been developed to measure RBC deformability and recent technical advances revolutionize the way we study RBCs and their roles in hematology. This chapter reviews a variety of tools for measuring RBC deformability. For each technique, we seek to provide insights how these deformability measurement techniques can improve the study of RBC pathophysiology.

2. Deformability of RBCs

RBCs are the most deformable cell in the human body. RBC deformabiltiy is an intrinsic mechanical property determined by (1) its geometry, (2) cytoplasmic viscosity, mainly attributed to hemoglobin (Hb) solution in the cytoplasm, and (3) viscoelastic properties of RBC membrane cortex structure.

2.1. RBC geometry

Mature human RBCs have a biconcave disc shape and they do not contain nucleus or subcellular structures but mainly consist of Hb solution in the cytoplasm (Fig. 1a). A typical human RBC has a thickness of 2-3 μm, diameter of 6-8 μm, cell volume of 90 fl, and surface area of approximately 136 μm^2 (Kenneth,2010). Depending on species, RBC shape and size vary. In mammals, RBCs develope from nucleated progenitor cells in bone mellow but RBCs discard their nucleus as they mature, whereas RBCs of other vertebrates have nuclei. Throughout their life span of 100-120 days, human RBCs circulate the body delivering oxygen from the lungs to tissues. RBCs gradually lose their deformability with age and eventually rupture in spleen. The biconcave shape of normal RBCs has advantages in having deformability. Compared to a spherical shape, RBCs with biconcave shape have less volume for a given surface area, which can decrease bending energy associated with the membrane (Canham,1970).

2.2. Membrane cortex structure

The unique deformability of RBCs is mainly determined by the structures of RBC membrane cortex. The membrane of human RBC is a multicomponent structure comprised of three layers: (1) an external carbohydrate-rich layer, (2) the phospholipid bilayer with 4-5 nm thickness, embedded with transmembrane proteins, and (3) a 2-D triangular mesh-like spectrin cytoskeleton network attached to the surface bilayers. The mesh size of the spectrin network is 60-80 nm. The spectrin network is anchored to the phospholipid bilayer via juntional complexes and ankyrin proteins. Junctional complexes and ankyrin proteins can diffuse in the lipid membrane.

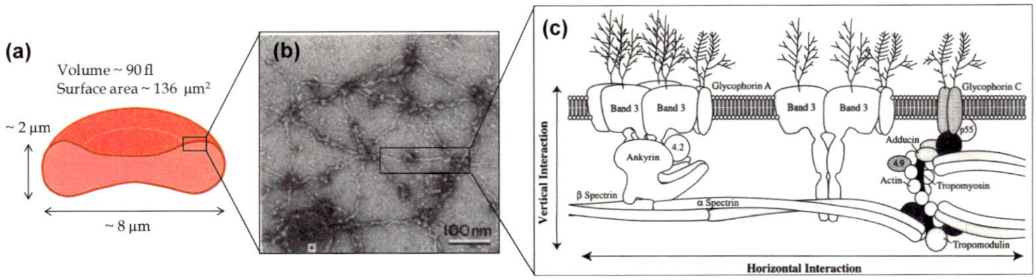

Figure 1. (a) RBC morphology. (b) Spectrin network measured by high resolution negative staining electron microscopy. (b) Schematic model of the red cell membrane. Reproduced, with permission, from (Liu, Derick et al.,1987; Tse and Lux,1999).

2.3. Viscoelastic properties of RBC

In a view of classical mechanics, soft biomaterials can be characterized by viscoelastic properties - exhibiting both energy-storing elastic and energy-dissipating viscous characteristics. RBC is a typical soft biomaterial showing unique viscoelastic properties (Hochmuth and Waugh,1987).

2.3.1. *Elastic property*

Elastic property chracterizes deformability of a material when a force is applied. Since RBC cytoplasm mainly consists of Hb solution, the elastic properties of RBC is determined by RBC membrane cortex structures. RBC membranes are only a few molecules thick, and they can be treated with a 2-D continuum model. Although the deformation of RBC membrane is highly complex, it can be simply explained by three fundamental deformation modes: area expansion, shear, and bend of the membrane (Fig. 2).

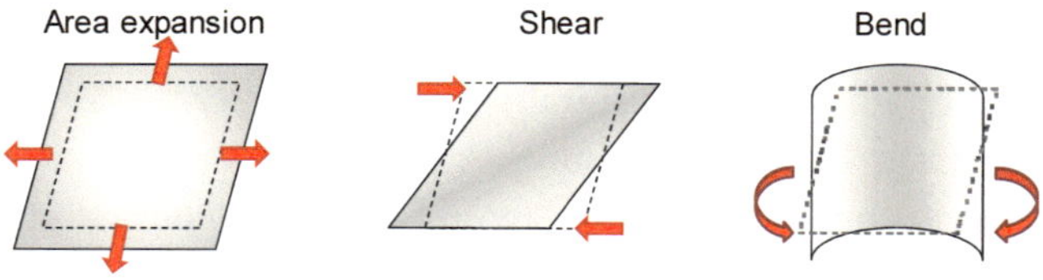

Figure 2. Schematic illustrations of area expansion, shear, and bend modes of a 2-D membrane.

The elastic property of a 2-D membrane cortex is characterized by three mechanical elastic moduli: area expansion modulus *K*, shear modulus μ, and bending modulus *B*. The detailed explanations for three elastic moduli are described as follow:

Area expansion modulus. The area expansion (or compression) modulus *K* reflects the elastic energy storage produced by an isotropic area dilation or compression of the membrane surface. The area expansion modulus *K* is described as

$$T_t = K\frac{\Delta A}{A_o}, \tag{1}$$

where T_t, A_0, and ΔA correpond to the isotopic tensile force, the original surface area, and the increase in surface area, respectively (Hochmuth and Waugh,1987). The area expansion modulus of RBC membranes is mainly dominated by the elasticity of the bilayer. Interestingly, the lipid bilayer itself is highly inextensible; the stand-alone lipid bilayer area compression modulus was given in the range of 200-300 mN/m (Rawicz, Olbrich et al.,2000). However, RBC membranes exhibit significant area extensibility. There is a wide range of measured values for *K* of RBCs that fall into two groupings. (1) Values reported from micropipette-based studies are in the range of 300-500 mN/m (Evans,1973; Waugh and Evans, 1979). (2) Recently, measurements based on dynamic membrane fluctuations report *K* of RBC membranes in the range of 10-100 μN/m (Gov, Zilman et al.,2003; Betz, Lenz et al., 2009; Park, Best et al.,2010; Park, Best et al.,2011; Byun, Higgins et al., in press). These two techniques sample mechanical responses of the RBC under very different loading conditions and they involve different components of the cell; micropipette-based studies mainly probes lipid-bilayer dominated behavior while membrane fluctuation measurements primarily analyze spectrin network dominated behavior. In addition, the area expansion modulus *K* of RBC membranes can be changed by temperature; the micropipette asiperation techniques measured *K* at 25 °C is 450 mN/m and the temperature dependency of *K* was found to be -6 mN/m°C. (Waugh and Evans,1979).

Shear modulus. The shear modulus μ of a 2-D structure reflects the elastic energy storage associated with extension of the membrane surface with the same membrane area. The shear modulus μ is described as

$$T_s = \frac{\mu}{2}\left(\lambda^2 - \lambda^{-2}\right), \tag{2}$$

where T_s is the shear force and λ is the the extension ratio (Evans,1973). Shear modulus of lipid bilayers is essentially zero due to its fluidity nature; shear modulus of RBC is mainly contributed from the spectrin network. The shear moduli of RBC membranes have been extensively measured by micropipette aspiration; the values for μ are in the range of 6-10 μ N/m (Evans and La Celle,1975; Chien, Sung et al.,1978; Waugh and Evans,1979; Evans, Mohandas et al.,1984). Techniques based on optial tweezers (Lenormand, Hénon et al.,2001; Dao, Lim et al.,2003), magnetic twisting cytometry (Puig-de-Morales-Marinkovic, Turner et al., 2007), and dynamic membrane fluctuation measurements (Park, Best et al.,2010; Park, Best et al.,2011) have also reported consistent values for μ. The shear modulus μ is sensitive to the environment condition of the membrane. The shear modulus decreased as temperature increased from 5 to 45°C (Waugh and Evans,1979). Decreasing pH significantly increase the shear modulus of RBC membranes, but increasing pH above 7.2 does not cause a significant change (Crandall, Critz et al.,1978). More interestingly, bimodal distributions in the values for μ were observed in independently reported data (Lenormand, Hénon et al., 2001; Park, Best et al.,2010), suggesting the nonlinear stiffening of spectrin network (Park, Best et al.,2011). Malaria invasion cause significant increases in shear moduli values (Mills, Diez-Silva et al.,2007).

Bending modulus. Bending modulus (or fluxural modulus) B of a membrane is determined by the energy needed to deform a membrane from its original curvature to some other curvature. The bending modulus B of a 2-D membrane is described as

$$M = B\left(C_1 + C_2 - C_3\right) \tag{3}$$

where M is the bending momemt. C1 and C2 are two principle curvatures, and C3 is the curvature in the stress-free state (Helfrich,1973; Evans,1974). Bending of a 2-D structure involves both area compression and expansion. For a lipid bilayer structure, the bending modulus, area expansion (or compression) modulus, and the thickness of the bilayer are related by B=h2K/4, where h is the bilayer separation distance, and K is the compressibility of the bilayer (Helfrich,1973; Evans,1974). The elastic bending moduli B of lipid bilayer is determined by chemical compositions of the lipids, and there is a broad range of reported bending moduli for lipid bilayers (Boal,2002). The elastic bending moduli B of RBC membranes have been measured with various techniques. The values for the bending modulus measured by micropipette-based studies are in the range of 50 kbT (~ 10-19 Nm) where kb is Boltzmann constant, and T is the temperature (Evans,1983). The bending modulus B of RBCs does not significantly change with temperature (Nash and Meiselman,

1985) or cell Hb concentration for both normal and sickle cells (Evans, Mohandas et al., 1984). The recent experiments (Betz, Lenz et al., 2009; Yoon, Hong et al., 2009) have also measured that the bending modulus of RBCs is of the order of 50 kbT. However, several other techniques have measured lower bending moduli of RBC membranes. Studies based on measurements of RBC membrane fluctuations reported membrane bending moduli in the range of 10 kbT (~ 10-22 J) (Brochard and Lennon,1975; Zilker, Engelhardt et al.,1987; Zilker, Ziegler et al.,1992; Park, Best et al.,2010; Park, Best et al.,2011).

2.3.2. *Viscous property*

While the elasticic property of RBC membranes characterizes its resistance to deformation, the viscous property characterized its resistance to *a rate* of deformation (Hochmuth and Waugh, 1987). The viscous properties of RBC membranes can be determined by 3-D cytoplasmic viscosity and 2-D membrane viscosity.

Cytoplasmic viscosity. The values for the 3-D viscosity of blood plasma and cytosolic Hb solutions are ~ 1 mPa·s and ~ 5 mPa·s, respectively (Cokelet and Meiselman,1968). Cytosolic viscosity depends on the concentration and viscosity of Hb. By measuring the dynamic contour fluctuations of RBC membrane, the cytoplasmic viscosity has been obtained in the range of 2-5 mPa·s (Yoon, Hong et al.,2009). Recently, the dynamic membrane fluctuation measurements retrieved the cytoplasmic visocity of the RBCs at physiological osmotic pressure as 5-6 mPa·s, and the cytosol viscosity increases monotonically from with increasing osmolality (Park, Best et al.,2011).

Membrane viscosity. The major source of viscous dissipation in RBC membranes is the membrane viscosity. During the recovery process after large deformation of RBCs, 2-D membrane viscosity dominates energy dissipation (Evans and Hochmuth,1976). The 2-D viscosity of lipid membranes η_{2D} can be qualitatively related to a 3-D bulk visosity of phospholipid η_{3D} as $\eta_{2D} \sim \eta_{3D} \cdot d$ where d is the thickness of the 2D structure. For a typical lipid bilayer, $\eta_{3D} \sim 10^3$ mPa·s and $d \sim$ 1-10 nm, and thus $\eta_{2D} \sim 10^{-10}$-10^{-9} Ns/m. Reported surface viscosities for lipid bilayers are of the order of 10^{-10}-10^{-9} Ns/m (Waugh,1982; Evans and Yeung,1994). Considering viscous dissipation due to a 2-D membrane viscosity, the modified version of the shear force from Eq. (2) is described as

$$T_s = \frac{\mu}{2}\left(\lambda^2 - \lambda^{-2}\right) + 2\eta_{2D}\frac{\partial \ln \lambda}{\partial t}, \tag{4}$$

where t is time (Evans and Hochmuth,1976). Assuming the RBC membrane follows Kelvin-Voigt model, Eq. (4) can be simply expressed as

$$t_c = \eta_{2D} / \mu. \tag{5}$$

where t_c is the recovery time after large deformation of RBC membranes (Evans and Hochmuth,1976). Typically, t_c ~ 0.06 s at 37°C (Hochmuth, Buxbaum et al.,1980), and thus if

μ ~ 1-10 μN/m, η ~ 0.06 – 0.6 μNs/m. The 2-D surface viscosity of RBC membranes has been measured by several experiments. Tether experiments performed on model membrane systems, where cytoskeleton structure was absent, obtained a resultant upper bound of 5×10^{-3} μN·s/m for η_{2D} (Waugh,1982). The diffusion constant of membrane-bound proteins can be used to calculate the membrane viscosity (Saffman and Delbrück,1975). Using this method, the 2-D membrane viscosity values of RBC membranes have been reported in the range of (0.5-14)x10^{-9} Ns/m with various technqiues including fluorescence photobleaching recovery (Golan and Veatch,1980), fluorescence photo-bleaching technique (Kapitza and Sackmann, 1980), and restriction of the lateral motion of membrane embedded proteins (Tsuji and Ohnishi,1986).

2.4. Mathematical models and simulations

Using mathematical models, the mechanics of the membrane cortex structures has been simulated. Using a worm-like-chain model with surface and bending energy, the force-displancement relations for the spectrin network of RBCs have been described (Discher, Boal et al.,1998; Dubus and Fournier,2006). The viscoelastic properties of the RBC membrane was described using an effective continuum membrane model that simulates a finite-thickess 2-D continuum plane model with in-plane shear modulus and bending modulus (Dao, Lim et al.,2003). Recently developed numerical models accurately describes the complex viscoelastic properties of RBCs deformabilty (Fedosov, Caswell et al.,2010).

3. RBC deformability and blood microcirculation

The RBC deformability can influence blood microcirculation since viscosity and flow can be significantly changed by the viscoelastic properties of RBCs.

3.1. Blood viscosity

Viscosity of liquid characterizes its resistance to flow under certain deforming force, especially shear stress. Under laminar flow conditions where particles move parallel to adjacent neighbors with minimal turbulence, the fluidity is classified by the dependence of viscosity to shear strain or shear stress: (1) Newtonian fluid, if the viscosity is independent of shear stress or shear strain so that shear stress is linearly proportional to shear strain, (2) non-Newtonian fluid whose viscosity either decrease (shear-thinning) or increase (shear-thickening) depending on the changes of shear stress (Merrill,1969).

Blood is non-Newtonian fluid which exhibits shear-thinning behavior. Blood viscosity decreases at high shear stress due to the deformation of RBCs, while it increases at low shear stress because RBCs aggregate with each others and form stacked coin structure, called rouleaux (Shiga, Maeda et al.,1990). For normal blood at 37°C, blood viscosity at high shear rate (100~200 s^{-1}) is measured as 4 ~ 5 cP, while it increases rapidly up to 10 cP as shear stress decreases less than 10 s^{-1} (Rand, Lacombe et al.,1964).

Whole blood is a two-phase liquid consisting of a liquid medium (plasma) and formed elements such as RBCs, white blood cells, and platelets. Thus, its viscosity is mainly determined by (1) viscous properties of plasma, (2) the fraction of RBCs in the blood (hematocrit, normal range is 42 – 47%), and (3) viscoelastic properties of the formed elements.

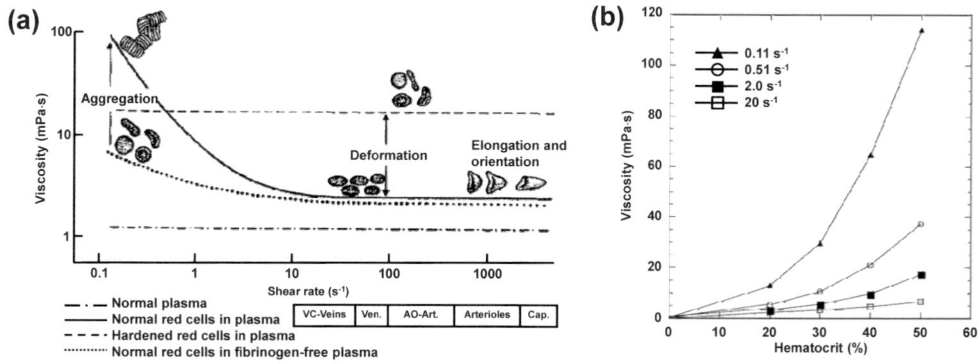

Figure 3. (a) Apparent viscosity of blood as a function of shear rates. (b) Hematocrit effects on blood as a function of shear rates. Modified, with permission, from (Somer and Meiselman,1993; Baskurt,2007)

- Plasma is a Newtonian fluid which viscosity in normal condition varies 1.10 ~ 1.35 cP at 37°C, while the viscosity of pure water is 1.0 cP at 20°C (Lowe, Drummond et al.,1980). Plasma proteins such as fibrinogen are thought to cause RBC aggregation by facilitating binding between RBCs. Elevated levels of fibrinogen concentration in plasma enhance RBC aggregation and thus it increases blood viscosity.
- Formed elements in the stream lines of laminar flow of blood can be considered as the source of turbulence which significantly increases blood viscosity. Among formed elements, RBCs cause the most significant effects since RBCs concentration is the highest among the formed elements in blood. The blood viscosity increases as hematocrit increases; the hematocrit effect becomes more severe when shear stress decreases since more aggregation of RBCs takes place (Dormandy,1970; Baskurt,2007).

3.2. Blood flow in microcirculation

Microcirculation transports blood to the small vessels in the vasculature embedded within organs. The arterial side of vessels in the microcirculation, surrounded by smooth muscle cells, has the inner diameter of ~ 10 – 100 μm. Capillaries, parts of the microcirculation, have only one RBC thick, having the diameter of ~ 5 – 10 μm. Blood flow in microcirculation has low Reynold number and thus it is governed by Stoke's law (Baskurt,2007). Flow dynamics in microcirculation requires deep consideration of (1) fluid dynamics in capillaries, (2) interaction between formed elements with vessel walls, and (3) the structure and network of microvessels. Blood flow in microcirculation is not only determined by the geometric features of blood vessels and hydrostatic blood pressure, but also affected by the rheological properties. RBC deformability can significantly alter blood flow in microcirculation (Chien,

1987). The reduction in RBC deformability under certain physiological or pathological conditions results into the retardation of blood-flow thourgh the microcirculation, which plays important roles in the stages of peripheral vascular insufficiency (Reid, Dormandy et al.,1976); reduced RBC deformability in sickle cell disease and malaria results into occlusions in the microcirculation.

4. Measurement techniques for individual RBCs

4.1. Micropipette aspiration

Micropipette aspiration techniques have been extensively used to measure the mechanical properties of RBC membranes (Evans and La Celle,1975; Shiga, Maeda et al.,1990; Hochmuth, 2000). Micropipette aspiration uses a glass micropipette, having inner diameter of 1~3 μm, to apply negative pressure onto RBC membranes. When negative pressure is applied, RBC membrane is aspirated into the micropipette and the amount of aspiration depends on the viscoelastic properties of cell membrane. Detailed measurement techniques vary depending on the mechanical property of interest (Fig. 4): (1) measuring pressure necessary to aspirate the membrane when the aspirated distance is equal to the radius of the pipette; (2) measuring the ratio between aspirated length of membrane and the radius of the pipette in given pressure; (3) measuring pressure required to aspirate whole RBC inside the micropipette (Evans,1973; Evans and La Celle,1975). The area expansion modulus of RBC membranes can be measured by using micropipette aspiration based on Eq. (1); the measured value for K for normal RBCs at room temperature was 450 mN/m (Evans and Waugh, 1977). In order to measure the shear modulus of RBC membranes, the second method (Fig. 4b) can be used and the shear modulus μ of the RBCs can be related to the aspirated length (or "tongue length") of membrane D_p as,

$$D_p / R_p \sim pR_p / \mu, \tag{6}$$

where R_p is the radius of the micropipette, p is the applied pressure (Evans,1973; Chien, Sung et al.,1978). Using micropipette aspiration, the value for μ was measured as 9±1.7 μN/m (Evans, Mohandas et al.,1984).

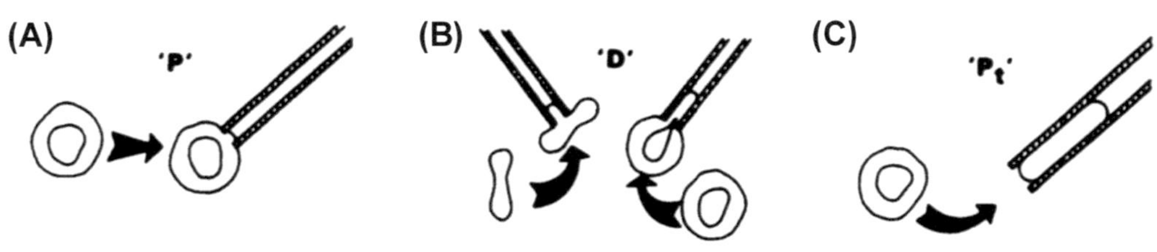

Figure 4. Various methods for micropipette aspiration. (A) Measuring pressure P to aspirate the distance same with the micropipette radius. (B) Measuring the ratio between the aspirated length of membrane D and the micropipette radius at a certain negative pressure. (C) Measuring pressure P_t necessary to aspirate a whole RBC into the pipette. Reproduced, with permission, from (Evans and La Celle,1975)

Micropipette asperation technique can measure the bending elastic modulus B of RBC membranes (Evans,1983; Shiga, Maeda et al.,1990). The value for B depends directly on the magitude of the aspiration pressure when RBCs start to buckle and inversely on the pipette area; measuring negative pressure with varying radius of the pipette can measure B of RBCs. The measured value for B was 43.5 k_BT (Evans,1983). By measuring the time for recovering original shape from releasing negative pressure, the 2-D viscosity of RBC membranes can also be obtained by Eq. (5).

4.2. Atomic force microscopy

Atomic force microscopy (AFM) is a tip-scanning technique that images topographies of materials in atomic or molecular scale (Binnig, Quate et al.,1986). It uses a cantilever with a sharp tip as a probe. Depending on the amount of force to apply or sensitivity, diverse tip shapes are used such as triangular, parabolic, or cylindrical shapes (Weisenhorn, Khorsandi et al.,1993). As a tip scans over a sample with physical contact, the vertical motion of the tip is monitored by photodiodes which precisely detect small changes in laser beam position reflected from the tip. As shown in Figs. 5a-b, the topographic images of RBCs can be obtained in high spatial resolution; cytoskeleton structure of membrane can even be revealed (Kamruzzahan, Kienberger et al.,2004).

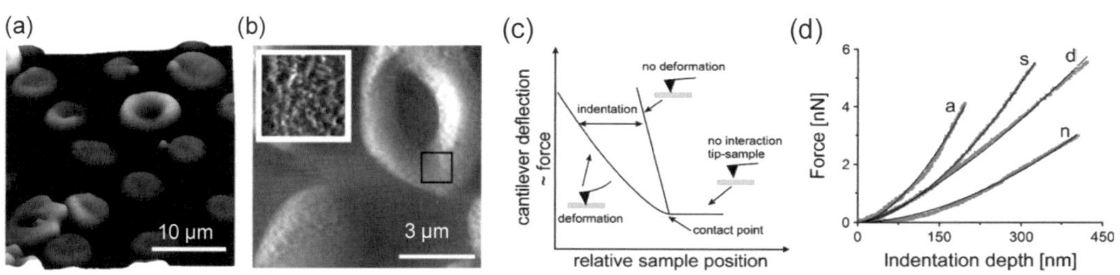

Figure 5. AFM measures RBC topography and deformability. (A) Topogram of normal RBCs. (B) Detailed texture of the RBC membrane surface. (C) Indentation depth measurement. (D) Different force-versus-indentation depth curves of RBCs in various conditions: a. anisocytosis; s. hereditary spherocytosis; d. G6PD deficiency; and n. normal condition. Reproduced, with permission, from (Kamruzzahan, Kienberger et al.,2004; Dulinska, Targosz et al.,2006)

Since AFM can apply forces to sample surfaces at the nN scales, it can measure mechanical properties of soft materials such as RBCs. The displacement of the stage required for the same deflection of the tip is different between solid- and soft-materials, from which applied forces can be calibrated. For a parabola-shaped or a spherical tip having the radius of curvature R_c, the indentation depth Δz relates an applied force F and a relative Young's modulus E^* (Weisenhorn, Khorsandi et al.,1993):

$$F = \frac{4\sqrt{R_c}}{3} E^* (\Delta z)^{3/2}. \tag{7}$$

The relative Young's modulus E^* is defined as:

$$\frac{1}{E^*} = \frac{1-\gamma_1^2}{E_1} + \frac{1-\gamma_2^2}{E_2} \cong \frac{1-\gamma_1^2}{E_1} \text{ for } E_1 << E_2, \tag{8}$$

where E_1, E_2, γ_1, and γ_2 are the Young's moduli and Poisson ratios for the simple and the tip, respectively. Since typical value of E_2 (~150 GPa for Si_3N_4 tip) is much greater than that of biological samples (1 ~ 100 kPa), the rightmost equation is valid for biological samples (Radmacher,1997). The Poisson ratio is 0.5 for a perfectly incompressible and elastic material deformed elastically; the Poisson ratio of soft tissues varies with 0.490 ~ 0.499 (Fung,1993). Young's moduli of RBCs at various pathophysiological conditions have been measured using AFM. Young's moduli of healthy RBCs have been obtained to be is 4.4 ± 0.6 kPa (Dulinska, Targosz et al.,2006). RBCs from hereditary spherocytosis, thalassemia (Dulinska, Targosz et al.,2006) and diabetes mellitus (Fornal, Lekka et al.,2006), and sickle cell traits (Maciaszek and Lykotrafitis,2011) have measured.

4.3. Optical tweezers

Optical tweezers use highly focused laser beams that transfer linear or angular momentum of light, in order to optically trap µm- and nm-sized dielectric spherical particles (Ashkin, 1970). Light refraction at a sample induces linear momentum change, resulting into trapping forces (Fig. 6). High numerical aperture (NA) objective lens is used to generate a tightly focused optical trap, and its trapping force is governed by the refractive indices of sample and surrounding medium, laser power, and sample size; optical force to trap particles much smaller than laser wavelength can be described by Rayleigh scattering theory, while trapping samples much larger than laser wavelength belongs to Mie scattering regime (Ashkin, Dziedzic et al.,1986; Svoboda and Block,1994). Optical tweezers have been widely used in many fields such as biophysics and soft matter sciences, where manipulation of µm sized particles (e.g. cells or microspheres) with a small force (pN scale) is required (Grier, 2003; Lee and Grier,2007).

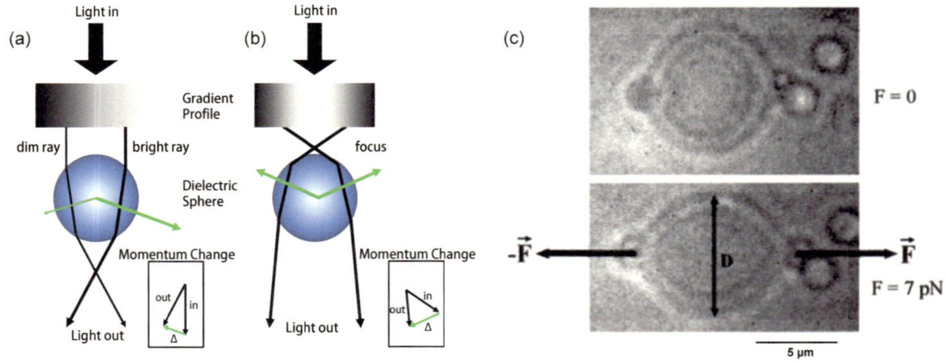

Figure 6. Principles of optical tweezers. (A) Laser beam with gradual intensity transfers linear momentum to a microsphere to escape from the beam center. (B) Focused Gaussian beam exerts trapping force. (c) Deformation of a RBC by exerting various optical forces to microspheres attached on the RBC membrane. The change of diameter *D* in response of optical force *F* is converted to shear modulus of the RBC. Modified, with permission, from (Svoboda and Block,1994; Henon, Lenormand et al.,1999).

Since optical tweezers can apply forces at the pN level, it has been employed for measuring the deformability of RBCs. Measurements of the mechanical properties of RBCs with optical tweezers can be done either by applying optical force to microspheres attached to RBCs (Henon, Lenormand et al.,1999; Dao, Lim et al.,2003) or stretching RBCs by diverging beams from opposite directions (Guck, Ananthakrishnan et al.,2001). In the former approach, two silica beads are attached to the opposite sides of a RBC, then these beads are trapped with a Nd:YAG laser beam (λ = 1064 nm) with maximum power of ~ 605 mW, corresponding maximum optical force is 80 pN (Henon, Lenormand et al.,1999). The change in the projected diameter of the RBC in response of optical force is converted to shear modulus of the RBC using mathematical membrane models. The shear modulus of discotic RBCs were measured as ~ 10 μN/m (Dao, Lim et al.,2003). Using optical twezers system with a high power laser, the shear modulus values of RBCs under large deformation (corresponding to 400 pN) was measured as 11-18 μN/m while initial values were 19-30 μN/m, showing hyperelastic constitutive response (Lim, Dao et al.,2004). Optical stretcher, a variant of optical tweezers, uses two diverging laser beams from opposite directions (Guck, Ananthakrishnan et al.,2001). Linear momentum changes by two laser beams apply stretching force to the RBC along the optical axis, and the RBC deformations under varying optical force are measured from which mechnical properties are retrieved. Optical tweezers can also be used for detecting membrane fluctuation dynamics of RBCs by imposing a deformation (Yoon, Kotar et al.,2011).

4.4. Magnetic twisting cytometry

Magnetic twisting cytometry (MTC) applies both static and oscillating magnetic field to ferromagnetic microbeads attached to the surface of cell membrane (Wang, Butler et al.,1993). Depending on the applied magnetic field, the microbeads exhibit both translational and rotational motion, which applies torques to the cell membrane. The motion of beads is recorded by a CCD camera, and the stiffness G' and loss modulus G'' of the membrane can be obtained by analyzing the displacement of bead in response to applied torque. By varying oscillating frequency (0.1 to 100 Hz) and the magnitude of applied magnetic field (~ 1 - 10 Gauss), the stiffness and loss modulus of RBC membranes are measured at different driving frequencies (Puig-de-Morales-Marinkovic, Turner et al.,2007).

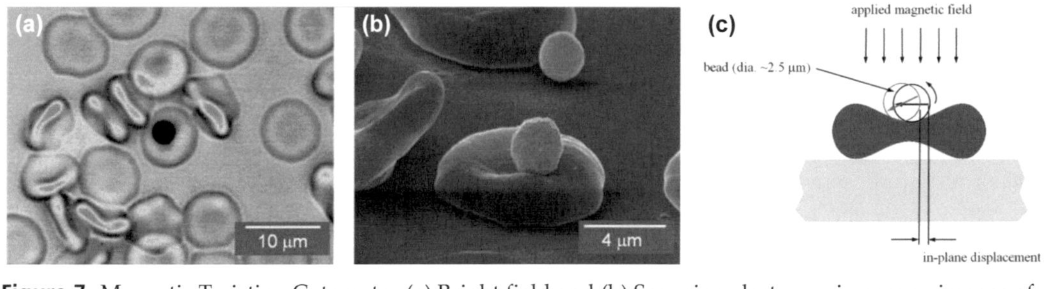

Figure 7. Magnetic Twisting Cytometry (a) Bright field and (b) Scanning electron microscopy images of RBCs with ferromagnetic beads attached. (c) Principles of magnetic twisting cytometry. Reproduced, with permission, from (Puig-de-Morales-Marinkovic, Turner et al.,2007)

The torsional stiffness modulus is independent of frequency, whose value is ~ 10^{-3} Pa/nm at sinusoidal magnetic field of 1 G, while the loss modulus increases as frequency increases; these values correspond to the bending moduli in the range of 0.2 - 0.8 pN·µm and the shear moduli in the range of 6-12 µN/m (Puig-de-Morales-Marinkovic, Turner et al.,2007). MTC technique also revealed dramatic increases in the stiffness of malaria-infected RBC at the febrile temperature (41°C) (Marinkovic, Diez-Silva et al.,2009).

4.5. Quantitative phase imaging

Quantitaitve phase imaging technqiues measure the electric field, i.e. amplitude and phase images whereas conventional brightfield microscopy only images light intensity (Fig. 8) (Popescu, 2011). Employing the principle of laser interference, electric field information of target sample is modulated onto intereferograms recorded by a CCD camera. By using appropriate field retrieval algorithms, the field information can be retrieved from the measured holograms (Debnath and Park, 2011). Typical interferogram and quantitative phase image of a RBC are shown in Fig. 8b-c. Quantitative phase imaging techniques can measuring dynamic membrane fluctuations of RBCs (Popescu, Ikeda et al.,2005; Popescu, Park et al.,2008; Park, Best et al.,2011) as well as cellular dry-mass (Popescu, Park et al.,2008). Dynamic membrane fluctuation, consisting of submicron displacement of the membrane, has a strong correlation with deformability of RBCs and can be altered by biochemical changes in protein level (Waugh and Evans,1979). By measuring membrane fluctuation of RBCs, bending modulus and tension factor of RBCs were calcualated (Popescu, Ikeda et al., 2006).

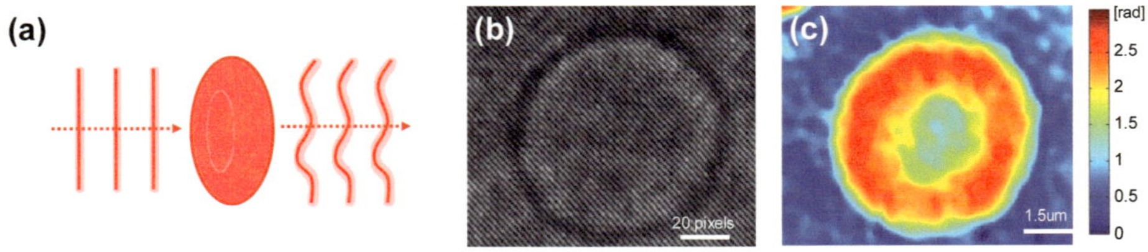

Figure 8. Quantitative phase imaging. (A) Schematic of the principle of quantitative phase imaging. (B) Measured interferogram and (C) retrieved phase image of a RBC using quantitative phase imaging. Reproduced, with permission, from (Park, Best et al.,2011).

Diffraction phase microscopy (DPM), a highly stable technique for quantitative phase imaging, has been widely used for investigating the deformability of RBCs. Employing common-path laser interferometry, DPM provides full-field quantitative phase imaging with unprecedented stability (Park, Popescu et al.,2006; Popescu, Ikeda et al.,2006). DPM measured spatiotemporal coherency in dynamic membrane fluctuations (Popescu, Park et al.,2007), shear modulus for the RBCs invaded with malaria-inducing parasite *Plasmodium falcifarum* (*Pf*-RBCs) (Park, Diez-Silva et al.,2008), and effective viscoelastic properties of RBCs (Wang, Ding et al.,2011). Recently, integrated with a mathematical model, DPM provide the mechanical properties of individual RBCs from membrane fluctuations: shear modulus, bending modulus, area expansion modulus, and cytoplasmic viscosity (Park, Best et al.,2010). Several alterations in the deformability of RBCs have been studied using DPM, including the effects of ATP (Park, Best et al.,2010; Ben-Isaac, Park et al.,2011), the nonlinear behavior of RBC deformability in response to different osmotic pressure (Park, Best et al., 2011), and malaria egress mechanism (Chandramohanadas, Park et al.,2011). Employing spectroscopic quantitative phase imaging, cytoplasmic Hb concentration that is tightly related to the cytoplasmic viscosity, can also be simultaneously quantified (Park, Yamauchi et al.,2009; Jang, Jang et al.,2012). In addition, polarization-sensitive quantitative phase microscopy will be potentially used for the study of sickle cell disease and its implications to RBC deformability (Kim, Jeong et al.,2012).

4.6. Dynamic light scattering

Dyanmic light scattering signals provide rheological information about RBCs (Tishler and Carlson, 1987; Amin, Park et al.,2007). Although dynamic light scattering have been extensively used in combination with ektacytometry, it provides averaged signals from many RBCs. Thus it is difficult to access the deformability of individual RBCs.

Fourier transform light scattering (FTLS) provides both static and dynamic light scattering signal from individual cells. Light field, measured by quantitative phase microscopy or digital holographic microscopy, contains both amplitude and phase information, and thus far-field light scattering pattterns can be directly calculated by numerically propagating the measured field – technically applying Fourier transformation (Ding, Wang et al.,2008). FTLS technique can provide both morphological and rheological information about individual biological cells. By analyzing dynamic light scattering signals measured by FTLS, one can qualitatively access the membrane surface tension and viscosity of individual RBCs (Park, Diez-Silva et al.,2010). Due to its capability of measuring light scattering signals from individual cells with high signal-to-noise ratio, FTLS has been employed to study several pathophysiological effects to the deformabiltiy of RBCs, including malaria infection (Park, Diez-Silva et al.,2010), depletion of ATP (Park, Best-Popescu et al.,2011), and sickle cell disease (Kim, Higgins et al.,2012).

5. Measurement techniques for blood rheology

5.1. Blood viscometer and ektacytometry

Blood viscometer measures the viscosity of blood over a wide range of shear rates. Blood viscometer controls either shear stress or shear rate of blood using rational objects. Stress-controlled blood viscometer applys a constant torque which corresponds to constant rotational speed in a well-designed rotational rheometer. In a rate-controlled system, applied torque is controlled by a stress-sensing device so that a constant rotational speed is achieved. Viscometers can be classified by the cylinder shape: a concentric cylinder, a cone plate, and a parallel plate viscometer (Fig. 9).

Cylinder-type viscometer uses two concentric cylinders: a rotational inner cup and a stationary outer cylinder. Time-independent shear rate can be precisely measured by concentric cylinder viscometer (Nguyen and Boger,1987). Cone and plate viscometer rotates an inverted cone having very shallow angle (~ 5°); the shear rate under the plate is maintained consistently and independent of a flow curve. Parallel plate viscometer is a simplified version of the cone and plate viscometer and has a advantage of flexible space between two parallel plates. The viscous fluid can confined and rotated in narrow space between two circular parallel plates (Gent,1960).

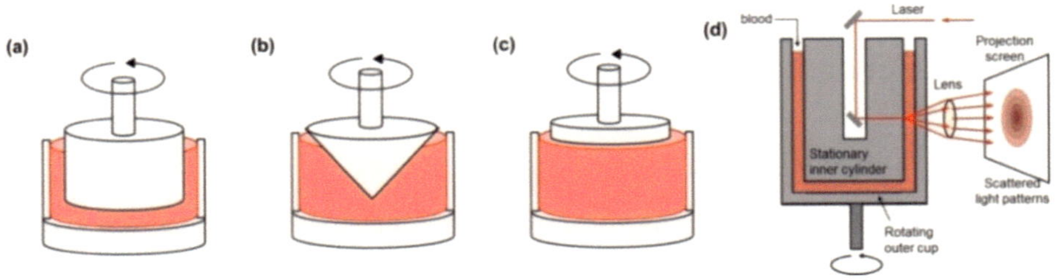

Figure 9. Schematic diagrams of typical viscometers. (a) Concentric cylinder viscometer (or Couette viscometer), (b) cone and plate viscometer, and (c) parallel plate viscometer. (d) Experimental setup of ektacytometer.

Ektacytometer employes a laser diffraction technique with blood viscometer in order to measure RBC deformabiltiy. Conventional blood viscometer applys controlled shear stress to the RBCs in the blood viscometer, and deformability of RBCs can be measured from laser diffraction pattern. Ektacytometer consists of a concentric rotational outer cup and a stationaly inner cylinder; outer cup produces varying shear stress field on blood (Fig. 9d). Through the measurement of diffraction patterns of the laser passing through the blood, RBC deformability can be obtained. The RBC deformation is quantitatively calculated from the scattered laser beam intensity pattern. Under a certain shear rate, isointensity curves in the intensity pattern of the scattered beam will show elliptical shapes, which represent elliptically deformed RBC population (Bessis, Mohandas et al.,1980). From the measured isointensity curves, a deformaion index (DI) of RBCs is calculated as

$$DI = \frac{l-s}{l+s}, \tag{9}$$

where l and s are distances along the long- and short- axes in the elliptical isointensity curves. DI values are measured at different angular velocities (and thus different shear rate) of the outer cyliner in the ektacytometer. Ektacytometer is a simple and effective technique to measure the deformability of RBC population, and it has been widely used for the study pathophysiology of RBCs. Abnormal deformability in RBCs from patients with hereditary pyropoikilocytosis, hereditary spherocytosis, and Hb CC disease were studies by ektacytometer (Mohandas, Clark et al.,1980).

5.2. Microfluidic device technique

Microfluidic device has emerged as a promising tool to precisely control fluids with small volumes of fluid containing samples and reagents in channels with dimensions of 10-100 μm. Microfludic device reduced space, labor, and measurement time on numerous experiments, and also enabled precise control and manipulation of the small volume of samples. Microfludic device has been used to study the deformabiltiy of RBCs. Microfluidic channel with a few micrometer diameter mimics micro-capillary structure in blood circulation system. Rheological behaviors of *Pf*-RBCs were studies in microfludic devices (Shelby, White et al.,2003). Microfludic device was used to induce large deformation of RBCs and its mechanical behavior was studied (Fig. 10) (Li, Lykotrafitis et al.,2007) .

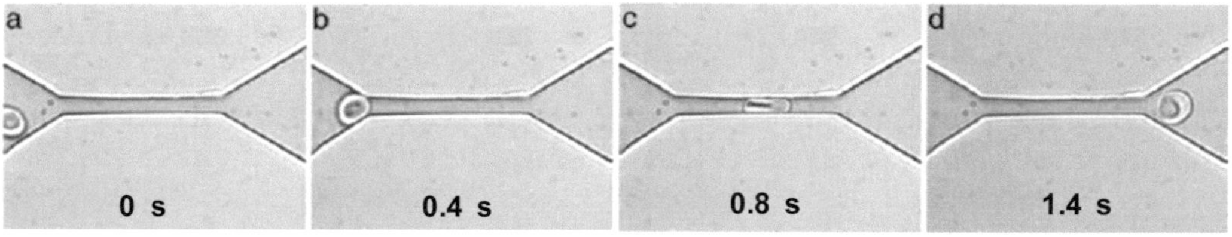

Figure 10. (a-d) Snapshot showing the fluidization of a healthy RBC when it passes through a microfluidic channel. Reproduced, with permission, from (Li, Lykotrafitis et al.,2007).

For the study of sickle cell disease, microfluidic device has been used to measure the resistance change rate of blood flow under the sudden change of oxygen concentration (Wang, Ding et al.,2011). Recently, microfludic channels with obstracles have measured the deformabiltiy of malaria infected RBCs in high throughput (Bow, Pivkin et al.,2011; Diez-Silva, Park et al.,in press).

5.3. Filtration test

Filtration test measures RBC deformabiltiy using a membrane filter with holes of diameter of 3-5 μm (JANDL, SIMMONS et al.,1961). By applying a negative pressure, whole blood is subject to pass through holes in the membrane filter. The deformability of RBCs can affect the speed of flow. RBC deformabiltiy can be calculated from either the flow time or the volume of blood filteres in a certain amount of time (~1 min). Since the filteration test requires for a relatively simple instrument and provides clinically relevant results with high reproducibility, it has been widely used in various studies related to RBC deformability, including the effects of diabetes (Juhan, Buonocore et al.,1982), spesis (Baskurt, Gelmont et al.,1998), sickle cell disease (JANDL, SIMMONS et al.,1961), and oxygen radical (Srour, Bilto et al.,2000).

6. Pathophysiological coditions affecting RBC deformability

Mechanical properties of RBCs is crucial for cell physiology of RBCs. This essential deformability is in turn affected by various physiological and pathological cues.

6.1. Temperature

Temperature plays important roles in RBC deformabilty. The elastic properties of RBC membrane were investigated as function of temperature using the micropipette aspiration technique (Waugh and Evans,1979). Over the temperature range of 2-50°C, both the shear modulus and the area expansion modulus decrease as temperature increased; the changes were -6×10^{-2} μN/m°C and 6×10^{3} μN/m°C, respectively. Due to the structual transitions of proteins occuring at certain critical tempertures, RBC deformabiltiy exhibits complex behaviors. At the transition temperature, RBCs undergo a sudden change from blocking to passing through a micropipette with a diameter of ~ 1 μm (Artmann, Kelemen et al.,1998). Body temperature or febril temperature are particularly important in various pathophysiology of RBCs. Membrane fluctuation measurements using DPM revealed that the shear modulus of *Pf*-RBCs significantly increases as temperature increases from body temperature to febrile temperature whereas healthy RBCs do not show noticible changes (Park, Diez-Silva et al., 2008). MTC study also reported that *Pf*-RBCs becomes significantly stiffened with temperature compared to the healthy RBCs (Marinkovic, Diez-Silva et al.,2009).

6.2. Morphology

RBCs exhibit diverse morphological features depending on pathophysiological conditions (Diez-Silva, Dao et al.,2010). A healthy human RBC shows a smooth and biconcave disc shape (discocyte). However, atypical shapes of RBCs can be found under abnormal pathophysiological conditions, including acanthocyte, stomatocyte, schizocyte, and tear drop cells (Kenneth,2010). Our understanding of what determines RBC morphology and how RBC morphologies are related to the mechanics of RBCs still remains incomplete. One of the hypotheses describing RBC morphology is the bilayer-couple hypothesis (Sheetz and Singer,1974); small changes in the relaxed area difference between two layers of phospholipids. Later, this model can be used for explaning stomatocyte–discocyte–echinocyte morphological transitions (Lim HW, Wortis et al.,2002).

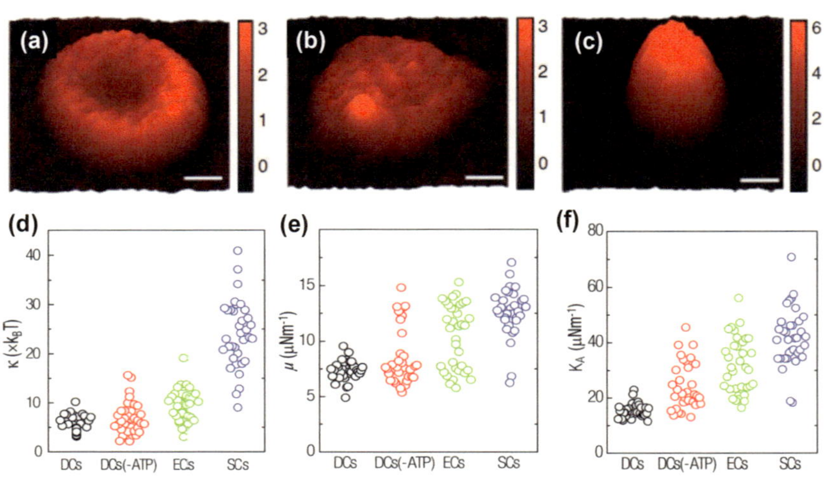

Figure 11. (a-c) Topographies of (a) discocyte, (b) echinocyte, and (c) spherocyte. (d-f) Retrieved mechanical properties: (d) bending modulus κ, (e) shear modulus μ, and (f) area modulus K_A of discocytes (DCs), ATP-depleted discocytes [DCs (-ATP)], echinocytes (ECs), and spherocytes (SCs). Reproduced, with permission, from (Park, Best et al.,2010)

Increased deformability of RBCs in abnormal shapes has been reported with various experimental methods. Ektacytometer measured increased DI values for SCs and ECs that were induced by 2,4-dinitrophenol treatment (Meiselman,1981). Recently, using DPM, the mechanical properteis of RBCs in different morphologies were quantified from dynamic membrane fluctuations (Park, Best et al.,2010). Bending modulus and area expansion modulus of ECs and SCs showed significantly high values compared to normal DCs. The shear moduli values show bimodal distributions (Fig. 11e), suggesting two independent conformations of the spectrin network: a soft configuration ($\mu \sim 7$ μN/m) and a stiff one ($\mu \sim$ 12 μN/m). Aging of RBCs also cause significant morphological alterations: aged RBCs exhibit decreased surface area and volume (Waugh, Narla et al.,1992). The aged RBCs were found by ektacytometry to have decreases shear modulus mainly because of decreased surface area and increased cytoplasmic viscosity.

6.3. Osmotic pressure

Different osmolalities of extracellular medium can bring significant changes in RBC shape and thus deformability. At normal physiological condition (295mOsm/kg), RBCs maintain their biconcave shapes. In hypotonic medium, RBCs are swollen due to water intake. At the osmotic pressure less than 100mOsm/kg, most of RBCs are lysed. In the hypertonic case, RBCs lose its volumes, which result in significant cell shrinkage. Although the total amount of Hb molecules in RBCs, or the mean corpuscular Hb (MCH), does not significantly change at different osmolality, Hb concentration can be considerably changed due to water influx and efflux. RBCs exhibit the maximum deformability at physiological condition; under either hypertonic or hypotonic condition, the deformability of RBCs decreases (Mohandas, Clark et al.,1980).

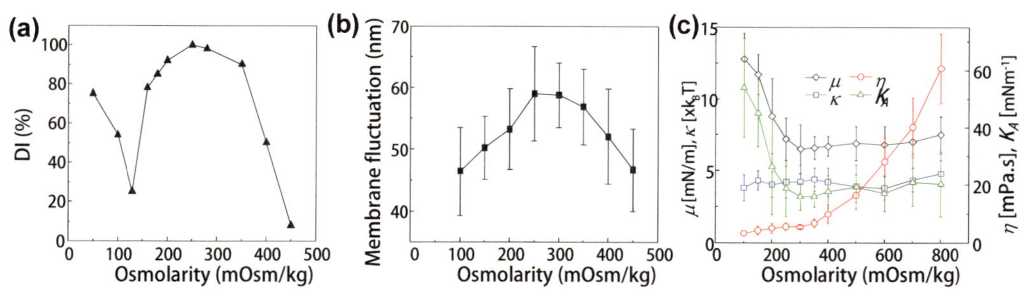

Figure 12. (a) DI of RBCs as a function osmolality, measured by ektacytometer. Modified, with permission, from (Mohandas, Clark et al.,1980). (b) Membrane fluctuations of RBCs as a function of osmotic pressure, measured by DPM. (c) Retrieved mechanical properties of RBCs from membrane fluctuations. 20 individual RBCs were measured at each osmotic pressure. Modified, with permission, from (Park, Best et al.,2011).

A recent study, based on membrane fluctuation measurements, retrieved mechanical properties of RBC membrane under diffferent osmolarities (Park, Best et al.,2011). Although membrane fluctuation or deformability decreases either in hypotonic or hypertonic case; the reasons for the decreased deformability are different. Under hypotonic cases, both shear moduli and area expansion moduli increase, suggesting nonlinear stiffening in streached membrane structure. Under hypertonics cases, other mechanical parameters are not significantly changed except that cytoplasmic viscosity increases.

6.4. ATP effect

The presence of adenosine 5'-triphosphate (ATP) is important in maintaining the biconcave shape of RBCs and also significantly affects the RBC deformability. In the absence of ATP, RBCs loss its biconcave shapes and become flattened echinocytes (Sheetz and Singer,1977). The metabolic state of RBCs, determined by the level of ATP, is crucial for maintaining cellular deformability. When celullar ATP level decreases, the stored RBCs significantly lose the deformability (Weed, LaCelle et al.,1969). Micropipette aspiration technqiue measured mechanical properties of RBCs upon ATP depletion; shear modulus and elastic area compression modulus increase by 17% and 14%, respectively (Meiselman, Evans et al.,1978). Decreased membrane fluctuation in the absence of ATP was first observed by using dark-field microscopy (Tuvia, Levin et al.,1998). Membrane fluctuation measurements studied the effects of ATP to the mechanical properties of RBCs (Betz, Lenz et al.,2009; Park, Best et al.,2010). Analysis on dynamic membrane fluctutions further showed non-Gaussian dynamics in the presence of ATP, suggesting the metabolic remodelling in the lipid membrane and spectrin network structure (Park, Best et al.,2010). ATP-dependent RBC deformability has been also studied using theoretical models (Gov and Safran,2005; Ben-Isaac, Park et al.,2011).

6.5. Malaria: Parasite invasion

Pathogenesis of malaria causes structural and mechanical modifications to the host RBCs. During intra-erythrocytic development, the malaria-inducing parasite exports proteins that interact with the host cell membrane and spectrin cytoskeletal network (Simmons, Woollett et al.,1987). Parasite-exported proteins modify material properties of host RBCs, resulting in altered cell circulation. Despite the genetic and biochemical approaches identified, proteins exported by parasites have remained elusive as well as the mechanism and effect of these proteins on the host cells.

Pf-RBCs exhibits significantly decreased deformability. Microfluidic technique demonstrated the occlusion of small channels by infected RBCs (Shelby, White et al.,2003). Optical tweezers technique measured that membrane shear modulus continuously increases as the disease progesses during the intraerythrocytic cycle (Suresh, Spatz et al.,2005). Employing genetic knock-out assay, the effects of RESA protein to the host RBC deformabiltiy has been studied (Mills, Diez-Silva et al.,2007). Membrane fluctuation measurement also showed increased shear modulus of malaria-invaded RBCs (Park, Diez-Silva et al.,2008). Recently, the loss of deformability in the malaria-invaded RBCs has been simulated using multiscale numerical models (Fedosov, Lei et al.,2011).

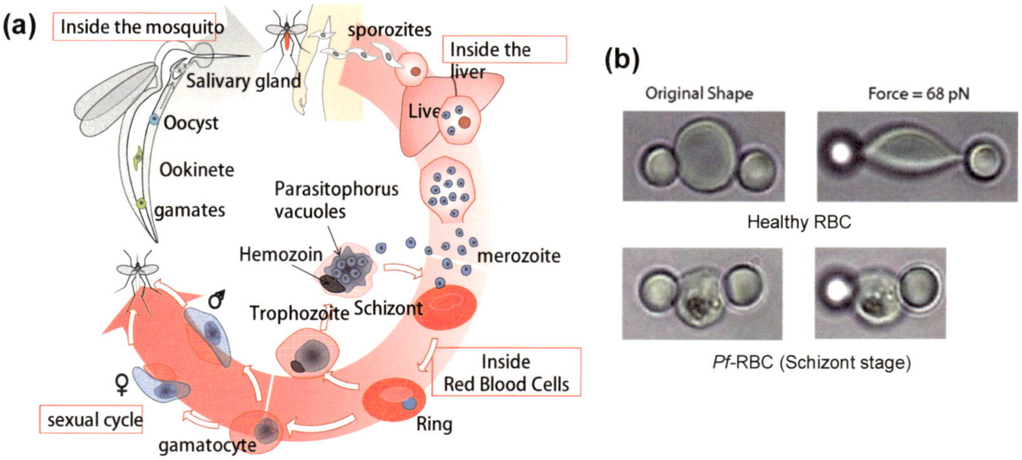

Figure 13. Malaria parasite life cycle in human body. Reproduced, with permission, from (Cho, Kim et al.,2011). (b) Optical images of a healthy RBC and a *Pf*-RBC (schizont stage) stretched by optical tweezers. Reproduced, with permission, from (Suresh, Spatz et al.,2005).

6.6. Genetic diseases: sickle cell disease

Sickle cell disease, characterized by abnormal rheological properties and a sickle-shape of RBCs, is an autosomal recessive inherited blood disorder. A point mutation in β-globin gene encoding Hb results in the production of sickle Hb (HbS) instead of normal Hb (HbA) (Barabino, Platt et al.,2010). Under deoxygenated conditions, HbS molecules becomes self-assembled and grows to fibers inside RBCs up to a few micrometer lengths. Due to these highly stiff HbS fibers, sickle RBCs have elongated- and crescent-shape at deoxygenated conditions and the deformabiltiy of sickle RBCs significantly decreases.

Sickle RBCs have different morphologies depending on its density (Kaul, Fabry et al.,1983; Evans, Mohandas et al.,1984). After repeated sicklings, a fraction of RBCs becomes irreversibly sickled cells and they exhibit the most significant loss in deformability. While Hb concentrations does not affect static rigidity of normal RBCs, static rigidity of sickle RBCs depends on Hb concentration (Evans, Mohandas et al.,1984). Earlier studies using ektacytometry and filteration techniques reported decreased deformability of sickle RBCs even under oxygenated conditions (Chien, Usami et al.,1970; Klug, Lessin et al.,1974).

Quantitative phase microscopy measured decreased membrane fluctuations for sickle RBCs (Shaked, Satterwhite et al.,2011). FTLS showed significantly altered elastic and viscous membrane properties in sickle RBCs (Kim, Higgins et al.,2012). Recently, four important mechanical properties of sickle RBCs were retrieved with memebrane fluctuations measurements (Byun, Higgins et al.,under review). Using AFM technique, decresed deformability was measured in sickle RBCs (Maciaszek, Andemariam et al.,2011). RBCs in sickle cell trait, having only one abnormal allele of the Hb beta gene, also exhibit decreased deformability compared to healthy RBCs (Maciaszek and Lykotrafitis,2011).

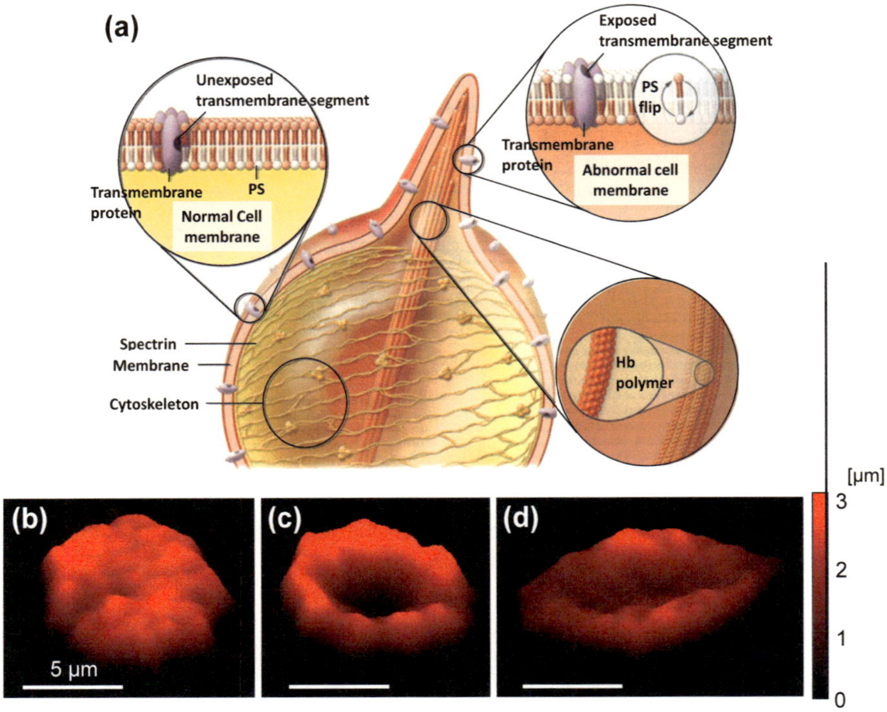

Figure 14. (a) Illustration showing structural modifications inside a sickle RBC. Modified, with permission, from (Barabino, Platt et al.,2010). (b-d) Typical morphologies of sickle RBCs measured by DPM; (b) echinocyte, (c) discocyte, and (d) crescent-shaped irreversibly sickled cell. Reproduced, with permission, from (Kim, Higgins et al.,2012).

6.7. Other conditions altering RBC deformability

There are still many pathophysiological conditions that affect the deformabiltiy of RBCs, which are not covered in the above sections. Several hereditary disorders associated with formation of RBC membrane structures and Hb protein can result into altered RBC deformability. Thalassemias, causing the formation of abnormal Hb molecules due to the limited synthesis of the globin chain, results into loss of RBC deformability. Thalassemia is thus often accompanied by the destruction of a large number of RBCs in spleen, accompanying with the enlargement of spleen. In addition, abnormal Hb molecules in thalassemia often caues the formation of Heinz bodies, inclusions within RBCs composed of denatured Hb, and it causes the local rigidification of RBC membrane (Reinhart, Sung et al., 1986). Ektacytometer study measured that RBCs in hereditary spherocytosis showed markedly diminished deformability while their surface/volume ratio was normal (Nakashima and Beutler,1979). RBCs from the patients with homozygous hereditary elliptocytosis exhibits marked abnormalities in deformability and membrane fragility; these changes are closely related to the reduced levels of band 4.1 proteins (Tchernia, Mohandas et al.,1981). Since band 4.1 plays an important role in the modulation of spectrin-actin interaction, it has been suggested to be closely related to the maintenance of normal membrane shape and deformability. In addition, it will be possible to study RBC deformability in vivo in the near future, by directly imaging and manipulating RBCs through highly scattering skin tissues. Recent works have demonstrated that it is indeed possible to control and suppress multiple light scattering (Vellekoop, Lagendijk et al.,2010; Vellekoop and Aegerter,2010; Mosk, Lagendijk et al.,2012; Park, Park et al.,2012; Park, Park et al.,2012). In diabetes mellitus, RBCs exhibit reduced deformability (McMillan, Utterback et al.,1978), which has been attributed to the changes in lipid composition of the membranes. This impaired RBC deformability in diabetes occurs before significant histological vascular changes (Diamantopoulos, Kittas et al.,2004). RBCs from the patients with diabetes mellitus undergoes substantial alterations in the lipid composition, membrane proteins, and Hb molecules. Saturated fatty acid levels in diabetes mellitus were significantly elevated compared to normal RBCs while the amount of polyunsaturated fatty acids were decreased in diabetes (Prisco, Paniccia et al.,1989).

7. Conclusion and outlook

We have highlighted techniques for studying RBC deformabilty. Due to various deformability test techniques developed in the last years, our understandings on pathophysiology of RBCs have been significantly improved. Recent advances have enabled the precise measurements of various biomechanical properties of RBCs under systemically controlled conditions that mimic complex *in vivo* physiological environments. However, three major technical issues should be resolved in order to bring a much significant impact. First, the molecular mechanisms on RBC deformability should be directly accessed and studied. Employing biochemical assays such as molecular imaging and genetic knock-out methods, the relation between molecule-level changes and cellular-level deformability alterations can be studied. Second, such measurements should be performed at individual cell levels. Profiling mechanical, chemical, and biological properties at the cellular levels and their correlations may allow accessing to unexplored regimes of diseases mechanisms. Third, interactions between cell-to-protein, cell-to-cell, and cell-to-vessel should be considered, since these interactions can be affected and *in turn* modify RBC deformability. As more knowledge is gained about the pathophysiology of RBCs and their circulation through biomechanical studies, the potential for the development of novel diagnostic and treatment strategies for various RBC-related disease will become real and answer to important questions in hematology.

Author details

Youngchan Kim, Kyoohyun Kim and YongKeun Park
Department of Physics, Korea Advanced Institute of Science and Technology, Daejeon, South Korea

Acknowledgement

The authors wish to acknowledge supports from KAIST, KAIST Institute for Optical Science and Technology, Korean Ministry of Education, Science and Technology (MEST) grant No.

2009-0087691 (BRL), and National Research Foundation (NRF) (2011-355-c00039, 2012R1A1A1009082). YKP acknowledges support from TJ ChungAm Foundation. KHK is supported by Global Ph.D. Fellowship from NRF of Korea.

8. References

Amin, M., Y. Park, et al. (2007). "Microrheology of red blood cell membranes using dynamic scattering microscopy." *Opt Express* 15(25): 17001-17009.

Artmann, G., C. Kelemen, et al. (1998). "Temperature transitions of protein properties in human red blood cells." *Biophysical Journal* 75(6): 3179-3183.

Ashkin, A. (1970). "Acceleration and trapping of particles by radiation pressure." *Physical Review Letters* 24(4): 156-159.

Ashkin, A., J. M. Dziedzic, et al. (1986). "Observation of a Single-Beam Gradient Force Optical Trap for Dielectric Particles." *Opt Lett* 11(5): 288-290.

Barabino, G. A., M. O. Platt, et al. (2010). "Sickle cell biomechanics." *Annual review of biomedical engineering* 12: 345-367.

Baskurt, O. K. (2007). *Handbook of hemorheology and hemodynamics*, Ios Pr Inc.

Baskurt, O. K., D. Gelmont, et al. (1998). "Red blood cell deformability in sepsis." *American journal of respiratory and critical care medicine* 157(2): 421-427.

Ben-Isaac, E., Y. K. Park, et al. (2011). "Effective Temperature of Red-Blood-Cell Membrane Fluctuations." *Physical Review Letters* 106(23): 238103.

Bessis, M., N. Mohandas, et al. (1980). "Automated ektacytometry: a new method of measuring red cell deformability and red cell indices." *Blood cells* 6(3): 315.

Betz, T., M. Lenz, et al. (2009). "ATP-dependent mechanics of red blood cells." *Proc. Natl. Acad. Sci. U. S. A.* 106(36): 15312–15317.

Binnig, G., C. F. Quate, et al. (1986). "Atomic force microscope." *Physical Review Letters* 56(9): 930-933.

Boal, D. (2002). *Mechanics of the Cell*, Cambridge Univ Pr.

Bow, H., I. V. Pivkin, et al. (2011). "A microfabricated deformability-based flow cytometer with application to malaria." *Lab on a chip*.

Brochard, F. and J. F. Lennon (1975). "Frequency spectrum of the flicker phenomenon in erythrocytes." *J. Physique* 36: 1035-1047.

Byun, H.-S., J. Higgins, et al. (in press). "Non-invasive measurement of biomechanical properties of individual erythrocytes from sickle cell anemia patients." *Acta Biomat.*

Canham, P. B. (1970). "The minimum energy of bending as a possible explanation of the biconcave shape of the human red blood cell*." *Journal of Theoretical Biology* 26(1): 61-81.

Chandramohanadas, R., Y. K. Park, et al. (2011). "Biophysics of Malarial Parasite Exit from Infected Erythrocytes." *PLoS ONE* 6(6): e20869.

Chien, S. (1987). "Red Cell Deformability and its Relevance to Blood Flow." *Annual. Rev. Physiol.* 49(1): 177-192.

Chien, S., K. Sung, et al. (1978). "Theoretical and experimental studies on viscoelastic properties of erythrocyte membrane." *Biophysical Journal* 24(2): 463-487.

Chien, S., S. Usami, et al. (1970). "Abnormal rheology of oxygenated blood in sickle cell anemia." *Journal of Clinical Investigation* 49(4): 623.

Cho, S., S. Kim, et al. (2011). "Optical imaging techniques for the study of malaria." *Trends in biotechnology* 30(2): 71-79.

Cokelet, G. R. and H. J. Meiselman (1968). "Rheological comparison of hemoglobin solutions and erythrocyte suspensions." *Science* 162(3850): 275-277.

Crandall, E., A. Critz, et al. (1978). "Influence of pH on elastic deformability of the human erythrocyte membrane." *American Journal of Physiology-Cell Physiology* 235(5): C269-C278.

Dao, M., C. Lim, et al. (2003). "Mechanics of the human red blood cell deformed by optical tweezers." *Journal of the Mechanics and Physics of Solids* 51(11-12): 2259-2280.

Debnath, S. K. and Y. Park (2011). "Real-time quantitative phase imaging by spatial phase shifting algorithm." *Optics Letters* 36(23): 4677-4679.

Diamantopoulos, E., C. Kittas, et al. (2004). "Impaired erythrocyte deformability precedes vascular changes in experimental diabetes mellitus." *Hormone and metabolic research* 36(3): 142-147.

Diez-Silva, M., M. Dao, et al. (2010). "Shape and biomechanical characteristics of human red blood cells in health and disease." *MRS bulletin* 35(05): 382-388.

Diez-Silva, M., Y. Park, et al. (in press). "Pf155/RESA protein influences the dynamic microcirculatory behavior of ring-stage Plasmodium falciparum infected red blood cells." *Scientific Reports*.

Ding, H. F., Z. Wang, et al. (2008). "Fourier Transform Light Scattering of Inhomogeneous and Dynamic Structures." *Physical Review Letters* 101(23).

Discher, D. E., D. H. Boal, et al. (1998). "Simulations of the erythrocyte cytoskeleton at large deformation. II. Micropipette aspiration." *Biophys. J.* 75(3): 1584-1597.

Dormandy, J. A. (1970). "Clinical significance of blood viscosity." *Ann R Coll Surg Engl* 47(4): 211-228.

Dubus, C. and J. B. Fournier (2006). "A Gaussian model for the membrane of red blood cells with cytoskeletal defects." *EPL (Europhysics Letters)* 75: 181.

Dulinska, I., M. Targosz, et al. (2006). "Stiffness of normal and pathological erythrocytes studied by means of atomic force microscopy." *Journal of Biochemical and Biophysical Methods* 66(1-3): 1-11.

Evans, E. (1973). "New membrane concept applied to the analysis of fluid shear-and micropipette-deformed red blood cells." *Biophysical Journal* 13(9): 941-954.

Evans, E., N. Mohandas, et al. (1984). "Static and dynamic rigidities of normal and sickle erythrocytes. Major influence of cell hemoglobin concentration." *Journal of Clinical Investigation* 73(2): 477.

Evans, E. and R. Waugh (1977). "Osmotic correction to elastic area compressibility measurements on red cell membrane." *Biophysical Journal* 20(3): 307-313.

Evans, E. and A. Yeung (1994). "Hidden Dynamics in Rapid Changes of Bilayer Shape." *Chemistry and physics of lipids* 73(1-2): 39-56.

Evans, E. A. (1974). "Bending resistance and chemically induced moments in membrane bilayers." *Biophysical Journal* 14(12): 923-931.

Evans, E. A. (1983). "Bending elastic modulus of red blood cell membrane derived from buckling instability in micropipet aspiration tests." *Biophysical Journal* 43(1): 27-30.

Evans, E. A. and R. M. Hochmuth (1976). "Membrane Viscoelasticity." *Biophys J* 16(1): 1-11.

Evans, E. A. and P. L. La Celle (1975). "Intrinsic material properties of the erythrocyte membrane indicated by mechanical analysis of deformation." *Blood* 45(1): 29-43.

Fedosov, D. A., B. Caswell, et al. (2010). "A multiscale red blood cell model with accurate mechanics, rheology, and dynamics." *Biophysical Journal* 98(10): 2215-2225.

Fedosov, D. A., H. Lei, et al. (2011). "Multiscale Modeling of Red Blood Cell Mechanics and Blood Flow in Malaria." *PLoS computational biology* 7(12): e1002270.

Fornal, M., M. Lekka, et al. (2006). "Erythrocyte stiffness in diabetes mellitus studied with atomic force microscope." *Clin Hemorheol Microcirc* 35(1-2): 273-276.

Fung, Y. (1993). *Biomechanics: mechanical properties of living tissues*, Springer.

Gent, A. (1960). "Theory of the parallel plate viscometer." *British Journal of Applied Physics* 11: 85.

Golan, D. E. and W. Veatch (1980). "Lateral Mobility of Band 3 in the Human Erythrocyte Membrane Studied by Fluorescence Photobleaching Recovery: Evidence for Control by Cytoskeletal Interactions." *Proc. Natl. Acad. Sci. U. S. A.* 77(5): 2537-2541.

Gov, N. and S. Safran (2005). "Red blood cell membrane fluctuations and shape controlled by ATP-induced cytoskeletal defects." *Biophysical Journal* 88(3): 1859-1874.

Gov, N., A. G. Zilman, et al. (2003). "Cytoskeleton Confinement and Tension of Red Blood Cell Membranes." *Phys. Rev. Lett.* 90(22): 228101.

Grier, D. G. (2003). "A revolution in optical manipulation." *Nature* 424(6950): 810-816.

Guck, J., R. Ananthakrishnan, et al. (2001). "The optical stretcher: a novel laser tool to micromanipulate cells." *Biophysical Journal* 81(2): 767-784.

Helfrich, W. (1973). "Elastic properties of lipid bilayers: theory and possible experiments." *Z. naturforsch* 28(11): 693-703.

Henon, S., G. Lenormand, et al. (1999). "A new determination of the shear modulus of the human erythrocyte membrane using optical tweezers." *Biophys J* 76(2): 1145-1151.

Hochmuth, R., K. Buxbaum, et al. (1980). "Temperature dependence of the viscoelastic recovery of red cell membrane." *Biophysical Journal* 29(1): 177-182.

Hochmuth, R. and R. Waugh (1987). "Erythrocyte membrane elasticity and viscosity." *Annual review of physiology* 49(1): 209-219.

Hochmuth, R. M. (2000). "Micropipette aspiration of living cells." *J Biomech* 33(1): 15-22.

JANDL, J. H., R. L. SIMMONS, et al. (1961). "Red cell filtration and the pathogenesis of certain hemolytic anemias." *Blood* 18(2): 133-148.

Jang, Y., J. Jang, et al. (2012). "Dynamic spectroscopic phase microscopy for quantifying hemoglobin concentration and dynamic membrane fluctuation in red blood cells." *Optics Express* 20(9): 9673-9681.

Juhan, I., M. Buonocore, et al. (1982). "Abnormalities of erythrocyte deformability and platelet aggregation in insulin-dependent diabetics corrected by insulin in vivo and in vitro." *The Lancet* 319(8271): 535-537.

Kamruzzahan, A. S. M., F. Kienberger, et al. (2004). "Imaging morphological details and pathological differences of red blood cells using tapping-mode AFM." *Biological Chemistry* 385(10): 955-960.

Kapitza, H. G. and E. Sackmann (1980). "Local measurement of lateral motion in erythrocyte membranes by photobleaching technique." *Biochim Biophys Acta* 595(1): 56-64.

Kaul, D. K., M. Fabry, et al. (1983). "Erythrocytes in sickle cell anemia are heterogeneous in their rheological and hemodynamic characteristics." *Journal of Clinical Investigation* 72(1): 22.

Kenneth, K. (2010). *Williams hematology*, McGraw-Hill New York:.

Kim, Y., J. M. Higgins, et al. (2012). "Anisotropic light scattering of individual sickle red blood cells." *Journal of Biomedical Optics* 17: 040501.

Kim, Y., J. Jeong, et al. (2012). "Polarization holographic microscopy for extracting spatio-temporally resolved Jones matrix." *Optics Express* 20(9): 9948-9955.

Klug, P. P., L. S. Lessin, et al. (1974). "Rheological aspects of sickle cell disease." *Archives of Internal Medicine* 133(4): 577.

Lee, S. H. and D. G. Grier (2007). "Holographic microscopy of holographically trapped three-dimensional structures." *Opt. Express* 15(4): 1505-1512.

Lenormand, G., S. Hénon, et al. (2001). "Direct measurement of the area expansion and shear moduli of the human red blood cell membrane skeleton." *Biophysical Journal* 81(1): 43-56.

Li, J., G. Lykotrafitis, et al. (2007). "Cytoskeletal dynamics of human erythrocyte." *Proc. Natl. Acad. Sci. U. S. A.* 104(12): 4937.

Lim, C. T., M. Dao, et al. (2004). "Large deformation of living cells using laser traps." *Acta Materialia* 52(7): 1837-1845.

Lim HW, G., M. Wortis, et al. (2002). "Stomatocyte–discocyte–echinocyte sequence of the human red blood cell: Evidence for the bilayer–couple hypothesis from membrane mechanics." *Proc Natl Acad Sci U S A* 99(26): 16766.

Liu, S. C., L. H. Derick, et al. (1987). "Visualization of the hexagonal lattice in the erythrocyte membrane skeleton." *The Journal of cell biology* 104(3): 527-536.

Lowe, G. D. O., M. M. Drummond, et al. (1980). "Relation between Extent of Coronary-Artery Disease and Blood-Viscosity." *British Medical Journal* 280(6215): 673-674.

Maciaszek, J. L., B. Andemariam, et al. (2011). "Microelasticity of red blood cells in sickle cell disease." *The Journal of Strain Analysis for Engineering Design* 46(5): 368.

Maciaszek, J. L. and G. Lykotrafitis (2011). "Sickle cell trait human erythrocytes are significantly stiffer than normal." *Journal of biomechanics* 44(4): 657-661.

Marinkovic, M., M. Diez-Silva, et al. (2009). "Febrile temperature leads to significant stiffening of Plasmodium falciparum parasitized erythrocytes." *American Journal of Physiology-Cell Physiology* 296(1): C59-C64.

McMillan, D., N. Utterback, et al. (1978). "Reduced erythrocyte deformability in diabetes." *Diabetes* 27(9): 895.

Meiselman, H. J. (1981). "Morphological determinants of red cell deformability." *Scandinavian Journal of Clinical & Laboratory Investigation* 41(S156): 27-34.

Meiselman, H. J., E. A. Evans, et al. (1978). "Membrane mechanical properties of ATP-depleted human erythrocytes." *Blood* 52(3): 499-504.

Merrill, E. W. (1969). "Rheology of blood." *Physiol Rev* 49(4): 863-888.

Mills, J. P., M. Diez-Silva, et al. (2007). "Effect of plasmodial RESA protein on deformability of human red blood cells harboring Plasmodium falciparum." *Proc Natl Acad Sci U S A* 104(22): 9213-9217.

Mohandas, N., M. R. Clark, et al. (1980). "Analysis of factors regulating erythrocyte deformability." *Journal of Clinical Investigation* 66(3): 563.

Mosk, A. P., A. Lagendijk, et al. (2012). "Controlling waves in space and time for imaging and focusing in complex media." *Nature photonics* 6(5): 283-292.

Nakashima, K. and E. Beutler (1979). "Erythrocyte cellular and membrane deformability in hereditary spherocytosis." *Blood* 53(3): 481-485.

Nash, G. and H. Meiselman (1985). "Alteration of red cell membrane viscoelasticity by heat treatment: effect on cell deformability and suspension viscosity." *Biorheology* 22(1): 73.

Nguyen, Q. and D. Boger (1987). "Characterization of yield stress fluids with concentric cylinder viscometers." *Rheologica acta* 26(6): 508-515.

Park, J. H., C. Park, et al. (2012). "Dynamic active wave plate using random nanoparticles." *Optics Express* 20(15): 17010-17016.

Park, J. H., C. H. Park, et al. (2012). "Active spectral filtering through turbid media." *Optics Letters* 37(15): 3261-3263.

Park, Y., C. A. Best, et al. (2010). "Metabolic remodeling of the human red blood cell membrane." *Proc Natl Acad Sci U S A* 107(4): 1289-1294.

Park, Y., M. Diez-Silva, et al. (2010). "Static and dynamic light scattering of healthy and malaria-parasite invaded red blood cells." *Journal of Biomedical Optics* 15(2): 020506.

Park, Y., M. Diez-Silva, et al. (2008). "Refractive index maps and membrane dynamics of human red blood cells parasitized by Plasmodium falciparum." *Proc Natl Acad Sci U S A* 105(37): 13730-13735.

Park, Y., T. Yamauchi, et al. (2009). "Spectroscopic phase microscopy for quantifying hemoglobin concentrations in intact red blood cells." *Optics Letters* 34(23): 3668-3670.

Park, Y. K., C. A. Best-Popescu, et al. (2011). "Light scattering of human red blood cells during metabolic remodeling of the membrane." *Journal of Biomedical Optics* 16: 011013.

Park, Y. K., C. A. Best, et al. (2010). "Measurement of red blood cell mechanics during morphological changes." *Proceedings of the National Academy of Sciences* 107(15): 6731.

Park, Y. K., C. A. Best, et al. (2011). "Measurement of the nonlinear elasticity of red blood cell membranes." *Physical Review E* 83(5): 051925.

Park, Y. K., C. A. Best, et al. (2011). Optical Sensing of Red Blood Cell Dynamics. *Mechanobiology of Cell-cell and Cell-matrix Interactions*, Springer: 279.

Park, Y. K., G. Popescu, et al. (2006). "Diffraction phase and fluorescence microscopy." *Optics Express* 14(18): 8263-8268.

Popescu, G. (2011). *Quantitative Phase Imaging of Cells and Tissues*, McGraw-Hill Professional.

Popescu, G., T. Ikeda, et al. (2005). "Erythrocyte structure and dynamics quantified by Hilbert phase microscopy." *J. Biomed. Opt.* 10: 060503.

Popescu, G., T. Ikeda, et al. (2006). "Diffraction phase microscopy for quantifying cell structure and dynamics." *Optics Letters* 31(6): 775-777.

Popescu, G., T. Ikeda, et al. (2006). "Optical Measurement of Cell Membrane Tension." *Physical Review Letters* 97(21): 218101.

Popescu, G., Y. Park, et al. (2008). "Imaging red blood cell dynamics by quantitative phase microscopy." *Blood Cells, Molecules, and Diseases* 41(1): 10-16.

Popescu, G., Y. Park, et al. (2008). "Optical imaging of cell mass and growth dynamics." *Am. J. Physiol.: Cell Physiol.* 295(2): C538.

Popescu, G., Y. K. Park, et al. (2007). "Coherence properties of red blood cell membrane motions." *Physical Review E* 76(3): 31902.

Prisco, D., R. Paniccia, et al. (1989). "Red blood cell lipid alterations in type II diabetes mellitus." *Thrombosis research* 54(6): 751-758.

Puig-de-Morales-Marinkovic, M., K. T. Turner, et al. (2007). "Viscoelasticity of the human red blood cell." *Am J Physiol Cell Physiol* 293(2): C597-605.

Radmacher, M. (1997). "Measuring the elastic properties of biological samples with the AFM." *Engineering in Medicine and Biology Magazine, IEEE* 16(2): 47-57.

Rand, P. W., E. Lacombe, et al. (1964). "Viscosity of normal human blood under normothermic and hypothermic conditions." *journal of applied physiology* 19(1): 117-122.

Rawicz, W., K. Olbrich, et al. (2000). "Effect of chain length and unsaturation on elasticity of lipid bilayers." *Biophysical Journal* 79(1): 328-339.

Reid, H., J. Dormandy, et al. (1976). "Impaired red cell deformability in peripheral vascular disease." *The Lancet* 307(7961): 666-668.

Reinhart, W. H., L. A. Sung, et al. (1986). "Quantitative Relationship between Heinz Body Formation and Red-Blood-Cell Deformability." *Blood* 68(6): 1376-1383.

Saffman, P. and M. Delbrück (1975). "Brownian motion in biological membranes." *Proceedings of the National Academy of Sciences* 72(8): 3111.

Shaked, N. T., L. L. Satterwhite, et al. (2011). "Quantitative microscopy and nanoscopy of sickle red blood cells performed by wide field digital interferometry." *Journal of Biomedical Optics* 16: 030506.

Sheetz, M. and S. Singer (1977). "On the mechanism of ATP-induced shape changes in human erythrocyte membranes. I. The role of the spectrin complex." *Journal of Cell Biology* 73(3): 638-646.

Sheetz, M. P. and S. Singer (1974). "Biological membranes as bilayer couples. A molecular mechanism of drug-erythrocyte interactions." *Proceedings of the National Academy of Sciences* 71(11): 4457.

Shelby, J. P., J. White, et al. (2003). "A microfluidic model for single-cell capillary obstruction by Plasmodium falciparum infected erythrocytes." *Proc Natl Acad Sci U S A* 100(25): 14618-14622.

Shiga, T., N. Maeda, et al. (1990). "Erythrocyte Rheology." *Critical Reviews in Oncology/Hematology* 10(1): 9-48.

Simmons, D., G. Woollett, et al. (1987). "A malaria protein exported into a new compartment within the host erythrocyte." *EMBO J.* 6(2): 485-491.

Somer, T. and H. J. Meiselman (1993). "Disorders of Blood-Viscosity." *Annals of Medicine* 25(1): 31-39.

Srour, M., Y. Bilto, et al. (2000). "Exposure of human erythrocytes to oxygen radicals causes loss of deformability, increased osmotic fragility, lipid peroxidation and protein degradation." *Clinical hemorheology and microcirculation* 23(1): 13-22.

Suresh, S., J. Spatz, et al. (2005). "Connections between single-cell biomechanics and human disease states: gastrointestinal cancer and malaria." *Acta Biomaterialia* 1(1): 15-30.

Svoboda, K. and S. Block (1994). "Biological applications of optical forces." *ANNUAL REVIEW OF BIOPHYSICS AND BIOMOLECULAR STRUCTURE* 23(1): 247-285.

Tchernia, G., N. Mohandas, et al. (1981). "Deficiency of skeletal membrane protein band 4.1 in homozygous hereditary elliptocytosis. Implications for erythrocyte membrane stability." *Journal of Clinical Investigation* 68(2): 454.

Tishler, R. and F. Carlson (1987). "Quasi-elastic light scattering studies of membrane motion in single red blood cells." *Biophysical Journal* 51(6): 993-997.

Tse, W. T. and S. E. Lux (1999). "Red blood cell membrane disorders." *British journal of haematology* 104(1): 2-13.

Tsuji, A. and S. Ohnishi (1986). "Restriction of the lateral motion of band 3 in the erythrocyte membrane by the cytoskeletal network: dependence on spectrin association state." *Biochemistry* 25(20): 6133-6139.

Tuvia, S., S. Levin, et al. (1998). "Mechanical fluctuations of the membrane-skeleton are dependent on F-actin ATPase in human erythrocytes." *J. Cell Biol.* 141(7): 1551-1561.

Vellekoop, I., A. Lagendijk, et al. (2010). "Exploiting disorder for perfect focusing." *Nature photonics* 4(5): 320-322.

Vellekoop, I. M. and C. M. Aegerter (2010). "Scattered light fluorescence microscopy: imaging through turbid layers." *Opt. Lett* 35(8): 1245-1247.

Wang, N., J. P. Butler, et al. (1993). "Mechanotransduction across the Cell-Surface and through the Cytoskeleton." *Science* 260(5111): 1124-1127.

Wang, R., H. Ding, et al. (2011). "Effective 3D viscoelasticity of red blood cells measured by diffraction phase microscopy." *Biomedical optics express* 2(3): 485-490.

Waugh, R. and E. A. Evans (1979). "Thermoelasticity of red blood cell membrane." *Biophysical Journal* 26(1): 115-131.

Waugh, R. E. (1982). "Surface viscosity measurements from large bilayer vesicle tether formation. II. Experiments." *Biophysical Journal* 38(1): 29-37.

Waugh, R. E., M. Narla, et al. (1992). "Rheologic Properties of Senescent Erythrocytes - Loss of Surface-Area and Volume with Red-Blood-Cell Age." *Blood* 79(5): 1351-1358.

Weed, R. I., P. L. LaCelle, et al. (1969). "Metabolic dependence of red cell deformability." *Journal of Clinical Investigation* 48(5): 795.

Weisenhorn, A. L., M. Khorsandi, et al. (1993). "Deformation and height anomaly of soft surfaces studied with an AFM." *Nanotechnology* 4: 106.

Yoon, Y. Z., H. Hong, et al. (2009). "Flickering analysis of erythrocyte mechanical properties: dependence on oxygenation level, cell shape, and hydration level." *Biophysical Journal* 97(6): 1606-1615.

Yoon, Y. Z., J. Kotar, et al. (2011). "Red blood cell dynamics: from spontaneous fluctuations to non-linear response." *Soft Matter* 7(5): 2042-2051.

Zilker, A., H. Engelhardt, et al. (1987). "Dynamic reflection interference contrast (RIC-) microscopy: a new method to study surface excitations of cells and to measure membrane bending elastic moduli." *Journal De Physique* 48(12): 2139-2151.

Zilker, A., M. Ziegler, et al. (1992). "Spectral analysis of erythrocyte flickering in the 0.3-4 mm^{-1} regime by microinterferometry combined with fast image processing." *Phys. Rev. A* 46(12): 7998-8001.

Chapter 11

Use of Microfluidic Technology for Cell Separation

Hisham Mohamed

Additional information is available at the end of the chapter

http://dx.doi.org/10.5772/50382

1. Introduction

1.1. Motivation for cell sorting

The cell is the basic functional unit within a tissue or an organ. Methods that can be used to probe the cell, so as to understand, or even manipulate its interrelated processes, pathways, and/or overall functioning, are of great scientific and commercial value. Research efforts in molecular biology, biochemistry, and biotechnology over the last two decades have created high demand for efficient, cost-effective, cell enrichment, isolation, and handling methods. Cell studies can be performed on continuously growing cell lines, many of which are commercially available, in tissue culture, or on cells obtained from intact tissues or isolated from blood [1-3].

Mammalian cells are highly heterogeneous in structure, function, and characteristics. However, many types of biochemical, pharmaceutical, and clinical studies, such as immunophenotyping, studies of the cell cycle, cell proliferation, or apoptosis, and other specialized cell analyses require a homogenous population consisting of a single cell type; as the analyte. Only then can the results deemed accurate and specific to the cell type under investigation [4, 5]. Accordingly, techniques to separate cell types in a heterogeneous cell population are of immense practical value. Any such efforts are further complicated when the target cell is rare within a population such as in many cancer and prenatal diagnosis applications. The more stringent the requirements for specific and precise cell separation, the greater the degree of accuracy and reproducibility required in the technology that underlies the separation method [6-8].

Recent progress in microfabrication, technologies developed and utilized by the integrated circuits (ICs) industry, is being exploited to biomedicine, spawning a relatively new field of research that has become known as BioMEMS. Microfabricated devices have already had a broad range of biomedical and biological applications [9, 10]. These devices can be manufactured with a reproducible accuracy of less than 1 micrometer (1/100th the diameter of a human hair). In the last decade, microchips have been used in a huge range of devices and contexts: microscale sensors for surgical instruments, monitoring of physiological activities, drug discovery and delivery, DNA amplification, and electrophoresis, as well as cell sorting, the application discussed in this chapter [11-16].

Microfluidic technology, a subcategory of BioMEMS, is a set of techniques and processes for making devices to precisely control and manipulate fluid in a geometrically small channels; sub- to few hundred- micrometers in size. Microfluidic is multi-disciplinary; developing a device with biological utility requires the integration of knowledge and techniques from the fields of engineering, biology, physics, and chemistry. Such microfabricated devices are used to study biological systems and to generate new insights into how these systems work. Conversely, the biological knowledge gained through micro/nano - scale analyses can lead to further improvements in device design. BioMEMS is a challenging field because the materials, and chemistries, important for biological microfluidics applications are so diverse [17, 18].

The objective of the present chapter is to introduce the principals of cell sorting by microfluidic technology, and to discuss its strengths, current limitations, and current and potential applications, with illustrative examples from the literature and from the author's laboratory.

1.2. Challenges in cell sorting

Cells of different types have characteristic sizes, shapes, densities, and arrays of surface molecules that can be exploited for sorting. For example, red blood cells (RBCs) are the cells responsible for delivering oxygen to the tissues. RBCs have to squeeze through capillaries and therefore are relatively small, approximately 6-8 μm in diameter, and flexible. Mature RBCs are anucleate; the maturing cells lose their nuclei before leaving the bone marrow. Loss of the nucleus leads to cell membrane collapse, conferring the characteristic biconcave shape of RBCs, and giving the cell a greater surface area to volume ratio than of spherical cells. These physical features allow easier movement of oxygen (O_2) and carbon dioxide (CO_2) through the membrane. RBCs are composed mainly of hemoglobin, whose iron atoms temporarily bind O_2 molecules in the lungs, and then release the molecules throughout the body. RBCs have the highest density of any cell type in blood. All of the above characteristics can be used for separation: for example size can be used to separate RBCs since they are smaller and more flexible than white blood cells (WBCs). RBCs' high density causes them to spin down to the bottom of a test tube after density gradient centrifugation. The high iron content gives RBCs intrinsic magnetic properties and can be used for magnetic separation [19].

In other cases, a cell changes its shape or size as a result to a disease or change in function. In sickle-cell disease, a genetic blood disorder, RBCs assume an abnormal, rigid, sickle shape. The change in shape and the increased rigidity of the RBCs lead to obstruction of capillaries, thereby restricting blood flow to organs, causing anemia and other "sickle cell crisis", and decreasing life expectancy. Cancer is a second example of such changes [20]. Malignant tumor cells differ from benign tumor cells in structure, growth rate, invasiveness, and their ability to metastasize. Benign tumor cells grow slowly, pushing neighboring tissues away while staying well encapsulated. In contrast, malignant tumor cells grow rapidly, invade neighboring tissues, and may metastasize [21]. Furthermore, they generally are irregular in shape, and exhibit a more "rugged" or "ruffled" surface appearance than do normal cells [22, 23]. Cancer is detected and diagnosed based on physical changes present in tissues and cells. Nuclear changes such as an increase in size, deformation, and a change in internal organization are among the most universal criteria for detecting malignancy [24-25]. These changes may reflect alterations in the nuclear matrix and the connections of the nuclear matrix to or via the cytoskeleton. Cancer cells modify their morphology, principally by increasing the size of the nucleus, before they become invasive, i.e., in dysplasia and carcinoma *in situ*. The nucleus of a dysplastic cell can be up to four times as large as that of a non-dysplastic cell. Accordingly, light scattering microscopy has been used to distinguish normal, dysplastic, and cancerous epithelial cells in a range of tissues including esophagus, colon, bladder, and oral cavity [26]. However, this technique can only succeed if a sufficient number of cells are available for analysis.

Additionally, most cell types have characteristic complements of surface molecules. Among the most useful for identification is the cluster of differentiation (CD), or cluster of designation. CD molecules have roles in signaling and adhesion processes, and the specific compliments of CD molecules is a determinant of the specific function of the cell. Cell populations are usually denoted by a pattern of "+" or a "-"scorings; indicating the presence or absence of specific CD molecules. For example, a nomenclature of $CD34^{+}$, $CD31^{-}$ denotes a cell that expresses CD34 but not CD31. Use of more than one marker can make the cell selection very specific. However, not all cell types have a known specific surface marker [27].

For some cells such as cancer cells, not many cell-surface markers have been identified. In such a situation, some techniques have used a surface marker directed against surface membrane antigens that are expressed in tissue of origin, which is most often epithelial. Thus, detection of these tissue-specific surface markers in the blood stream is suggesting that cancer cells have detached from the tumor. Some techniques attempting to isolate circulating tumor cells (CTCs) from whole blood have used EpCAM, an epithelial cell adhesion molecule that is overexpressed in epithelial carcinomas such as colon and breast. However, published studies have shown inconsistent frequency of EpCAM expression in breast cancer, from as low as 35% to as high as 100% [28-31]. Thus, EpCAM cannot be considered a CTC specific marker. Additional bio-molecules such as DAPI (nucleic acid stain) and antibodies against cytokeratin (expressed on the epithelial cell membrane) and CD45 (expressed on the majority of hematopoietic cells) must be used if captured cells are to be positively identified as CTC. Therefore a cell with the phenotype $EpCAM^{+}$, $DAPI^{+}$, CK^{+}, and $CD45^{-}$ is considered a CTC.

The number of available cells of interest poses and additional challenge; in some applications such as the isolation of CTCs from cancer patient or fetal nucleated red blood from maternal circulation, only 1-2 cell are available per milliliter (mL) of whole blood. Specificity is problematic for either method, due to the lack of a cell-specific surface marker/antibody to exclusively detect CTCs or fetal cells [32].

Despite great successes, cell sorting techniques are not ideal and therefore remain an active area of research. In addition to sensitivity and specificity requirements, an ideal technique should not be overly labor intensive, should be automated and quantitative, the results should predict clinical outcome, and help the physician personalize therapeutic options. Automating sample preparation and handling would minimize human errors. Integration of preparation, cell sorting, and post processing will lead to more cost-effective instruments, and alleviate the need for trained personnel and infrastructure. Microfluidic technology enables the precise control over the cell microenvironment during separation, scales down the analyses to very small volume of blood, and has the potential for high-throughput to cell separation and analyses.

2. Microfluidic technology

2.1. What microfluidic has to offer?

Microfabrication enables the deposition and etching of thin layers (angstrom to micrometer) of different materials on silicon or glass substrates. These layers can be patterned with accuracy and high resolution, down to the nanometer level using lithography. Lithography is the technique used to transfer a pattern from a mask to the substrate to control the location of the deposition of the next layer or the etching of an existing layer on the substrate.

Microfabricated devices have been used in a broad range of biomedical and biological applications. In the last decade, microchips have been used in microscale sensors for surgical instruments, to monitor physiological activities, in microfluidics applications such as drug discovery and delivery, cell sorting, DNA amplification, electrophoresis, etc. Of relevance to this chapter are the microchips for blood fractionation and cell sorting.

Micromachining consists of a series of robust, well controlled, and well characterized processes that enable the fabrication of microfluidic devices. Such devices can be made cost-effective by the use of any of a wide range of biocompatible polymers or plastics and bulk processing (mass production). The miniaturization of reactions and assays confers many advantages over "macro" scale techniques beyond the obvious reduction in quantities of reagents and materials required per test. The scaling down of volumes results in higher surface to volume ratio: a cube with side length L will scale down by a factor of L^3, while the surface area will scale down by only a factor of L^2. Thus, miniaturization results in higher reactivities, shorter diffusion distances, smaller heat capacities, faster heat exchange, shorter assay times, and better overall process control, as well as the capability to integrate multiple steps and to achieve massive parallelization on-chip. Additionally, microfluidic devices are safer than "macro" platforms due to the smaller chemical quantities used and hence the lower stored energies. A microfluidic device that performs one assay is typically referred to as Lab-on-a-chip, while a device that integrates more than one step is referred to as micro total analysis system (μTAS) [18].

2.2. Introduction to microfabrication

This section will briefly describe the basic concepts in the microfabrication of microfluidic devices. Microfabrication is the already subject of many textbooks and the interested reader can consult one of these for more in-depth details [33, 34]. Microfabrication is the technology developed by ICs industry to make devices and circuits with feature sizes as small as 14 nm in research, and 45 nm in production. Among these are the microprocessors and the electronic components found in computers, smart phones, television sets, and major other electronic products. Microfabrication is also used for MEMS devices (micro-electro mechanical systems), devices that include a movable part and can be used for sensing. The airbag sensor used to deploy an airbag in a vehicle, the pressure sensors inside car tires, and the electronic compass in a smart phone are all examples of MEMS devices that we unknowingly use every day. BioMEMS, microfluidic devices, and μTAS are all microfabricated devices similar to MEMS but customized for biological and chemical applications.

Creation of a a new microfluidic device includes design of the channel(s), fluid inlet(s) and outlet(s), using a CAD (computer-aided design) software. These softwares, such as CoventorWare® [35], ANSYS CFD [36], COMSOL Multiphysics® [37], can be also used for simulation of the various design parameters such as device dimensions, heat transfer, and flow conditions, therefore narrowing the design space range in which optimum performance should be obtained. The pattern of channels is laid out with the CAD software; this is the 2D design of the device. The depth of the channel will be determined by the etching time. The drawings are transferred to a mask, typically a glass or quartz plate (transparent to UV light), covered with chrome. The chrome is etched (removed) where the UV light will expose the photoresist. The mask, similar to a stencil, transfers the pattern to the photoresist. The device is built on a substrate, which is a silicon, glass or quartz wafer, or a regular glass slide. After substrate cleaning, the photoresist, a photosensitive polymer, is applied. Photoresist is dispensed onto the substrate and it is spun at high speed (2000-4000rpm) to create a thin (1-100 micrometer), uniform and smooth layer. The mask is placed in contact with the substrate and exposed to UV lights on a mask aligner. The photoresist is developed in a developer solution specific for it, and is removed from areas exposed to UV light (positive photoresist). The channels can be etched, with substrate material being removed from areas unprotected by the photoresist. Etching can be either wet (using chemicals) or dry (plasma etching). Deep reactive ion etching (DRIE) is a plasma etching technique typically used to achieve deep channels with vertical side walls. Use of DRIE is necessary if the etched substrate will serve as a template for molding devices in polymer such that the polymer mold can be peeled off the substrate. At this stage, the device can be sealed by the bonding of a top piece to the substrate. Top pieces are typically transparent, to permit observation under the microscope. Silicon can be bonded to glass by thermal or anodic bonding technique. Usually, however, microfluidic devices are constructed of polymer. Polymers are more cost effective, transparent, and biocompatible materials, many polymer devices can be molded from one silicon master, this is a key advantage because microfluidics devices are hard to clean and hence, can only be used for one or a few experiments.

Polydimethysiloxane (PDMS), PMMA, polyurethane, and polystyrene are all polymeric materials used for microfluidic devices. PDMS, the most frequently used, comes in the form of two liquid components that are mixed (1:10, w/w) and poured onto the substrate. The PDMS is degassed to remove all air bubbles and ensure that the liquid fills the smallest feature of the mold. PDMS is cured in a 60-80°C oven for 20 to 45 min to solidify. Once solid, it can be peeled off the master substrate. PDMS devices are sealed with glass cover slips to form the channels. Several alternatives to the above described processes exist that can accelerate fabrication. Masks can be printed on transparencies using high-resolution printers; this method is suitable for feature sizes of 100 μm or larger. SU8 is a photoresist that is used to create deep structures for molding eliminating the need for deep etching such as the utilization of DRIE. Utilization of a chrome mask and a well-equipped clean-room facility are necessary for making devices with very small features; sub-micrometer to a few micrometers. The development cycle from concept to prototype can take few weeks. For less fine featured devices, the use of transparencies, polymers, and/or SU8 can be reduce the cost and developmental time to one to few days from concept to prototype [38]. Figure 1a and 1b illustrates the typical processes involved in making channels in silicon and molding devices in PDMS respectively.

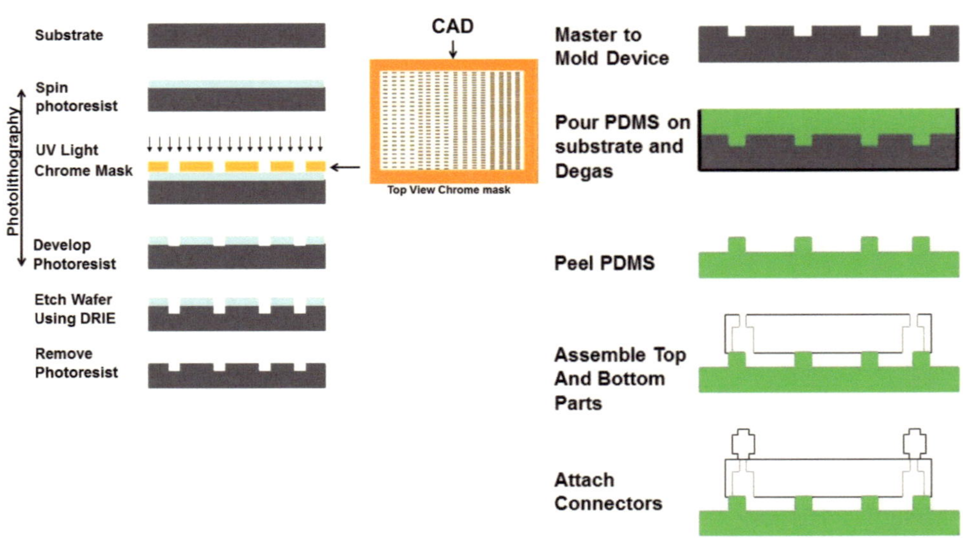

Figure 1. a: Schematic summary of the processes involved in making channel in a hard substaret such as silicon. b: Schematic summary of steps involved in making a PDMS mold from a hard master.

2.3. Types of flow: laminar versus turbulent

Two modes of fluid flow exist: laminar and turbulent. In laminar flow, the fluid moves with slow velocity and each particle of fluid moves in a straight trajectory parallel to the channel walls in the flow direction; and the velocity, pressure, and other flow properties at each point in the fluid remain constant. There are no cross-currents perpendicular to the flow direction, no eddies or swirls of current in laminar flow. Examples are oil flowing slowly through a tube, and blood flowing through a capillary. Turbulent flow in contrast is chaotic, with rapid, spatial and temporal variations of pressure and velocity. Examples of turbulent flow are the blood flow through in arteries, the flow of water through pumps and turbines, and the flow eddying seen in boat wakes and around the wing tips of aircraft [17, 33].

The relative turbulence of a flow can be determined by the dimensionless Reynolds number (Re), which is the ratio of inertial forces to the viscous forces:

$$R_e = \rho v \frac{L}{\mu}$$

Where:

ρ is the density of the fluid (kg/m^3),
V is the mean velocity of the object relative to the fluid (SI units m/s),
L is a characteristic linear dimension, (travelled length of the fluid, and
μ is the dynamic viscosity of the fluid (Pa·s or N·s/m^2 or kg/(m·s)).

Below a certain Re value the flow is laminar; above this threshold the flow becomes turbulent. For macroscopic structures such as pipes with a circular cross-section, the transition from laminar to turbulent flow has been empirically determined at Re of approximately 2300. For most microstructures, in contrast, the Re number is usually low (10^{-1} to 100) thus only laminar flow is relevant for microfluidic devices.

3. Fluid transport process

3.1. Poiseuille flow

A pressure-driven laminar flow inside a tube with a circular cross-section, away from the entrance, is commonly known as *Hagen-Poiseuille* flow or simply *Poiseuille* flow [17, 33]. This flow is governed by the *Navier-Stokes* equations, which are nonlinear, second-order, partial differential equations for describing incompressible fluids. These equations are derived from motion and conservation of mass equations. *Poiseuille* flow is a solution to the *Navier-Stokes* equation, and describes the fluid velocity at any point as a function of the viscosity, pressure, and radius of the tube:

$$V_z = \frac{1}{4\mu}\left(\frac{\partial p}{\partial z}\right)\left(r^2 - R^2\right)$$

Where:

V_z is the velocity distribution,
μ is the fluid viscosity,
(δp/δz) is the z component of the pressure gradient,
R is the distance from the center of the tube, and
R is the radius of the tube.

This equation reveals that the velocity distribution is parabolic, with the maximum velocity occurring at the center of the tube. **Figure 2a**

3.2. Electrokinetic Flow

Electrokinetic flow is the underlying basis of electro-osmosis, electrophoresis, streaming potential, and dielectrophoresis. In electro-osmosis, fluid is made to flow through, by the application of an electric field. The field induces the formation of an electric double layer (EDL). This EDL consists of (1) a compact liquid layer adjacent to the channel surface that has immobile balancing charges, and (2) a second *diffuse* liquid layer, composed of mobile ions. Most solid-liquid, and many liquid-liquid, interfaces have an electrostatic charge, and hence an electric field exists there. In the presence of an electric field, molecules of many dielectric materials, such as the glass or polymer used for making the microfluidic devices, will become permanently polarized, since the material has a dipole that comprises two opposite, but equal, charges, due to the asymmetrical molecular structure. The electrostatic charges on the channel surface, mainly negative charges in the case of glass or polymer, attract counter-ions from the liquid. This attraction creates the channel double layer; the first has immobile charges that balance the charges on the channel surface. The second *diffuse* layer has a higher concentration of counter-ions near the channel surface than does the bulk of the fluid. The net charge density gradually decreases to zero in the bulk liquid. The diffuse layer will move under the electric field. Surrounding molecules are pulled along by a viscous effect, resulting in bulk fluid motion or electro-osmotic flow. The diffuse layer is several nm to 1 or even 2 μm thick, depending on the ionic concentration and electrical properties of the liquid. The *Poisson-Boltzmann* equation describes the ion and potential distribution in the diffuse layer. The electro-osmotic flow velocity can be quantified by Li's equation [39]:

$$V_{av} = E_z \varepsilon_r \varepsilon_o \frac{\zeta}{\mu}$$

Where,

V_{av} is the average elelctro-osmotic flow velocity,
E_z is the applied electric field (V/m),
ε_r is the Dielectric constant of the medium,
ε_o is the permetivity of the vacuum,
ζ is the zeta potential at the shear plane, and

μ is the Viscosity.

This equation reveals that the velocity is linearly proportional to the applied electric field, such that all travel at the same speed inside the channel **Figure 2b**. This situation contrasts with the pressure-driven flow, in which the middle has the greatest velocity resulting, in a parabolic migration.

In conclusion, the velocity distribution being parabolic or flat can impact the microfluidic device performance. The electrokinetic flow is favored in applications such as DNA separation, proteomics, rapid mixing, and time dependent applications where sample homogeneity and reaction time need to be stringently controlled. The flow pattern is typically not an issue for cell separation since it happens in continuous flow without time dependence.

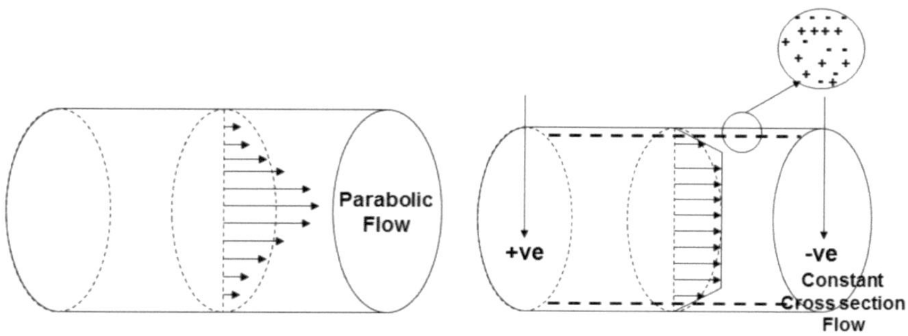

Figure 2. a: schematic of velocity distribution in Poiseuille flow.
b: schematic of velocity distribution in Electro-osmosis flow.

4. Technologies and on-chip mechanisms of separation

Cells are separated either in bulk or individually. In individual cell sorting, each cell is analyzed, and then the cells of choice are individually selected. This technique is rarely used, due to its very low throughput. Thus cells are generally sorted by bulk separation, in which a large number of cells are selected on the basis of shared characteristics such size, density, or the affinity of a receptor for a specific cell-surface target. The result of such bulk separation is enrichment rather than a true purified population [9].

The cells of interest are first identified, than separated, and finally collected. The initial step is to screen the cells of interest to identify one or more common specific characteristics to be used as the basis of sorting. Specific characteristics can be intrinsic such as size, density, response to electrical or magnetic fields, or resistance to chemical lysis. Alternatively, cells can be labeled using a specific cell surface target that binds to a monoclonal antibody conjugated to a fluorophore, or to magnetic particles for flow cytometric cell sorting.

Once the cells of interest have been identified, they can be separated from the other cell types. In some methods, the identification and separation occur simultaneously, e.g., affinity capture.

In other methods such as fluorescence-activated cell sorting, cells are identified on the basis of the presence or absence of one or more fluorescent tags then are then sorted into two or more separate containers. Sorting can either use negative or positive selection. In positive selection, the target cell itself is labeled; in negative selection, it is the background cells or other cells in the solution that are labeled.

4.1. Separation of cells on the basis of affinity

Affinity chromatography or separation of cells on the basis of their affinity is the fractionation of a cell mixture based on the use of specific immunologic targets. One or more of these specific targets are immobilized on a chip surface; there, they capture the cells of interest with high purity (positive selection), or alternatively they capture large number of background cells so as to enrich the remaining sample (negative selection). Microfluidic devices provide a high surface area to volume ratio, which is necessary for chromatography; to keep processing times manageable, many devices can be used in parallel.

Toner's group demonstrated affinity-based separation of cells based on two specific immunologic targets; CD5 and CD19 [40]. Two microfluidic devices were used for affinity separation: a *Hele-Shaw* device and a parallel flow chamber device. The chamber in the *Hele-Shaw* device was 57 μm deep and 50 mm long, and the inlet was 5 mm wide. The device was fabricated using PDMS and sealed with a glass cover slip. The chip surface was treated with silane solution in ethanol, followed by GMBS in ethanol (a water-soluble amine-to-sulfhydryl crosslinker with a short spacer arm), flushed by Neutravidin (strong affinity to biotin) solution in PBS, and incubated overnight. Antibody, anti-CD5 or anti-CD19, solution stocks were diluted in BSA and sodium azide, flowed through the chamber, incubated for 15 min and then flushed with PBS to remove unattached antibodies. Flow experiments were performed with human immature T-lymphoblasts (MOLT-3 cells) and human mature B-lymphocyte (Raji cells). MOLT3 cells, which express CD5 but not CD19, were stained with green cell-tracker dye. Raji cells, which express CD19 but not CD5, were stained with orange cell-tracker dye. Cells were flowed over the coated chip surface with a syringe pump, at flow rate of 30 or 50 μL/min. Flow rates were optimized for efficient capture to allow dynamic cell adhesion, shear stress was minimized in the axial direction permitting sufficient interaction between the cell and the coated surface so that binding can occur. A device coated with anti-CD19 was used to deplete a 50:50 MOLT-3/Raji cell mixture of Raji cells, producing a 100% pure MOLT-3 in less than 3 minutes. Obviously, this level of enrichment is exceptional and cannot be achieved with a heterogeneous ("real world") blood sample. Nevertheless enrichment by 10- to 2000-fold have been obtained using similar devices [41]. Sin and coworkers also used an alternative parallel flow serpentine chamber design, the effective increase in device length was intended to increase the number of cell capture and also to ensure constant shear stress throughout the device. In summary, Sin and coworkers have demonstrated the possibility of using dynamic cell attachment to antibody-coated microfluidic chambers in shear flow to enrich mixtures of MOLT-3 and Raji cells.

To further increase the chip surface area, Toner's group has developed a microfluidic platform "the 'CTC-chip" [42]. This device is composed of a two-dimensional array of round pillars.

These pillars are 100 μm in diameter and 100 μm deep; they are separated by 50 μm and each three rows are shifted from the previous three rows by 50 μm to maximize interaction (Figure 3). The chip was etched in silicon with DRIE to produce smooth straight pillars; the result was 78,000 pillars within a surface of 970mm². The pillars were coated with antibody (EpCAM). The chip is enclosed by a manifold. The group had optimized the flow rate allowing adequate cell-pillar interaction time, and to minimize shear forces, ensuring attachment of maximal number of cells to the pillars. The chip successfully identified CTCs in the peripheral blood of patients with metastatic lung, prostate, pancreatic, breast and colon cancer in 115 of 116 (99%), with a range of 5–1,281 CTCs per mL and approximately 50% purity (Figure 3).

Similarly, Chang and coworkers produced two chips with an array of pillars coated with E-selectin IgG chimera, to test the interaction of HL-60 and U-937 cells with these structures [43]. In one device, the square pillars were separated by 25 μm; each pillar was 25 μm wide by 25 μm long by 40 μm deep. In the second device, pillars were 10 μm wide by 35 μm long by 40 μm deep, and spaced 30 μm apart. In this second device each row of pillars was offset from the previous one by 15 μm so as to allow more cells to ne interrogated. Devices were fabricated in silicon by DRIE and were sealed with thin pyrex glass using anodic bonding. In the first device, HL-60 cells were enriched 400 fold over to the original concentration, while the second device achieved only 260-fold enrichment. Offsetting the pillars on the second device had been expected to improve the cell capture, however smaller size resulted in the flow being faster in the channels, thereby increasing shear stress on the cells and making them less likely to be captured on the surface.

It is possible to further increase cell surface interaction if the cells passed through a packed bed of antibody-conjugated beads. However, such a design is no longer attractive since cell crossing takes as long as 2 hr due to the retardation of the flow rate [44].

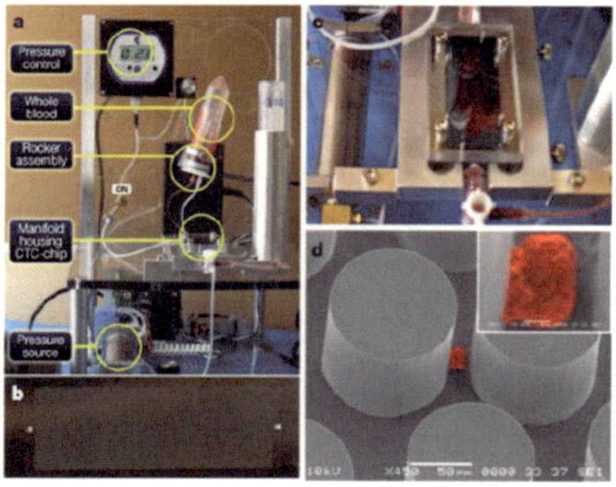

Figure 3. Isolation of CTCs from whole blood using a microfluidic device a, The workstation setup for CTC separation. The sample is continually mixed on a rocker, and pumped through the chip using a pneumatic-pressure-regulated pump. b, The CTC-chip with microposts etched in silicon. c, Whole blood flowing through the microfluidic device.d, Scanning electron microscope image of a captured NCI-H1650 lung cancer cell spiked into blood (pseudo coloured red). The inset shows a high magnification view of the cell (Reprinted with permission from Nature Publishing Group).

Malmstadt and coworkers developed an innovative approach that could benefit from the increased bed of beads area while avoiding its limitation [45]. The group used beads that were modified twice: (i) with the affinity moiety biotin, which binds streptavidin to function as chromatographic affinity separation matrix, (ii) with the temperature-sensitive polymer poly(N-isopropylacrylamide). At room temperature, a suspension of these beads flows through the channel. When the temperature is raised above a certain threshold, the beads aggregate. The sample is then introduced and the beads remain stable during sample flow, and the device functions as a chromatography affinity matrix. The temperature is then lowered below the threshold to allow the beads to dissolve and elute from the channel.

4.2. Separation of cells by flow cytometry

Flow cytometry is a technique that uses light scattering to measure various physicochemical characteristics of suspended cells. Cells are stained and then confined to flow in a single file through a fluidic system. The stream of cells passes at high speed through a focused laser beam. Light scattering and fluorescence data are collected from the individual cells and analyzed. A laser of one wavelength such as blue can be used for excitation; the instrument records fluorescence at multiple wavelengths such as red, orange, and green, in addition to the blue light scattering in the forward direction and right angle to the laser beam. This information is processed by a computer attached to the cell analytical instrumentation. Alternatively, flow cytometers can be equipped to sort cells of interest based on scattering properties, by use of an electric field, flow switching, or optical trapping.

The first key aspect of flow cytometry is the focusing of the cells in a single file so they can be individually interrogated by the optical detection system. This step is usually achieved by hydrodynamic focusing [46, 47]. A sheath flow surrounds the samples from both sides; the flow rate can be adjusted to make the middle stream as thin as required to carry cells in a single file **(Figure 4).** This also reduces cellular aggregation that can clog the device. Microfabricated channel structures are capable of stably delivering samples to a detection area with higher accuracy and better flow control than are glass capillary-based fluidic systems used in conventional flow cytometric equipment; this superior performance is a function of the small channel dimensions possible in microfluidics. The hydrodynamic focusing typically constrains the cells on both sides, but not in the z direction [48].

Miyake and coworkers have developed a multilayered sheath flow chamber that can generate a three-dimensionally focused narrow stream. The channel system was formed by the lamination of five separate silicon and glass plates; defining the three-dimensional geometry of a sample injection nozzle and a detection microchannel. A simpler, albeit less flexible or programmable, approach would be to use a shallow channel that confined the cells in the z direction to remain within the analysis window [49].

Sheath liquid-based hydrodynamic focusing, while being the standard technology in microfabricated flow cytometers, require continuous pumping of a large volume of sheath liquid at a high flow rate to pinch the middle stream down to single-cell width. Sheath liquid volume required can be up to 1000 time the sample volume. New types of microfluidic systems have been developed to minimize or eliminate the sheath liquid requirements and to further miniaturize flow cytometry. Huh and coworkers demonstrated the use of ambient air as an alternative sheath fluid in a disposable air–liquid two-phase microfluidic system [50]. The system produces a thin (>100 μm) liquid stream transporting cells focused by air-sheath flows in a rectangular microfluidic channel. To achieve this focusing, the authors had to conduct a detailed study of the PDMS surface wettability, and of the flow conditions so as to overcome the two-phase (air-liquid) instabilities.

In a contrasting approach, a V-shaped groove device was developed by Altendorf and coworkers to transport blood cells in a single file. The groove microchannel was fabricated by anisotropic wet etching of silicon [51]. The top of the groove was 20–25 μm, wide and the constriction channel geometry allowed the generation of a single-file stream of blood cells moving through the channel without the need for sheath fluid. Light scattering caused by the flow of the individual blood cell through the device was measured by optics based on a photomultiplier tube, photodiode detector, and laser source. The device was capable of differentiating between various cell populations such as RBCs, platelets, lymphocytes, monocytes and granulocytes, based on the intensity of scattering signals. This study demonstrated the potential utility of such a device for differential counting of blood cells.

The second aspect of a flow sorter system that is pertinent to our discussion is the system capability to sort cells at high speed. The requirement of rapid deflection after the cell has been identified by the optical system, can be achieved through redirection of the flow via high-speed valving or reverse electrokinetic flow, dielectrophoresis, ultrasonic transducer, or optical trapping.

Kruger and coworkers achieved switching by use of pressure-driven flow systems [46]. As a liquid sample stream that was hydrodynamically focused along the center of an input channel approach a junction, a small amount of buffer liquid is injected into or withdrawn from the side stream along a switch channel, causing the focused sample stream to be deflected and to flow into a collection channel.

Fu and coworkers demonstrated the use of electric field to quickly switch the flow from the waste to the collection channel, to isolate a cell of interest [52]. The disposable activated cell sorter consisted of three channels joined at a T shaped junction. Electro-osmotic flow drives cells or particles from the inlet to the junction where the flow is diverted to the waste or collection channels. The diversion is achieved by a switching of the electric field at the T junction to control the flow in a rapid manner. This device does not use sheath flow but rather a small-diameter channel, to constrain the cells in single file. When the fluorescently tagged bacterial cell of interest is detected, the sample stream flowing from an inlet to a waste port is quickly switched by reversed electric field, such that the flow is diverted direction to a collection port, selectively delivering the labeled target particles to a sample collector. Using this fluidic switching-based sorting technique, the authors demonstrated sorting of fluorescent microbeads and *E. coli* cells at a throughput of ~10 beads s−1 and ~20 cells s−1. The device was fabricated by softlithography in PDMS.

Similarly, Oakey and coworkers demonstrated the use of electric field for diverting the flow rather than switching since their device did not have hydrodynamic focusing [53].

Johansson and coworkers developed an ultrasound transducer that was placed in the middle of the channels at the intersection between the waste and collection channels. In the absence of ultrasound wave, cells migrated to the waste channel. When a cell of interest was identified, the transducer produced a radiation force acting on a density interface that caused fluidic movement, and the particles or cells on either side of the fluid interface were displaced in a direction perpendicular to the standing wave direction toward the collection channel [54].

Chun and coworkers demonstrated a polyelectrolytic salt bridge-based electrode, placed across the channel to replace the laser used for cell fluorescence analyses. The salt bridge produced impedance signals in proportional to cell's size to be used as basis for sorting to eliminate the need for the optical system that typically exist off-chip [55].

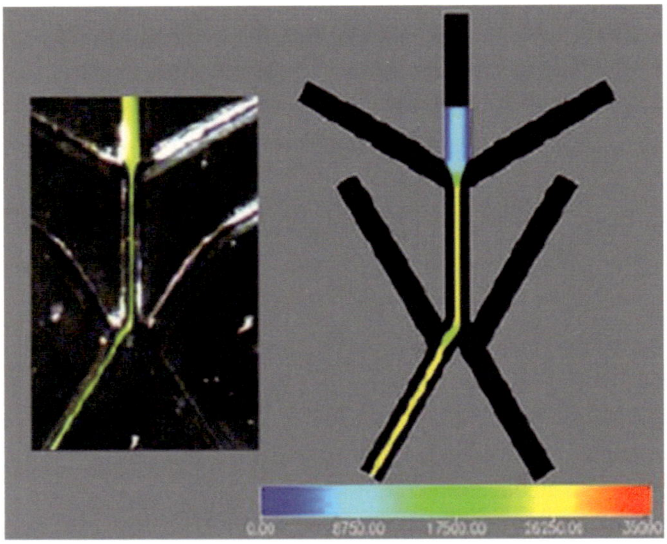

Figure 4. Left: Image of prototype device in operation. Right: Computational modelling of fluid dynamics in a microfluidic cell sorter structure. The performance of this structure was simulated using FlumeCAD (Microcosm Technologies), a finite element modelling (FEM) software package that uses full Navier–Stokes equations. (Printed with permission from Institute of Physics Publishing).

4.3. Separation of cells using immunologic targets

Magnetic separation can be achieved by using the cell's intrinsic magnetic properties or by attachment of a magnetic particle to a specific surface antigen that can later be exposed to a magnetic column for separation. Magnetic particles are typically composed of large numbers of superparamagnetic nanoparticles packed inside micrometer sized sphere made of polymer. The surface of each magnetic bead is then functionalized with antibody specific to an antigen found on the surface of one type of cell. The cells are incubated with the magnetic beads to allow interaction; the magnetic bead attaches specifically to the cell by the antibody-antigen recognition. The cells are transferred to the magnetic column of a separation device. The cells are then manipulated via a magnetic field generated by an internal patterned electromagnet or external macroscopic magnets. The cells attached to the magnetic beads stay on the column, while other cells, not expressing the antigen, and hence not attached to beads, flow through it. With this method, the cells can be separated positively or negatively with respect to the particular antigen(s). Positive selection results in the binding of the cells of interest to the column and they then need to be washed off of the column. In negative selection, the cell of interest do not bind, and are passed through the column enriched [56].

Han and coworkers have exploited the intrinsic differences in the magnetic properties of the RBCs and WBCs without use of magnetic beads, to separate the cell types in a one-stage or three-stage magnetophoretic microseparator [57]. Their single-stage device was able to separate 91% of RBCs out of whole blood; the three-stage device improved on this performance to separate 93.5% of RBCs and 97.4% of WBCs from the whole sample at 5 μL/hr flow rate. Qu and coworkers demonstrated identical separation efficiency [58]. Han's channels were 50 μm deep created by hydrofluoric acid etching of borofloat glass slides. The wire area, included to deform the magnetic field inside the channel and hence generated a high field gradient, was defined using photolithography, and a Ti/Cu/Cr seed layer was deposited by e-beam evaporation, followed by microelectroforming (a process for making thick metal structure) of the ferromagnetic nickel wire. The device was sealed with a second glass slide bythermal bonding. An external magnet provided the magnetic field.

Adams and coworkers developed a multi-target magnetic cell sorter to purify two types of target cells. They simultaneously sorted (i) multiple magnetic tags achieving >90% purity and >5,000-fold enrichment, and (ii) multiple bacterial cell types achieving >90% purity and >500-fold enrichment, with a throughput of 10^9 cells per hour [59]. Their device incorporates microfabricated ferromagnetic strips (MFS) to generate large and reproducible magnetic field gradients within its microchannel and utilizes a multistream laminar flow architecture to accurately control the hydrodynamic forces. This design enables continuous sorting to of multiple target cells into independent spatially addressable outlets with high purity and throughput.

The chip was fabricated in three layers: glass-PDMS-glass. The channel was 50 μm deep and 500 μm wide, and contained two sets of 20-200 nm thick nickel patterns that compose the MFS structures. (Figure 5) The two sets of MFS arrays are aligned at different angles with respect to the flow direction. The result is that two magnetophoretic forces that differ is amplitude and direction, act on the labeled cells. The labels are different in size and magnetization and thus require different forces to deflect them out of the stream of laminar flow. The magnetic field is created with a magnet made of a custom stack of neodymium-iron-boron (NeFeB) and placed underneath the chip.The MT-MACS sorting chip was used to sort two subtypes of *Escherichia coli* MC1061 cells. One type was labeled with label 1 with tag 1 (r = 2.25 μm, M =14 kA/m) and tag 2 (r =1.4μm, M = 30 kA/m), and was fluorescently labeled for observation under a fluorescent microscope. Using 5 mL/hr flow rate, each of the tags was enriched several thousand fold at its respective outlet after a single round of purification. At outlet 1, the population with tag 1 was enriched from 0.020% to 95.876% of the total population corresponding to a 5,000-fold enrichment. The impurities in this fraction consisted of 2.974% tag 2 and 1.150% nontarget beads. Similarly, the population with tag 2 in outlet 2 was enriched 15,000-fold, with contamination of 3.125% target 1 and 6.358% nontarget beads. The waste output consisted almost entirely of nontarget beads (99.997%), and contamination of 0.002% of tag 1 and 0.001% of tag 2.

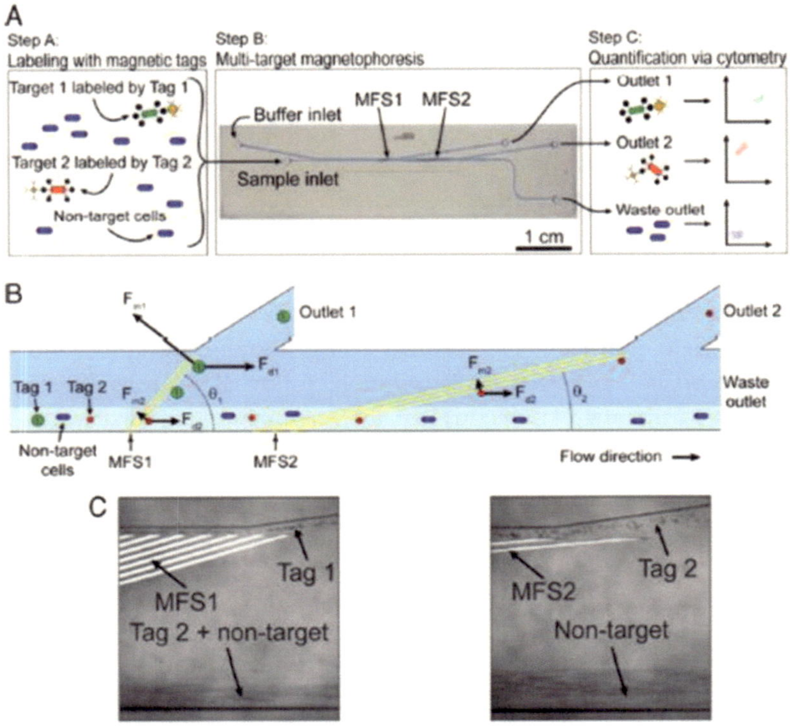

Figure 5. MT-MACS separation architecture. (*A*) (Step A) The sample contains an excess of nontarget cells and 2 different target cells (target 1 and target 2) that are labeled with 2 different magnetic tags (tag 1 and tag 2) by specific surface markers. (Step B) The sample is continuously pumped into the device where the 2 target cell types are sorted into spatially-segregated independent outlets. Separation occurs in 2 regions of high magnetic field gradient generated by the microfabricated ferromagnetic strip (MFS) 1 and MFS 2. (Step C) After sorting, the eluted fractions from each outlet are analyzed via flow cytometry. (*B*) A free-body diagram showing the balance of forces at the MFS structures. At MFS 1 (_1 _ 15°), tag 1-labeled target 1 cells are deflected and elute through outlet
1 because *Fm*1 _ *Fd*1 sin(_1). This is not the case for tag 2-labeled target 2 cells, which are instead deflected at MFS 2 (_2 _ 5°) because *Fm*2 _ *Fd*2 sin(_2), and elute through outlet 2. Nontarget cells are not deflected by either MFS and elute through the waste outlet. (*C*) Optical micrographs (magnification _ 100_) of the tags being separated at the 2 MFS structures at a total flow rate of 47 mL/h (sample _ 5 mL/h, buffer _ 42 mL/h). (*Left*) Tag 1 is deflected by the steep angled MFS 1. (*Right*) Tag 2 is deflected by MFS 2 (Reprinted with permission from PNAS).

Xia, Modak and coworkers used similar have demonstrated similar magnetic cells sorting design with the structure concentrating the magnetic field being adjacent to the flow channel but not exposed to the sample solution [60, 61].

Lee and coworkers demonstrated the use of patterned channels to magnetically manipulate single cell. Lee's device had a matrix of two separate layers of straight gold wires, each addressed independently, aligned perpendicular to each other, and covered with an insulating layer. A magnetic field was created by passing electrical current through the wires creating a programmable magnetic field to control the motion of individual cells in the fluid. Lee's device demonstrated the separation of viable from nonviable yeast cells attached to magnetic beads [62].

Saliba and coworkers demonstrated a 2D array of dots by deposited by microcontact printing of a magnetic ink acting as magnetic traps. Antibody-coated magnetic beads were injected in the channels and were submitted to a Brownian motion in the absence of any field. The application of an external vertical magnetic field induced the antibody-coated magnetic beads to assemble on the patterned dots creating columns [63].

Kose and coworkers demonstrated a novel device to use colloidal suspension of nonfunctionalized magnetic nanoparticles for manipulation and separation of microparticles. It is a size-based separation mediated by angular momentum transfer from magnetically excited ferrofluid particles to microparticles. The nanocytometer is capable of rapidly sorting and focusing two or more species, with up to 99% separation efficiency [64].

4.4. Separation of cells using chemotaxis phenomena

Chemotaxis is the process whereby a single cell, or multicellular organism, moves away or toward a certain chemical. This movement can be away from a poison (chemorepellent or negative chemotaxis) or toward food (chemoattractant or positive chemotaxis). For example, neutrophils leave the blood vessel and migrate toward the smell produced by bacteria in a cut of the skin in an effort to defend the body against infection. The influence of these gradients of molecules and cues cellular behavior in the surrounding microenvironment is an important biomedical focus of study. Chemotaxis, in particular, plays an important role in many biological and physiological processes such as creation of new tissues, wound healing, cancer metastasis, and embryogenesis.

To test a cell response to a certain chemical gradient, the cells are typically placed in a well, and the test substance or chemical is placed in a second well. The two wells are separated by a barrier such as a weir structure (Dunn chamber) or a filter (Boyden chamber), to ensure that the cell movement is due only to the signaling only and not random motion or diffusion.

The development of microfluidic devices for chemotaxis assays was motivated by the need to produce the gradient in a controllable and reproducible manner, and to minimize the quantities of test substance and cells required per assay [65].

Abboodi and coworkers have developed a hydrogel-based microfluidic chip for chemotaxis studies [66]. The device consists of three chambers in this study, the middle chamber is filled with a 3D porous hydrogel structure that contains the cell culture; here fibrosarcoma cell line HT1080 was used as an invasive cancer cell model. First, the left-hand chamber was filled with a cellulose enzyme solution and the right-hand one was filled with cell culture medium containing fetal bovine serum (FBS) (Figure 6). The cellulose enzyme solution diffuses into the hydrogel and degrades it, creating large pores in the structure closer to the left-hand reservoir. Pore size is progressively smaller as the solution migrates toward the right-hand reservoir. The result is that the cells, stained for observation by fluorescence microscopy, moved toward the large pores adjacent to the left-hand reservoir. After 3 days, the FBS –containing medium-FBS in the right-hand reservoir was replaced with pure FBS i.e., full strength chemoattractant. The cellulose enzyme solution in the left-hand reservoir was also replaced with a FBS-containing medium. In response, the cells reversed their motion and moved toward the right-hand reservoir containing the pure FBS, confirming that FBS is a chemoattractant for this cell type. The negative structure of the chambers of this device was fabricated with a 3D printer and a UV-curable polymer. The device was molded in PDMS from the polymer structure and sealed with a glass slide.

Agrawal and coworkers, in an effort to explore the sepsis complications that occur in burn patients, presumably as the result of improper activation of neutrophils, developed an assay on an advanced switching gradient device for monitoring the migration behavior of these cells following thermal injuries [67]. The device (i) integrates the isolation of neutrophils from whole blood, (ii) the provision of a controlled combinatorial chemotactic environment, and (iii) the monitoring of real-time migration of the captured neutrophils over different substrates all on-chip, thereby eliminating the need for preprocessing of the blood. The device was made with PDMS and was fabricated with standardized soft lithographic techniques. In a first trial, the capture was performed by a coating of the microfluidic cell chambers with P-selectin, E-selectin, or fibronectin substrate. A 10 μL drop of blood/heparin solution was loaded in the cell-capture device, and the cells were allowed to settle for 10 min; then flow was initiated (0.5 μL/min) and most of the unwanted cell population was washed away. In experiments repeated in the migration device, captured cells were exposed to a linear chemotactic gradient of the chemokines IL8 and fMLP. Migration patterns for both chemokines over each substrate were recorded with time lapse microscopy and were then compared.

The two chemoattractants, IL8 and FMLP, were used to create a gradient across each binding substrate. Neutrophils over P-selectin reacted similarly for the IL8 and fMLP gradients. However, for E-selectin, average 'y' displacements of 50 μm and 70 μm were observed within 30 min in the gradients of fMLP and IL8 respectively.

For fibronectin, the difference in migration was more significant: the cells migrated about 65 μm in fMLP gradient, but only 35 μm in the IL8 gradient over similar time courses. This system offers an efficient approach to the development of a simple diagnostic tool suitable for a variety of applications in addition to chemotactic studies such as genomic and proteomic analyses.

Chen and coworkers demonstrated a cell migration chip which can monitor chemotaxis at single cell resolution [68]. The chip is composed of weirs that captured individual cells. Once a cell is captured, the hydrodynamic force will push other cells to the next weir through a serpentine channel. A high capture rate over 94% is achieved by optimizing the geometry of capture sites and the length of serpentine structures. After capturing, cell migration experiments induced by chemotaxis were carried out using the fabricated platform, and the behavior of each single cell was successfully traced.

Englert, Walker, and coworkers focused their effort on generating reproducible gradients [69, 70]. Engelrt and coworkers device created reproducible chemoeffector gradients. Two gradients, to simulate competing conditions in nature, were created using a Laminar flow-based diffusive mixing and were tested on Escherichia coli. The sample containing the fluorescently stained Escherichia coli, for observation by microscopy, was introduced in a middle channel. Two side channels introduced the two gradients: quorum-sensing molecule autoinducer-2 (AI-2) and stationary-phase signal indole were introduced, one on each side of the sample. Results showed that the Escherichia coli was attracted by the AI-2 and repelled by the stationary-phase signal indole.

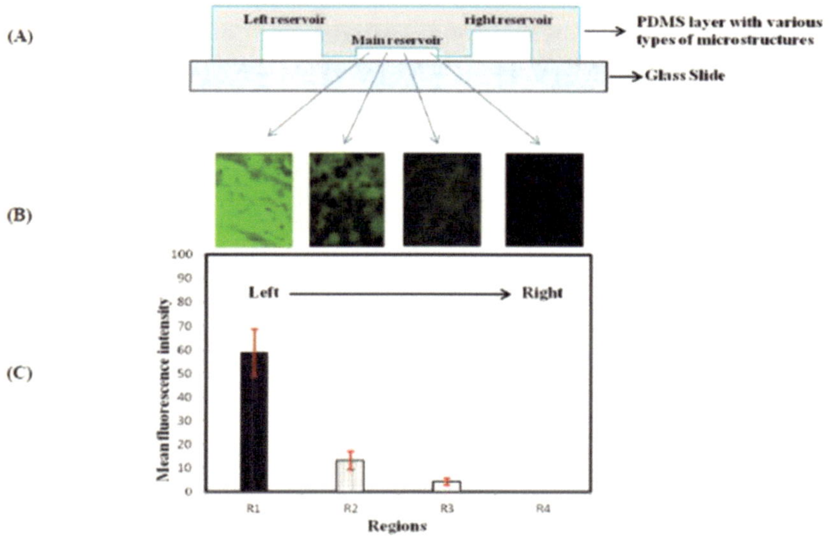

Figure 6. (A) Schematic for the device. (B) Image for each region in the main storage. (C) Average fluorescent intensity of FITC- BSA at four regions from left to right through the porous hydrogel in the main storage ± SD (Reprinted with permission from SPIE and A. Al Abboodi).

4.5. Separation of cells using optical methods and light traping

Optofluidics technology, which is the mating of optical trapping, switching, and microfluidic has been recently introduced as a new manipulation scheme. It has been motivated by its high selectivity, ability to maintain sterility, and how it allowed programmable manipulation of particles or fluids in microenvironments based on optically induced electrokinetics. While optical switching is often used with flow cytometry as the switching or sorting mechanism, it is here presented in a separate section to demonstrate its unique capabilities and potential. Typically, a focused laser beam provides a force to hold or move a microscopic dielectric particle. The dielectric particle is attracted to the strong electric field gradient at the narrowest point of the focused beam. This force is small, in the order of piconewtons, depending on the refractive index mismatch, and can be attractive or repulsive.

MacDonald and coworkers introduced a bow-tie like chip with four reservoirs linked in the middle by a flow channel (Figure 7). The two reservoirs on one side are for buffer (top) and sample (bottom) respectively. The two reservoirs on the other side are for waste (top) and sample collection (bottom). In the absence of any force, the cells migrated from their reservoir to waste, while the buffer passed to the collection reservoir. The two flows shared the channel but no mixing due to laminar conditions. When optical forces were focused on the flow of mixed particles as it passed through the lattice, selected particles were strongly deflected from their original trajectories into the collection reservoir, while others passed straight through, depending upon their sensitivity to the optical potential. The interaction with optical fields provided a selective means of removing material matching specific criteria from an otherwise laminar stream. The optical force was applied by the mean of a five-beam interference pattern created by a 1,070-nm laser beam that passed through a diffractive beam splitter, producing four beams diverging from the central, non-diffracted , in a cross shape. Collimating optics provided a parameter space to independently control the phase and amplitude of each of the five beams before being co-focused through an aspheric lens to produce a large, three-dimensional optical lattice through multibeam interference [71].

Kovac and coworkers introduced a microwell array that is passively loaded with mammalian cells via sedimentation. These cells were inspected using microscopy. After inspection, cells of interest were levitated from the well using a focused infrared laser into a passing stream to the collection reservoir. This is a simple device made of PDMS for the channels and the wells were sealed with glass slide [72].

Shirasaki and coworkers used optics to control a thermoreversible gelation polymer (TGP) as a switching valve. The chip has Y-shaped microchannels with one inlet and two outlets. The sample containing fluorescently labeled cells was mixed with a solution containing the thermoreversible sol-gel polymer. The fluorescently labeled target cells were introduced in the channels and observed using fluorescence microscopy. In the absence of a fluorescence signal, the collection channel was plugged through laser irradiation of the TGP and the specimens were directed to the waste channel. Upon detection of a fluorescence signal from the target cells, the laser beam was then used to plug the waste channel, allowing the fluorescent cells to be channeled into the collection reservoir. The response time of the sol-gel transformation was 3 ms, and a flow switching time of 120 ms was achieved. The TGP did not affect cell viability [73].

Lin and coworkers have demonstrated a microfluidic system based on a computer controlled digital image processing (DIP) technique and optical tweezers for automatic cell recognition and sorting in a continuous flow environment. In this system, the cells are focused electrokinetically into a narrow sample stream and are introduced into the channel where they are recognized and traced in real time. Synchronized control signals generated by the DIP system are then used to actuate a focused IR laser beam to displace the target cells from the main sample stream into a neighboring sheath flow, which carries them to a downstream collection [74].

In summary, Optoelectrofluidic technology, which has been recently introduced as a new manipulation scheme, allows programmable manipulation of particles or fluids in microenvironments based on optically induced electrokinetics. The behavior of particles or fluids can be controlled by inducing or perturbing electric fields on demand in an optical manner, which includes photochemical, photoconductive, and photothermal effects [75, 76].

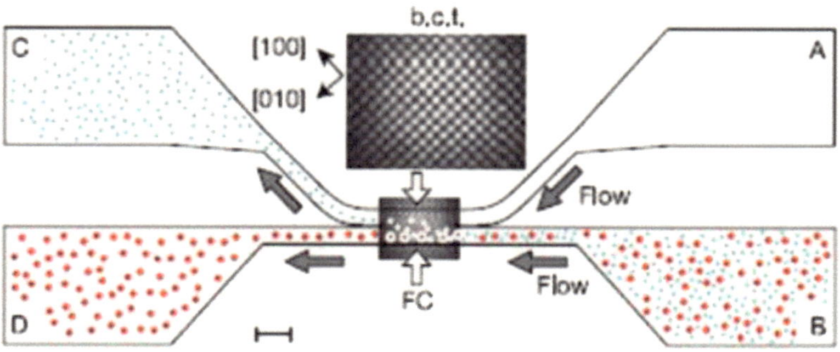

Figure 7. The concept of optical fractionation. Low Reynolds number flows will be laminar: without an actuator all particles from chamber B would flow into chamber D. Chamber A would typically introduce a 'blank' flow stream, although this could be any stream into which the selected particles are to be introduced. By introducing a three-dimensional optical lattice—in this case a body-centred tetragonal (b.c.t.) lattice—into the fractionation chamber (FC), one species of particle is selectively pushed into the upper flow field. The reconfigurability of the optical lattice allows for dynamic updating of selection criteria. For weakly segregated species, the analyte can be either recirculated through the optical lattice or directed through cascaded separation chambers. This latter option also allows the use of multiple selection criteria in a single integrated chip. The flow volume in our current sample cells is 100 mm thick; scale bar, 40 mm (Reprinted with permission from Nature Publishing Group).

4.6. Separation of cells using electrophoresis and dielectrophoresis

Dielectrophoresis (DEP), first described by Pohl in 1951, is a phenomenon in which a force is exerted on a dielectric (insulator that can be polarized) particle when subjected to a non-uniform electric field. This can take place in either direct (DC) or alternating (AC) electric fields. The strength of the force depends on the frequency of the electric field, the medium and particle electrical properties, and the particles size and shape. Varying the field's frequency can manipulate particles with different sizes with great selectivity, which is used for manipulating cells and nanoparticles.

Pommer and coworkers have used DEP phenomenon to separate platelets directly from diluted whole blood in microfluidic channels. Since platelets are the smallest cell type in blood, DEP-activated cell sorter (DACS) was used to perform size based fractionation of blood samples and continuously enrich the platelets [77].

Hu and coworkers used a comparable device to Pommer, but the difference in size-based separation was attributed to the size of the antibody-conjugated beads attached to the target instead of the cell's intrinsic size [78]. Pommer's device is composed of two identical purification stages, in each stage a buffer is introduced in the middle of the channel while the sample is loaded from both sides. The channel electrodes are at angle with the flow forming a funnel shape where the sample flows from the wide to the narrow side. The force exerted by the electric field on the cells has a cubic dependence on the radius ($\propto R^3$) and can be controlled by varying the applied voltage. The hydrodynamic drag force under laminar flow has a linear dependence on the particle radius ($\propto R^1$) and is controlled by varying the flow rate. Therefore, the resulting forces exerted on the cells has a square dependence ($\propto R^2$) and is used to deflect large cells (RBCs and WBCs) into the middle buffer stream to the waste collection reservoir while the platelets remain in the side flow and migrate to the collection reservoir. Post sorting cytometric analysis revealed that a single pass through the two-stage device yields 95% purity of platelets with minimal platelet activation. Two Borosilicate glass wafers were used to fabricate the top and the bottom of the device, the titanium-gold (20nm and 200nm respectively) electrodes were patterned and evaporated using e-beam, a polyimide layer was spun and patterned to form 20μm channel depth between the top and bottom wafer. The two wafers were aligned and bonded using thermal bonding (300°C) then 375°C to cure the ployimide.

Vahey et al have extended DEP to multiple electrodes creating an electric conductivity gradient to separate cells and particles. This is similar to using isoelectric focusing in analytical chemistry and proteomics with the conductivity replacing the pH gradient. Vahey et al have used this device to achieve label-free separation of multiple (>2) subpopulations from a heterogeneous background. The channel was 1mm wide and 20 μm deep molded in PDMS and sealed with pyrex wafer that has the evaporated electrodes. The six electrodes, 200nm gold on top of 10nm titanium (adhesion layer) are 60μm wide, separated by 15 μm, and are patterned at an angle with the flow direction. The electrical gradient was used to separate 1.6, 1.75, and 1.9 μm polystyrene beads from a mixture. Additionally the device was successfully used to separate similar size beads based on surface conductance due to different coating such as COOH modified and unmodified, as well as sorting nonviable from viable cells of the budding yeast Saccharomyces cerevisiae [79].

Lapizco-Encinas et al have used insulator-based (electrodeless) dielectrophoresis (iDEP), in which the nonuniform electric field needed to drive DEP is produced by insulators, avoiding problems associated with the use of electrodes [80]. This channel was 10.2mm long and contained a two dimensional array of 10μm deep pillars etched in borosilicate glass. The channel was thermally bonded with a drilled cover plate for fluid access. Two platinum wires, the only electrodes in the device, were placed in the inlet and outlet reservoirs, producing mean electric fields of up to 200 V/mm across the insulators. The insulator posts disturbed the electric field lines, squeezing them between the pillars. This created higher field strength between the pillars. Cell trapping and release were controlled by modifying the relative responses of electrokinetics and DEP by adjusting the magnitude of the applied voltage. Dead cells had significantly lower dielectrophoretic mobility than live cells but similar electrokinetic mobilities. Therefore, live cells were concentrated between the pillars. Cells were labeled with Syto 9 and propidium iodide for observation through a fluorescent microscope (Figure 8).

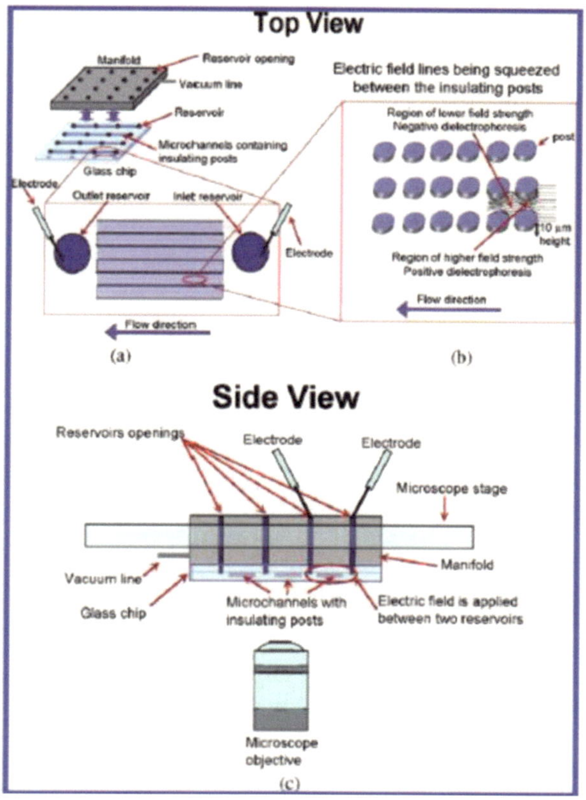

Figure 8. Schematic representation of the experimental setup: (a) top view, showing the manifold, glass chip, an enlargement of the flow microchannels; (b) cartoon showing the electric field lines being squeezed between the insulating posts; (c) side view showing the manifold and glass chip on the microscope stage (Reprinted with permission from ACS Publications).

4.7. Separation of cells by size

Size-based sorting has been our work's focus for a few years; we have successfully demonstrated the separation of WBCs, RBCs, or circulating tumor cells from whole blood, and fetal nucleated red blood cells (fNRBCs) from cord blood. Size- and density-based sorting has been demonstrated in open flow channels by Seki's group using "pinched flow fractionation" [81]. Enrichments up to 20 fold have been accomplished by the chip shown in

Figure 9. The sample is loaded into the 20 μm wide open channel, and a second solution, a buffer, is loaded from a second channel that is 200 μm wide. The buffer pinches the flow width against the channel wall down to 15 μm, forcing the cells to align along the channel wall, before the channel opens to a 350 μm wide area with 12 outlet ports. The separation occurs in the wider channel; the smaller, lower-density cells segregate and are dragged along the channel wall, while the larger, denser cells, tended to sediment earlier in the pinched region and occupy the outer stream that empties to a different outlet port. The device was fabricated by standard photolithographic techniques and was molded in PDMS, from an SU8 master. Wilding's group used weir-like structure to create a 3.5 μm space between the silicon bottom and a glass top of a device to separate WBCs from whole blood, they could then use the cell's DNA for amplification [82-84].

Austin's group has demonstrated cell sorting based on asymmetric bifurcation of a laminar flow around a periodic array of micrometer-scale pillars [85, 86]. Each row of pillars is offset horizontally with respect to the previous row by a fraction of the distance separating the pillars. This offset between successive rows forces particles to navigate around the obstacles and induces a lateral displacement proportional to their size. Therefore, cells or particles of different sizes exit the array at different locations and can be collected separately. The main advantage of such a device is that it never clogs, since the distance between the pillars is always larger than the cells or particles they separate. This device was used to fractionate a mixture of different-diameter beads; 0.8, 0.9, and 1.03 μm into three distinct streams. Additionally, this device was used to separate a mixture of DNA molecules, 61 and 158 kb, in two separate trajectories. In this case an electric field of 12V/cm was used to drive the flow.

Additionally, Austin group has used a variation of this chip to separate RBCs, WBCs, and platelets from blood plasma [87].

Our group has employed pillar configuration to create multiple sieving devices for size-based separation. With these devices, we have demonstrated the isolation of cultured cancer cells spiked into whole blood [88]. Our devices have successively narrower gap widths between the columns in the direction of flows with 20, 15, 10, and 5 μm spacings all on one device (**Figure 10**). The first 20 μm wide segment disperses the cell suspension and creates an evenly distributed flow over the rest of the device, whereas the other segments were designed to retain successively smaller cells [89]. The channel depth is constant across the device. Two types of devices were constructed, the first type was 10 μm deep and the second type was 20 μm deep. As cells traversed the device, they continued through each region until they were stopped at a gap width that prohibited passage due to their size. Experiments with human whole blood, from healthy individual, proved that channels 5 μm wide and 10 μm deep permitted all normal cell types to cross without resistance under our experimental flow conditions. Cultured cancer cell lines, mixed with whole blood and applied to the device, were retained inside the device while all other cells migrated to the output reservoir.

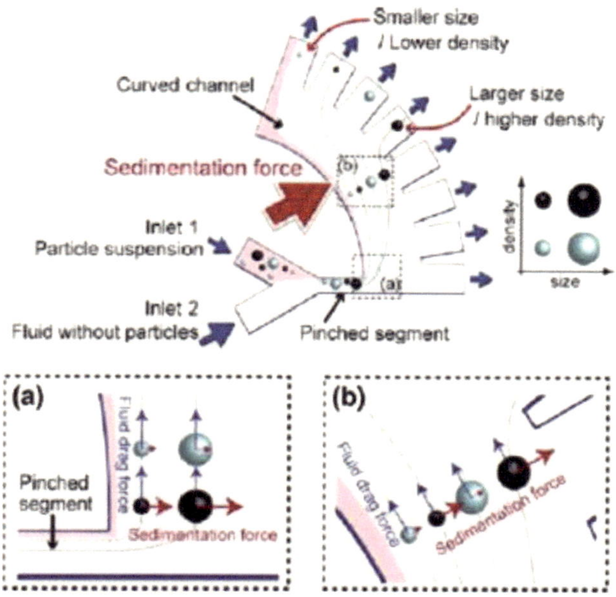

Figure 9. Schematic illustrations showing the separation mechanism of sedimentation pinched-flow fractionation. Images a and b show enlarged views of areas (a) and (b) of the upper image, respectively. In the pinched segment, particles are focused onto the upper sidewall regardless of size. By applying sedimentation force to the flowing particles in the curved channel, particles with a higher density (black) migrate beyond the streamline, achieving density-based sorting. (Reprinted with permission from Springer publisher.)

Eight different cancer cell line, brain neuroblasts (SK-N-MC, SK-N-AS, SK-N-SH, BE(2)-M(17), and SH-SY5Y), breast epithelial cells (MDA231), colon epithelial cells (SW620), and kidney epithelial cells (HEK293), were successfully isolated from whole blood by our device. Additionally, either intact cells, or DNA, could be extracted for molecular analysis. DNA was extracted by *in-situ* cell lysis. After the cancer cells had been retained, the device was flushed for 20 min, with medium used to remove all non-retained cells, followed by water to lyse the retained cells and release their DNA. DNA was collected from the output reservoir for 20 min (approximately 0.33 mL), purified, and tested, as a demonstration that the captured DNA was from the cancer cell line and not a contaminant DNA from the blood used for spiking.

Alternatively, retained intact cells were recovered by reversing the direction of the flow, using medium after allowing 20 min for them to migrate towards the outlet. Once flow was reversed, cells retained at the first row of transition at the 10 μm wide channels detached easily and traveled through the 15 μm and then the 20 μm segments, through the inlet reservoir, and into a collection tube. Cells were cultured from the collection tube and were able to proliferate, thus demonstrating the viability of the extracted cells.

Our device was made using standard photolithography techniques and was molded in PDMS, polystyrene, or polyurethane [90].

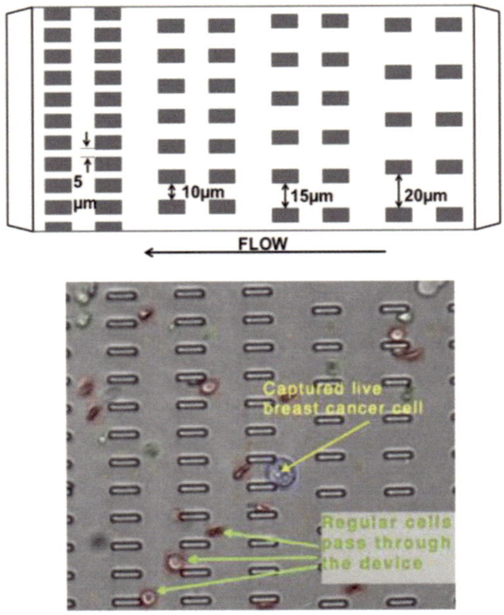

Figure 10. (top) Schematic showing flow direction and channel structure for the Second generation device having varying channel gap widths (20, 15, 10, and 5µm), cells separate based on size and deformability. Channel depths, constant over a single device are: 20 or 10µm. (Bottom) Adult blood cells spiked with MDA231 cells. All cells flow freely through the device except for the MDA231 cells, which are retained at the start of the 10µm wide channels

A derivative of the same design was utilized to separate fetal cells from cord blood [91]. The device has four segments of successively narrower channels along the flow axis; these have 15, 10, 5, and 2.5 µm spacings. Each segment is 30 mm wide and 15 mm long and has 375 rows of channels of the same width. Therefore, the entire device is 30mm wide and 60mm long, giving rise to over 3.5 million channels. The channels are formed between pillars separated by gaps rather than a continuous structure. This design was favored to allow the cells to deform and resume their normal shape as they traverse the device; further, if the cell flow is locally slowed or if a channel becomes clogged, a cell is able to migrate around the affected area. Currently, a one-step centrifugation is required for sample preparation, and only the mononuclear layer is used in the device. This step not only separates most of the mature RBCs before sample loading, but it also enriches for fNRBCs since mononuclear cells and fNRBCs have similar densities. To identify fNRBCs, we stained the buffy coat with fluorescein isothiocyanate-labeled monoclonal antibody to HbF (green) and SYTO red. Thus, fNRBCs should fluoresce green and red. Double-stained samples were applied to the device. When the mononuclear layer was tested in the device, WBCs were retained consistently at the start of the 2.5 µm wide segment, while fNRBCs and mature RBCs migrated to the output reservoir. Cells were removed from the output reservoir, and the DNA was extracted with DNA purification kit and was tested for X and Y chromosomal sequence by PCR. We used cord blood from mothers who delivered male babies, so the X and Y chromosome could be used to demonstrate that the isolated cells came from the baby and not the mother. Mature RBCs do not have a nucleus, and hence do not contaminate the DNA obtained [92].

5. Conclusion

In the last two decades, we witnessed many advances in microfluidic devices, and many of these devices are in advanced development stages or are commercially available. Microfluidic technology offers superior capability to precisely engineer and control the microenvironment to sort cells. Micro- and nano-fluidic technology will fulfill the sensitivity, specificity, and reproducibility requirements to bring cell sorting into clinical utility. The challenge remains to demonstrate that information acquired using microfluidic devices would change the way physicians diagnose, treat, and/or monitor diseases.

Author details

Hisham Mohamed
Egypt Nanotechnology Center (EGNC), Egypt

6. References

[1] Fisher D, Francis GE. and Rickwood D. Cell Separation. New York: Oxford; 1998.
[2] Wheeler AR, Throndset WR, Whelan RJ, Leach AM, Zare RN, Liao YH, Farrell K, Manger ID, Daridon A. Microfluidic Device for Single-Cell Analysis. *Anal. Chem.* 2003:*75* (14) 3581–3586.
[3] Horan PK, Wheeless LL. Quantitative single cell analysis and sorting Science 1977: (198) 149-157.
[4] Dino Di Carlo DD, Lee LP. Dynamic Single-Cell Analysis for Quantitative Biology. *Anal. Chem.* 2006: *78* (23) 7918–7925
[5] Anselmetti D. Single Cell Analysis. Hoboken: Wiley: 2009
[6] Iorgulescu DG, Kiroff GK. Minimal residual marrow disease: detection and significance of isolated tumour cells in bone marrow. ANZ J Surg. 2001: (71) 365-376.
[7] Engell HC. Cancer cells in the circulating blood. Acta Chir. Scand. 1955: (Suppl) (210), 1955.
[8] Vlems F A, Wobbes T, Punt CJ, Van Muijen GN. Detection and clinical relevance of tumor cells in blood and bone marrow of patients with colorectal cancer. Anticancer Res. 2003: (23) 523-530.
[9] Gomez FA. Biological Applications of Microfluidics. Hoboken:Wiley; 2008.
[10] Kumar CS. Microfluidic Devices In Nanotechnology. Hoboken: Wiley; 2010.
[11] Polla DL, Erdman AG, Robbins WP, Markus DT, Diaz-Diaz J, Rizq R, Nam Y, Brickner HT, Krulevitch P, Wang A. Microdevices in medicine. Annual Review of Biomedical Engineering 2000: (2) 552-572.

[12] Chou C, Austin RH, Bakajin O, Tegenfeldt JO, Castelino JA, Chan SS, Cox EC, Craighead, H, Darnton N, Duke T, Han J, Turner S. Sorting biomolecules with microdevices.. Electrophoresis 2000: *(21)* 81-90.

[13] Lee TMH, Hsing I, Lao AIK, Carles MC. A miniaturized DNA amplifier: its application in traditional chineses medicine. Anal Chem, 2000: (72) 4242-4247.

[14] Simpson JL, Elias S. Isolating fetal cells from maternal blood: Advances in prenatal diagnosis through molecular technology. JAMA 1993: (270) 2357-2361.

[15] McCormick RM, Nelson RJ, Alonso-Amigo MG, Benvegnu DJ, Hooper HH. Microchannel electrophoretic separations of DNA in injection-molded plastic substrates. Anal Chem. 1997: (69) 2626-2630.

[16] Lagally ET, Medintz I, Mathies RA. Single-molecule DNA amplification and analysis in an integrated microfluidic device. Anal Chem. 2001: (73) 565-570.

[17] Koch M, Evans A, Brunnschweiler A. Microfluidic Technology and Applications. Hertfordshire: Research Studies Press LTD: 2000.

[18] Saliterman SS. BioMEMS and Medical Microdevices. Bellingham: SPIE Press; 2006.

[19] Bunn HF, Aster JC. Pathophysiology of Blood Disorders. Boston: McGrawy Hill: 2010.

[20] Stuart M, Nagel R. Sickle-cell disease. The Lancet 2004: 364 (9442) 1343-1360

[21] Schaeffer CW, Partin AW, Isaacs WB, Coffey DS, Isaacs JT. Molecular and cellular changes associated with the acquisition of metastatic ability by prostatic cancer cells. Prostate 1994: (25) 249-265.

[22] Pienta KJ, Coffey DS. Nuclear-cytoskeletal interactions: evidence for physical connections between the nucleus and cell periphery and their alteration by transformation. J Cell Biochem. 1992: (49) 357-365.

[23] Nickerson JA. Nuclear dreams: the malignant alteration of nuclear architecture. J Cell Biochem. 1998: (70) 172-180.

[24] Pawlak G, Helfman D M. Cytoskeletal changes in cell transformation and tumorigenesis. Curr Opin Genet Dev. 2001: (11) 41-47.

[25] Konety BR, Getzenberg RH. Nuclear structural proteins as biomarkers of cancer. J Cell Biochem, Suppl 1999: (32-33) 183-191.

[26] Backman V, Wallace MB, Perelman LT, Arendt JT, Gurjar R, Muller MG, Zhang Q, Zonios G, Kline E, McGilligan JA, Shapshay S, Valdez T, Badizadegan K, Crawford JM, Fitzmaurice M, Kabani S, Levin HS, Seiler M, Dasari RR, Itzkan I, Van Dam J, Feld MS, McGillican T. Detection of preinvasive cancer cells. Nature 2000: (406) 35-36.

[27] Zola H, Swart B, Banham A, Barry S, Beare A, Bensussan A, Boumsell L, D Buckley C, Bühring HJ, Clark G, Engel P, Fox D, Jin BQ, Macardle PJ, Malavasi F, Mason D, Stockinger H, Yang X. CD molecules 2006--human cell differentiation molecules. J Immunol Methods 2007: 318 (1–2) 1–5.

[28] Went P, Lugli A., Meier S , Bundi M, Mirlacher M, Sauter G, Dirnhofer S. Frequent EpCam Protein Expression in Human Carcinomas. Human Pathology 2004: (35) 122-128.

[29] Gastl G, Spizzo G, Obrist P, Dunser M, Mikuz G. Ep-CAM overexpression in breast cancer as a predictor of survival. The Lancet 2000: (356) 1981-1082.

[30] Spizzo G, Gastl G, Wolf D, Gunsilius E, Steurer M, Fong D, Amberger A, Margreiter R, Obrist P. Correlation of COX-2 and Ep-CAM overexpression in human invasive breast cancer and its impact on survival. Br Jr Cancer 2003: (88) 574-587.

[31] Spizzo G, Went P, Dirnhofer S, Obrist P, Simon R, Spichtin H, Maurer R, Metzger U, Castelberg B, Bart R, Stopatschinskaya S, Kochli O, Haas P, Mross F, Zuber M, Dietrich H, Bischoff S, Mirlacher M, Sauter G, Gastl G. High Ep-CAM expression is associated with poor prognosis in node positive breast cancer. Breast Cancer Research and Treatment 2004: (89) 207-213.

[32] Talasaz AH, Powell AA, Huber DE. Berbee JG, Roh KH, Yu W, Xiao W, Davis MM, Pease RF, Mindrinos MN, Jeffrey SS, Davic RW. Isolating highly enriched populations of circulating epithelial cells and other rare cells from blood using a magnetic sweeper device. PNAS 2009: (106) 10 3970-3975.

[33] Kovacs GTA. Micromachined Transducers Sourcebook. Boston: McGraw Hill; 1998

[34] Madou MJ. Fundamentals of Microfabrication 2nd edn. Boca Raton: CRC Press: 2002.

[35] Coventor Inc. Http://coventor.com/ (accessed 29 April 2012).

[36] ANSYS. Http://ansys.com/ (accessed 29 April 2012).

[37] COMSOL. Http://comsol.com/ (accessed 29 April 2012).

[38] Mohamed H, McCurdy LD, Szarowski DH, Duva S, Turner JN, Caggana M.

[39] IEEE Trans. NanoBio. Sci. 2004: (3) 251-256.

[40] Sin A, Murthy SK, Revzin A, Tompkins RG, Toner M. Enrichment Using Antibody-Coated Microfluidic Chambers in Shear Flow: Model Mixtures of Human Lymphocytes. Biotechnology and Bioengineering 2005; 91(7) 817-826.

[41] Fu AY, Chou HP, Spence C, Arnold FH, Quake SR. An Integrated Microfabricated Cell Sorter. *Anal. Chem.* 2002: 74 (11) 2451–2457.

[42] Revzin A, Sekine K, Sin A, Tompkins RG, Toner M. Development of a microfabricated cytometry platform for characterization and sorting of individual leukocytes. Lab on a chip 2005: (5) 30-37.

[43] Chang WC, Lee LP, Liepmann D. Biomimetic technique for adhesion-based collection and separation of cells in a microfluidic channel. Lab on a chip 2005: (5) 64-73.

[44] Madrusov E, Houng A, Klein E, Leonard EF. Membrane-based cell affinity chromatography to retrieve viable cells. Biotechnol Prog 1995: (11) 208-213

[45] Malmstadt N, Yager P, Hoffman AS, Stayton PS. A Smart Microfluidic Affinity Chromatography Matrix Composed of Poly(*N*-isopropylacrylamide)-Coated Beads. Anal. Chem 2003: 75 (13) 2943-2949.

[46] Kruger J, Singh K, O'Neill A, Jackson C, Morrison A, O'Brien P. Development of a microfluidic device for fluorescence activated cell sorting. J. Micromech. Microeng. 2002: (12) 486–494.

[47] Dittrich PS, Schwille P. An Integrated Microfluidic System for Reaction, High-Sensitivity Detection, and Sorting of Fluorescent Cells and Particles. Anal. Chem. 2003: (75) 5767-5774.

[48] Chung TD, Kim HC. Recent advances in miniaturized microfluidic flow cytometry for clinical use. Electrophoresis 2007: (28) 4511–4520.

[49] Miyake R, Ohki H, Yamazaki I, Takagi T. Investigation of sheath flow chambers for flow cytometers (micromachined flow chamber with low pressure loss). JSME Int. J. B 1997: 40) 106–13.

[50] Huh D, Gu W, Kamotani Y, Grotberg JB, Takayama S. Microfluidics for flow cytometric analysis of cells and particles. Physiol. Meas. 2005: (26) R73–R98.

[51] Altendorf E, Zebert D, Holl M, Yager P. Differential blood cell counts obtained using a microchannel based flow cytometer. Transducers 1997: (97) 531–534.

[52] Fu AY, Spence C, Scherer A, Arnold FH, Quake SR. A microfabricated fluorescence-activated cell sorter. Nature Biotechnology 1999: (17) 1109-1111

[53] Oakey J, Allely J, Marr DWM. Laminar-Flow-Based Separations at the Microscale. Biotechnol. Prog. 2002: (18) 1439-1442.

[54] Johansson L, Nikolajeff F, Johansson S, Thorslund S. On-Chip Fluorescence-Activated Cell Sorting by an Integrated Miniaturized Ultrasonic Transducer. Anal. Chem. 2009: (81) 5188–5196

[55] Chun H, Chung TD, Kim HC, Cytometry and Velocimetry on a Microfluidic Chip Using Polyelectrolytic Salt Bridges. Anal. Chem. 2005: (77) 2490-2495.

[56] Pamme N. Magnetism and microfluidics. Lab on a chip 2006: (6) 24-38.

[57] Han KH, Frazier B. Paramagnetic capture mode magnetophoretic microseparator for high efficiency blood cell separations. Lab on a Chip 2006: (6) 265-273

[58] Qu BY,Wu ZY, Fang F, Bai ZM, Yang DZ, Xu SK. A glass microfluidic chip for continuous blood cell sorting by a magnetic gradient without labeling. Anal Bioanal Chem 2008: (392) 1317–1324.

[59] Adams JD, Kimb U, Sohb HT. Multitarget magnetic activated cell sorter. PNAS 2008: 105 (47) 18165–18170.

[60] Xia N, Hunt TP, Mayers BT, Alsberg E, Whitesides *GM*, Westervelt RM, Ingber DE. Combined microfluidic-micromagnetic separation of living cells in continuous flow. Biomed Microdevices 2006: (8) 299–308.

[61] Modak N, Datta A, Ganguly R. Cell separation in a microfluidic channel using magnetic microspheres. Microfluid Nanofluid 2009: (6) 647–660.

[62] Lee H, Purdon AM, Westervelta RM. Manipulation of biological cells using a microelectromagnet matrix. Applied Physics Letters 2004: (85) 1063-1065.

[63] Salibaa AE, Saiasa L, Psycharia E, Minca N, Simonb D, Bidardc FC, Mathiotd C, Piergac JY, Fraisierf V, Salamerof J, Saadag V, Faraceg F, Vielhg P, Malaquina L, Jean-Louis Viovya JL. Microfluidic sorting and multimodal typing of cancer cells in self-assembled magnetic arrays. PNAS 2010: (107) 33 14525-14529.

[64] Kose AR, Koser H. Ferrofluid mediated nanocytometry. Lab on a Chip 2012: (12) 190-196.

[65] Li, D Electrokinetics in microfluidics, 1st edition, vol. 2, Elsevier, Amsterdam (2004).

[66] Al-Abboodi A, Tjeung R, Doran P, Yeo L, Friend J, Chan P. Microfluidic chip containing porous gradient for chemotaxis study. Proc. of SPIE 2011: (8204) H1-H6

[67] Agrawal N, Toner M, Irimia D. Twelfth International Conference on Miniaturized Systems for Chemistry and Life Sciences: conference proceedings, October 12-16, 2008, San Diego, California, USA.

[68] Chen YC, Lou X, Ingram P, Yoon E. The 15th International Conference on Miniaturized Systems for Chemistry and Life Sciences: conference proceedings, October 2-6, 2011, Seattle, Washington.

[69] Englert DL, Manson MD, Jayaraman A. Flow-Based Microfluidic Device for Quantifying Bacterial Chemotaxis in Stable, Competing Gradients. Applied and Enviromental Microbiology 2009: (75) 4557–4564

[70] Walker GM, Sai J, Richmond A, Stremler M, Chung CY, Wikswo JP. Effects of flow and diffusion on chemotaxis studies in a microfabricated gradient generator. Lab on a Chip 2005: (5) 611-618.

[71] MacDonald MP, Spalding GC, Dholakia K. Microfluidic sorting in an optical lattice. Nature 2003: (426) 421-424.

[72] Kovac JR, Voldman J. Intuitive, Image-Based Cell Sorting Using Optofluidic Cell Sorting. Anal. Chem. 2007: (79) 9321-9330.

[73] Shirasaki Y, Tanaka J, Makazu H, Tashiro K, Shoji S, Tsukita S, Funatsu T. On-Chip Cell Sorting System Using Laser-Induced Heating of a Thermoreversible Gelatin Polymer to Control Flow. Anal Chem 2006: (78) 695-701.

[74] Lin CC, Chen A, Kin CH. Microfluidic cells counter/sorter utilizing multiple particle tracing technique and optically switching approach. Biomed Microdevices 2008: (10) 55-63.

[75] Hwang H, Park JK. Optoelectrofluidic platforms for chemistry and biology. Lab on a Chip 2011: (11) 33-47.

[76] Wang MM, Tu E, Raymond DE, Yang MJ, Zhang H, Hagen N, Dees B, Mercer EM, Forster AH, Kariv I, Marchand PJ, Butler W. Nature Biotechnology 2004: (23) 83-87.

[77] Pommer MS, Zhang Y, Keerthi N, Chen D, Thomson JA, Meinhard CD, Soh, HT. Dielectrophoretic separation of platelets from diluted whole blood in microfluidic channels. Electrophoresis 2008: (29) 1213-1218.

[78] Hu X, Bessette PH, Qian J, Meinhard CD, Daugherty PS, Soh HT. Marker-specific sorting of rare cells using dielectrophoresis. PNAS 2005: (102) 44 15757-15761.

[79] Vahey MD, Voldman J. An Equilibrium Method for Continuous-Flow Cell Sorting Using Dielectrophoresis. Anal Chem 2008: (80) 3135-3143.

[80] Lapizco-Encinas BH, Simmons BA, Cummings EB, Fintschenko Y. Dielectrophoretic Concentration and Separation of Live and Dead Bacteria in an Array of Insulators. Anal Chem 2004: (76) 1571-1579.

[81] Morijiri T, Sunahiro S, Senaha M, Yamada M, Seki M. Sedimentation pinched-flow fractionation for size- and density-based particle sorting in microchannels. Microfluid Nanofluid 2011: (11) 105-110.

[82] Wilding P, Kricka LJ, Cheng J, Hvichia G, Shoffner MA, Fortina P. Integrated cell isolation and polymerase chain reaction analysis using silicon microfilter chambers. Anal Biochem 1998: (257) 95-200.

[83] Yuen PK, Kricka LJ, Fortina P, Panaro PJ, Sakazume T, Wilding P. Microchip module for blood sample preparation and nucleic acid amplification reactions. Genome Res 2001: (11) 405-412.

[84] Panaro NJ, Lou XJ, Fortina P, Kicka LJ, Wilding P. Micropillar array chip for integrated white blood cell isolation and PCR. Biomed Eng 2005: (21) 157-162.

[85] Cabodi M, ChenYF, Turner SWP, Craighead HG, Austin RH. Continuous separation of biomolecules by the laterally asymmetric diffusion array with out-of-plane sample injection. Electrophoresis 2002: (23) 3496–3503.

[86] Huang LR. Cox EC, Austin RH, Sturm JC. Continuous Particle Separation Through Deterministic Lateral Displacement. Science 2004: (304) 987-990.

[87] Davis JA, Inglis DW, Morton KJ, Lawrence DA, Huang LR, Chou SY, Sturm JC, Austin RH. Deterministic hydrodynamics: Taking blood apart. PNAS 2006: 103 (40) 14779–14784.

[88] Mohamed H, McCurdy LD, Szarowski DH, Duva S, Turner JN, Caggana M. Development of a Rare-Cell Fractionation Device: Application for Cancer Detection. IEEE Transactions on NanoBioscience 2004: (3) 251-256.

[89] H. Mohamed, M. Murray, J. N. Turner, and M. Caggana, "Circulating tumor cells: capture with a micromachined device," Proceedings of the 2005 NSTI Bio Nano Conference, vol1, pp. 1-4, 2005.

[90] Mohamed H, Murray M, Turner JN, Caggana M. Isolation of tumor cells using size and deformation. Journal of Chromatography A 2009: (1216) 8289–8295.

[91] H. Mohamed, J. N. Turner, and M. Caggana. Bio Nano Conference: conference proceedings, May 7-11, 2006, Hynes Convention Center, Boston Massachusetts.

[92] Mohamed H, Turner JN, Caggana M. Bio Nano Conference: conference proceedings, May 20-24, 2007, Santa Clara, California.

[93] Murthy SK, Sethu P,Vunjak-Novakovic G, Toner M, Radisic M. Size-based microfluidic enrichment of neonatal rat cardiac cell populations. Biomed Microdevices 2006: (8) 231–237.

[94] Huang R, Barber TA, Schmidt MA, Tompkins RG, Toner M, Bianchi DW, Kapur R, Flejter WL. A microfluidics approach for the isolation of nucleated red blood cells (fNRBCs) from the peripheral blood of pregnant women. Prenat Diagn. 2008: (28) 892–899.

Section 3

Applications in Haematology

Chapter 12

Tigers Blood: Haematological and Biochemical Studies

A.B. Shrivastav and K.P. Singh

Additional information is available at the end of the chapter

http://dx.doi.org/10.5772/50360

1. Introduction

Tiger (*Panthera tigris tigris*) population in their historic ranges is critically endangered owing to habitat destructions, ruthless poaching and retaliatory killing. The tiger population now remains in few thousands located in about 150 fragments in 13 countries (Karanth and Gopal, 2005). However, declination is also associated with health related problems such as nutritional deficiencies and infectious diseases (Prater, 2005). Therefore, health monitoring and scientific health management, disease diagnosis and treatment should be made mandatory for conservation of wildlife as the tiger is a key stone species and important member of forest ecology (Shrivastav, 2001).

Haematological and biochemical studies are important tool for health evaluation and their interpretations to know the status of physiological functions of various organs. The concentration of biochemical constituents in tissues as well as in body fluid is fixed and during adverse conditions, it may be elevated or decreased (Douglas and Nelson, 1991). However, qualitative and quantitative analysis of corpuscles and chemical constituents of plasma or serum are closely linked with functional unit of the cell and their assessments may reflect the physiological disorders (Harvey, 1997).

Nevertheless, several factors involved to transmit infectious diseases either mechanically or biologically through contaminated water, food or vectors (Lice, Flea, Ticks and Mites) and the pathogens may alter the normal physiology (Shah, 1983). Viral, bacterial and parasitic diseases are very common in tigers which can affect the haematological and biochemical normal values (Rao and Acharyjo, 2002). Types of anaemia and significant blood loss may be estimated through complete blood count (CBC) and physiological function of different organs by biochemical parameters (Jain, 1986). Qualitative and quantitative reduction in the blood commonly observed in captive felid particularly in cubs those maintaining on milk alone. The values of liver function test, elevated on repeated immobilization by sedative drugs. It has been experienced that the values of serum enzymes increased after 72 hrs interval of 2nd immobilization by Ketamine and Xylazine mixture (personal communication, Shrivastav 2012). Sign of anemia such as pale mucous membranes weakness, fatigue and tachycardia may be observed depending on the severity of anemia. A variety of abnormalities may be noticed by analysis of blood, bone marrow cytology, serum chemistry and urine analysis.

Wild felids are commonly injured in territorial fight or sometimes serious injuries and internal hemorrhages occur during hunting. If blood loss is above the 50% of total volume in short period may be fetal and tiger may die due to hypovolumeic shock. Information on haematology and blood biochemistry is meagre in wild animals. However, several studies on selected haematological parameters of exotic species of captive Felids have been reported. Currier and Russell (1982) studied the higher pack cell volume in wild and captive mountain lions (*Felis concolor*) and Fowler (1986) has reviewed the haematological and biochemical profile of Felids including captive tigers whereas Jain (1986) reviewed the information of the genera *Panthera, Felis, Uncia* and *Acinonyx* concluded that blood parameters were almost similar to that of domestic cat with exception of higher concentration of plasma protein and Pack cell volume (PCV). Seal et al. (1987) have studied the haematological and biochemical profile of captive Bengal tigers with emphasis of anaesthetic effect on blood parameters. Chandranaik et.al. (2006) also studied the haematology of physically restrained tigers that were kept in squeeze cages without using anaesthetics. However, the haematological and biochemical studies were made in twelve apparently healthy tigers in free ranges of Central India (Shrivastav et.al. 2011).

Health monitoring, assessment of health during treatment and disease diagnosis in free range tigers needs baseline data on haemato-biochemical parameters. This baseline data is important especially for comparative health assessment of felids during out breaks of diseases between sylvatic and domestic cycle vice versa. It is also required, as the tiger is on top of the sylvatic food chain and to be protected for maintaining balances in ecosystem (Gopal, 1993).

2. Blood collection and investigation

The collection of blood for laboratory investigations is comparatively difficult in both free range and captive tigers and only possible when animal is sedated or restrained properly in squeeze cage.

Withstanding facts, chemical capture is comparatively safe, if accomplished by trained and experienced wildlife veterinarians. There are several drugs available for sedation. Each drug works in a different manner and is more suited to some species only. The time required for a drug to have an effect depends upon the factors such as route of administration, absorption rate, concentration and physiological status of the animal while it is difficult to generalize the choice of drug and doses (WII, 1985). It depends upon circumstances like species of the animal, age, sex, weight, location, temperature regimes in season, time of the day and emotional state. Shrivastav et.al.(2011) have used Xylazine hydrochloride + Ketamine hydrochloride as sedative drugs with the help of Tel-inject projectile syringe to immobilize the tigers of free range while Yohimbine hydrochloride was used as reversal drug.

Prior to collection of blood from immobilized animal, it is an essential protocol to obtain normal values only through free flow of the collected blood drawn from the animal either at rest or under conditions of least excitement to minimize the physiological variations in cell count (Jain, 1986). Normally the cephalic saphenous, femoral and jugular veins are used for collection of blood from dog, cat and non human primates while in tigers these sites are not convenient because the blood collector remained in front of face of the tiger. The caudal vein is convenient and safer site for blood collection (Shrivastav et.al.2011).

From sedated free range tigers, 2-5 ml of blood is drawn by venipuncture of the caudal vein through 18 no gauge disposal syringe in a tube containing Ethylenediaminetetraacetate (EDTA at 2 mg/ml of blood) as the anticoagulant (Shrivastav et.al. 2011). The blood samples should be processed as soon as possible after collection. If a delay is anticipated, it should be refrigerated at 4°C (Jain, 1986).The blood sample should be mixed several times before a portion is removed for test procedure (Shrivastav and Sharma, 2000). Automatic devices providing a continuous rocking or circular motion have been found satisfactory, but prolonged mixing should be avoided, particularly on a device with circular motion, to prevent a mechanical trauma to various blood cells, especially erythrocyte. In any event, blood smear must be made immediately after blood collection, either directly from fresh blood or after anticoagulation. Blood films should be dried quickly and protected from dust and flies till stained (Shrivastav and Sharma, 2005). Blood films can be made on glass slides and on cover slips.The haematological analysis needs precautionary measures and blood smear is stained with Romanowsky stains and at least 200 white cells should be examined for the differential leukocytes count. Simultaneously, the blood smears must be screened for parasitic blood protozoa, flagellates and rickettsial infections.

3. Haematology of Tiger

3.1. Erythrocytes

The morphology of erythrocytes varies with 2 to 7.6, 7.3 ± 0.45 μm in size; appears circular, discoid, central pallor with slight anisocytosis whereas the rouleaux formation(Plate- 2) is common in tiger's blood. Chandranaik, et.al. (2006) also reported the mild anisocytosis in physically restrained tigers. However, the range and mean (with one standard deviation) of total erythrocyte count (TEC) was 4.66 to 9.15, 7.9± 1.42 million /μl. Likewise haemoglobin concentration (Hb) was obtained 9.8 to13.5, 12.8 ±1.65 mg/dl in male and 7.8 to11.5, 10.8±1.05 mg/dl in female tigers (Shrivastav et.al. 2011).

Jain (1986) defined that the rouleaux formation is associated with erythrocyte sedimentation rate (ESR) and useful for evaluation of the disease status. Shrivastav et. al. (2011) encountered ESR (14 to 26, 21 ± 4.21 /hour) and PCV (36 to 45, 38 ± 4.45 %) in free range tigers (Table 1). The consequences of ESR and PCV up and downs mostly confined to erythrocyte osmotic fragility that increased in case of immune-mediated hemolytic anemia. Taketa et. al. (1967) have assessed the oxygen affinity of the haemoglobin is much lower in felines than that of other mammals including humans.

	Haematology	**Unit**	**Range**	**Mean**	**SE (±)**
1	Red blood corpuscles	(TEC) ×106/μl	4.66–9.15	7.90	1.42
2	Total Leukocytes Count	(TLC) ×103/μl	6.2–11.05	8.50	1.42
3	Haemoglobin	(Hb) g/dl	7.8–13.8	12.8	1.65
4	Haematocrit	(PCV) Ratio	36–45	38	2.54
5	Erythrocyte sedimentation rate	(ESR) Hours	14–26	21	4.21
6	Icterus index	(II) u/l	2– 5	2	1.51
7	Differential leukocyte count	%			
i	Neutrophils –		57–75	60	5.08
ii	Lymphocytes –		18–35	30	4.56
iii	Monocytes –		2– 6	0.5	1.21
iv	Eosinophils –		2–6	0.4	1.30
v	Basophils –		0–4	0.1	1.21
	Blood plasma biochemistry				
1	Albumin (ALB)	g/dl	2.1–4.6	3.50	0.99
2	Total protein (TPROT)	g/dl	3.7–8.7	6.40	1.88
3	Total bilirubin TBIL)	mg/dl	0.4–3.2	1.90	1.21
4	Creatinine (CRE)	mg/dl	1.6–4.6	2.90	1.03
5	Blood urea nitrogen (BUN)	mg/dl	6.5–48.2	27.90	13.77
6	Alanine Aminotransferase (ALT)	IU/L	21.2–109.0	67.88	27.84
7	Aspertate Aminotransferase (AST)	IU/L	14.4–84.0	57.96	17.27

Table 1. Haematological and Biochemical Values of Bengal tigers (*Panthera tigris tigris*)

Jain (1986) reviewed the haematological parameters of big cats including *Panthera, Felis, Uncia* and *Acinonyx* and found that the blood composition were almost similar. Among all cats few erythrocytes had single refractile structure (Heinz body) when stained with new methylene blue stain. The Heinz body appearance in erythrocytes is the unique feature of the family Felidae (Plate -1) while they are not visible usually in blood films with Romanowsky stain (Jain,1986). The reduction in erythrocyte count (TEC) and haemoglobin concentration (Hb) are generally associated with anaemia and classified on the basis of erythrocyte morphology, pathogenetic mechanism and bone marrow erythroid response (Jain, 1986).In wild animals the clinical signs and their magnitude depends on habitat and availability of nutritive materials. Prolonged nutritional deficiencies of protein vitamins and minerals essential for erythrocytes production lead to anaemia. The type of anaemia varies with the nutritional deficiency, blood loss and the animal species involved. Despite the nutritional consequences the blood loss may be encountered through traumatic injuries, complication in blood vascular system, thrombocytopenia, and coagulation disorders. A normocytic – nonchromatic, non responsive anaemia is commonly found in association with chronic infections, chronic infectious inflammatory conditions and some type of malignancies though microcytic-hypochromic is the sign of iron deficiencies (Jain and Kono 1975).

Several blood sucking parasites produce blood loss anaemia in tigers like Ancylostomes, Toxoscaris that may cause haemolytic anaemia while Trypanosomes, Babesia and Haemobartonella (*Mycoplasm haemofelis*) may alter the total blood as well as plasma volumes with acute blood loss. Chronic blood loss may lead to gastrointestinal lesions, ulcers, heavy parasitism like coccidiosis, neoplasm with bleeding into body cavity, deficiency of Vitamin K and prothrembin etc.

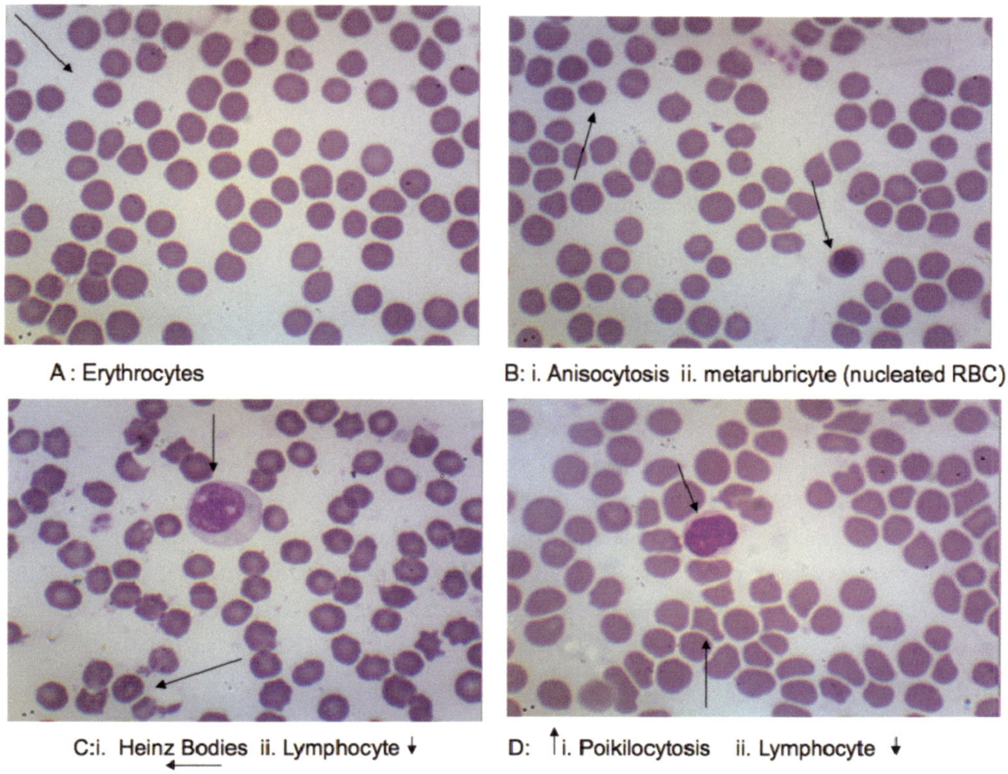

Plate 1. Tiger Blood smear stained with Modified Wright Stain x1000.

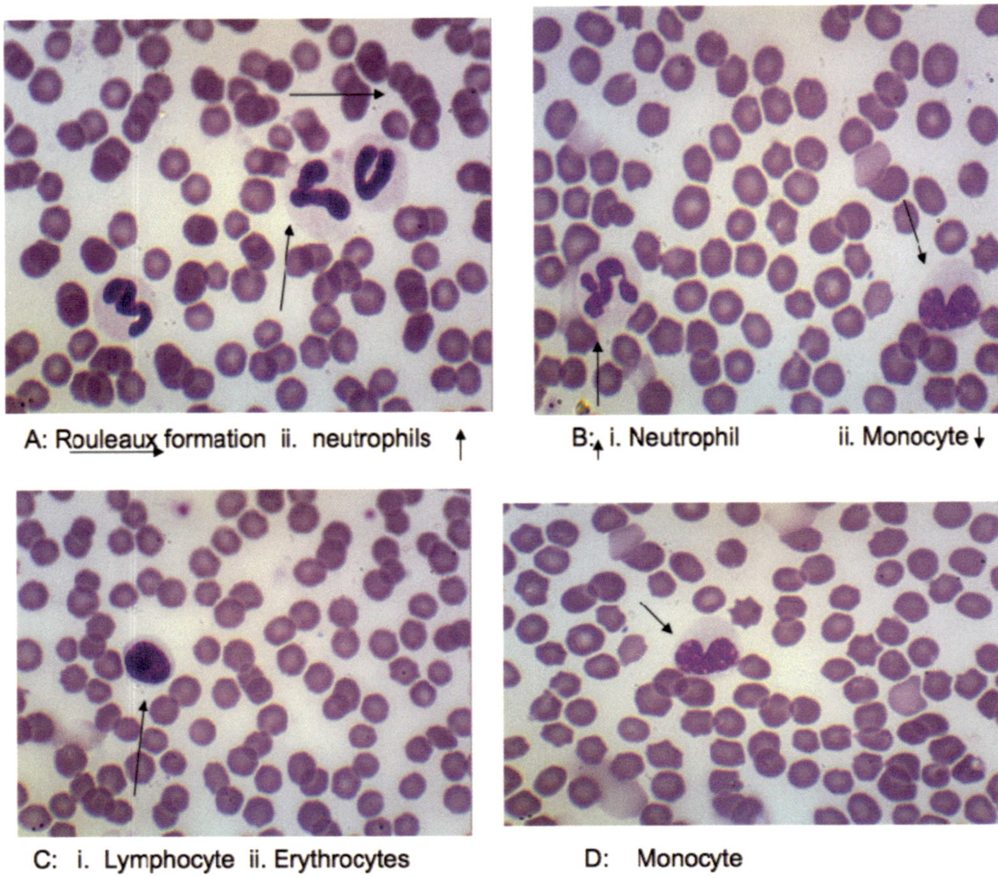

Plate 2. Tiger Blood smear stained with Modified Wright Stain x1000.

4. Leukocytes

The total leukocytes count (TLC) and differential leukocytes count are important parameters to judge the body response against diseases. The TLC was 6.2 to 11.05, 8.5 ±1.42 thousand/µl in free range tigers while differential leukocyte counts (DLC) reflect the information of infectious manifestations. A leukocytosis may be physiologic mediated by endogenous release of epinephrine or corticosteroids or it may be pathologic response to a diseases process (reactive leukocytosis) or a result of a neoplastic change in the haematopoiesis (proliferative leukocytosis) while leucopenia is always pathologic event. Quantitative and qualitative changes in a particular type of leukocyte indirectly reflect the nature of disease process and the body response to it.

Jain (1986) reported physiologic factors such as fright and "emotional" disturbances as an immediate effect on TLC and DLC and may confined to interpretation of conditions. The normal response to the stress is decrease in lymphocytes and eosinophil numbers. In "emotional" leucocytosis, lymphocyte numbers are increased and equal or exceed neutrophil numbers while eosinophil commonly not affected. Meyers-Wallen et. al. (1984) observed the young cats normally have high lymphocyte counts and hence a greater tendency to develop lymphocytosis than the adults. This observation may also be attributed in the case of tigers as they belong to the member of same family with wild habitat as an escape behavior. Increases in neutrophil numbers due to physiologic influences are more pronounced in felines than in canines because of the difference in the intravascular distribution of neutrophils. Prasse et. al.(1973) have observed 3 times mean marginal pool of neutrophils of clinically healthy cats than the circulating pool whereas in dog it was about equal or slightly greater.

4.1. The neutrophils

Neutrophils considered as first line of defense against microbial infections and are important participants in inflammatory reactions. Shrivastav, et.al. (2011) encountered 57 to 75, 60 ±5.08 % with multi-lobed nuclei of 3-5 lobes while sometimes mono-lobed nuclei with pale to slightly pink granules in the cytoplasm in free range tigers(Plate3). Chandranaik, et.al. (2006) has also reported the segmented or multi lobed nuclei while Jain (1986) studied the sex chromatin in few neutrophils as the drumstick lobe in the female cats.

The changes in blood neutrophil differential count (Haden, 1935) is associated with many consequences related to infectious diseases. Several functions have been suggested for the contents of granules, as neutrophils are phagocytic cells and regulating adhesiveness and aggression hydroxyl radical formation and generation of compliment derived chemotactic factors while azurophilic granules are involved in modulation of inflammatory process (Gallin, et. al.1982). Condensation of nuclear chromatin leads to formation of darker-staining plaques separated by delicate, light-staining areas with slight brown colour cytoplasm.

4.2. The eosinophils

Shrivastav et.al. (2011) observed eosinophils contained small, uniformly round bright eosinophilic granules almost occupying the entire and clear cytoplasm (Plate 3). These cells were encountered 2 to 6, 4 ±1.21 % in free range tigers (Table 1). The nuclei of the cells were generally less lobulated than those of the neutrophils. The eosinophils are slightly larger than neutrophils. Chandranaik, et.al. (2006) also observed the larger eosinophils larger than neutrophils and lobulated nuclei with orange cytoplasm in tigers. Jain (1986) reported the granules of the eosinophil are rod-like in domestic cats and Cheetah (*Acinonyx jubatus*) while round granules in the eosinophils of Lion and Leopard. The eosinophils are commonly seen in prolonged parasitic infections or allergic disorders.

4.3. The basophiles

The basophile is a numerically insignificant but functionally important leukocyte that resemble with mast cells and it believed to share similar function as it is associated with allergic reaction, inflammatory process and immunocompitancy to the body fluids. Galli et.

al. (1982) reported basophiles of cats have a limited capacity to phagocytised. Chadranaik et.al. (2006) have reported smaller basophiles than eosinophils with pale lavender pink stained cytoplasmic granules in physically restrained tigers. Jain (1986) observed the mature basophiles contains numerous small, round, lightly stained (pinkish or orangish) granules in light gray cytoplasm in experimental cats. The basophiles were rarely observed up to the size with 0 to 0.4 0.1 ±1.21 5 % in free range tigers.

4.4. The lymphocytes

The lymphocytes are comparatively smaller than eosinophils with round to oval nucleus occupying most space with spherical nucleus (Plate 3). Small and large lymphocytes were also seen in the blood smear. Some lymphocytes contained a few azurophilic granules in their cytoplasm.Jain (1986) reported small lymphocytes is common in cats with patchy nucleus and dense clumps of heterochromatin. In tigers, Shrivastav et.al.(2011) have report lymphocytes from 18 to 35, 30 ±4.56 % (Table 1& Plates 2).

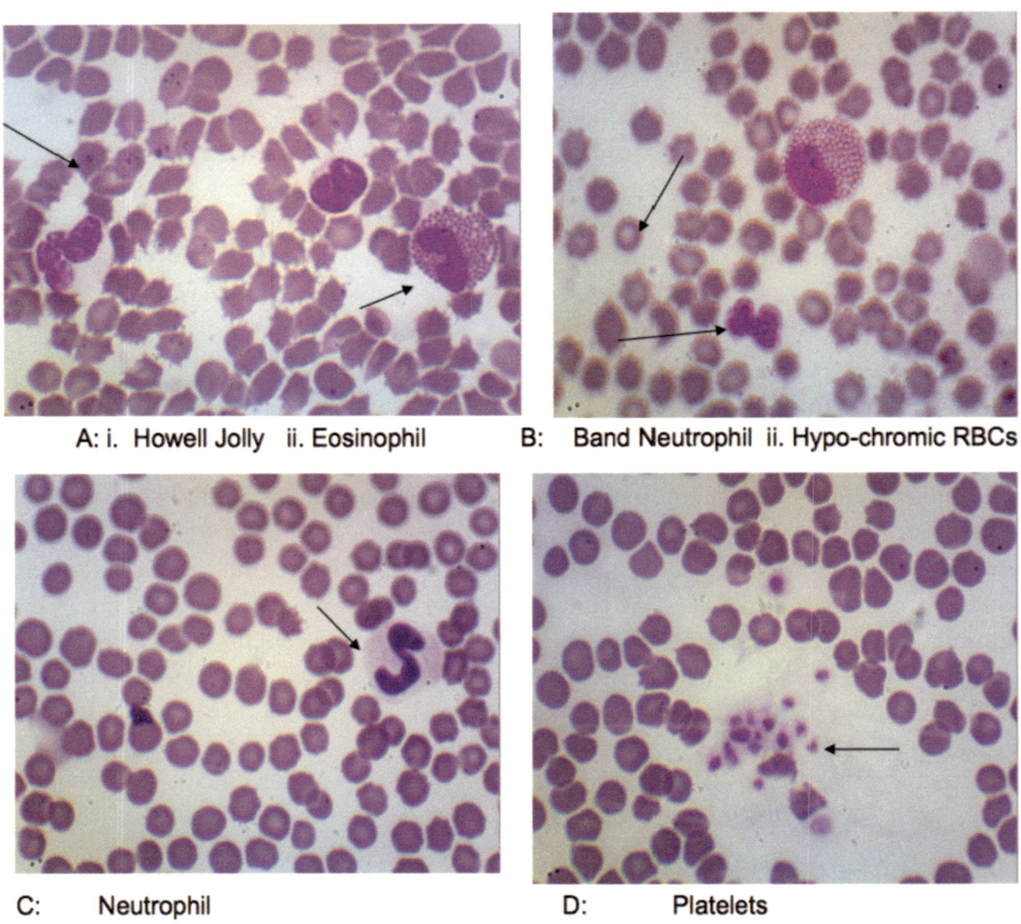

Plate 3. Tiger Blood smear stained with Modified Wright Stain x1000.

4.5. The monocytes

The monocytes are usually larger than lymphocytes. Shrivastav et.al. (2011) encountered 2 to 6, 5 ± 1.21% monocytes in free range tigers with distinguishing feature of the reddish grey nucleus and well defined vacuoles, the nucleus of the monocytes reported amoeboid and some time noticed horseshoe shaped nucleus while cytoplasm stained slightly blue and appeared foamy – vacuolated. (Plate 3). Jain (1986) has also observed similar monocytes in experimental domestic cats.

The monocytes are associated with phagocytosis principally against intracellular bacteria, viruses, fungi and protozoa. The cells perform regulation of the immune response, phagocytic removal of tissue debris (affected cells, antibody coated cells and other foreign materials) as scavenger (Jain, 1986).

Rao and Acharjyo, (2002) have emphasized that macrophages, B-lymphocytes and bone marrow precursor cells are targeted cells for viral replication and commonly observed in Feline Pan-leucopenia (FPL), Feline Viral Rhinotracheitis (FVR), Immunodeficiency Syndrome (FIDS), Canine Distemper (CD) and Inclusion Body Hepatitis (IBH) etc. The body immune system is badly affected and gradually reduced.

4.6. The platelets

Platelets are abundant in blood smear and usually distributed in small to large clumps. Shrivastav et.al.(2011) reported that individual platelets are pleomorphic with rounded to elongated shapes with a central cluster of azurophilic granules (Plate 3). Jain (1986) has observed the clumping platelets in cat blood and emphasized that the platelets of the cats clump readily during excitement of 3 minutes caused a sudden increase in platelet counts. A slight decrease occurred in sympathectomized cats and a somewhat greater decrease reported in splenectomized cats.

4.7. Blood biochemistry

The concentration of biochemical compounds in tissues and body fluid can be measured in a colorimetery, as it is capable of absorbing light of a particular wave length (Singh, 2004). Thus the health status of animal can be assessed by evaluation of Blood gases, acid base balances, electrolytes, metabolic intermediates, inorganic ions, enzymes and hormones.

Shrivastav, et.al. (2011) have conducted blood biochemical analysis of free range tigers for Albumin, Total protein, Total bilirubin, glucose, creatinine, Blood urea nitrogen (BUN), Glutamic oxalo-transaminase (GOT/AST), Glutamic pyruvic transaminase (GPT/ALT) by using an ERBA Chem-5 plus auto-analyzer (Transasia Bo-medicals Ltd.) with standard ERBA reagent kits for respective plasma constituents. The statistical analysis of obtained data is expressed in range, mean and standard deviation.

4.8. Icterus index

Jain (1986) reported an increase in the values of Icterus index in plasma is an indicative of an absolute increase in bilirubin concentration due to removal of aged erythrocytes from the circulation by the reticuloendothelial and liver. Shrivastav, et.al. (2011) reported 2 to 5, ± 2.1.5 units. in apparently healthy tigers of free range.

4.9. Total plasma protein

Protein in plasma can provide information reflecting functional status of various organ and systems as blood is composed of approx 20 % of protein excluding haemoglobin. However, the total protein values gives the information on nutritional consequences or severe organ diseases as they transported the carrier of most of the constituents of the plasma, maintains the colloid osmotic pressure, act as catalysts in biochemical reaction and play important role in formation of fibrin polymers during clot formation (Richard, 1991). The total plasma protein in tigers was estimated 3.7-8.7 to 6.4, ± 1.88g /dl. The values are commonly increases in haemoconcentration and reduced in malnutrition, hepatopathy, less intake of protein and in neoplastic condition etc.

4.10. Plasma albumin

The liver produces all the albumin and globulins while a small amount of globulins is produced by reticuloendothelial tissue (Benjamin, 1979).Liver synthetic capacity or protein-losing nephropathy can be measured by albumin estimation in the blood plasma or serum. It also can interpret high or low calcium and magnesium level since albumin binds about one half of each of the ions (Richard, 1991). However, it appears to be a direct correlation between albumin turnover and body size because it is clinically significant. It is usually constituted with two third of total plasma protein and also serve as mobile amino acids for the liver (Mc Pherson, 1991). Generally hypoalbuminism is observed in malnutrition, increased protein catabolism, nephropathy and chronic enterophathy. Shrivastav et. al. (2011) reported plasma albumin level 2.1 to 4.6, ± 3.5 g /dl, in free range tigers. Reduction in total albumin values is observed in malnutrition , liver diseases, stress, kidney dysfunction etc.

4.11. Total bilirubin

Bilirubin is a breakdown product of heme about 70 percent of which is derived from senescent red cells (Crawford et. al., 1988) however, 15 percent comes from hepatic cytoplasm and mitochondrial cytochromes and some from renal and other cytochromes, and some from defective red blood cell broken down in the bone marrow before release. Shrivastav et. al. (2011) reported 0.4 to 3.2, 1.90, ± 1.21mg /dl, total bilirubin in free range tigers. The yellow color of serum or plasma is due chiefly to the pressure of bilirubin. Increased concentration of bilirubin is commonly seen in haemolysis hepatocellular damage, biliary obstruction prolonged fasting reduced intake fluids etc.

4.12. Creatinine

Creatinine is important in muscles metabolism in that it provides storage of high energy phosphates through synthesis of phosphocreatine (Benjamin,1979).It was estimated in tigers as 1.6 to 4.6, 2.9, ±1.03 mg /dl. Serum or plasma creatinine concentration and urinary creatine secretion are increased significantly by skeletal muscles necrosis or atrophy and defect in renal functions (Pennington, 1971)

4.13. Blood urea nitrogen

Urea is the end product of protein and amino acids and is generated in the liver through urea cycle (Woo and Cannon, 1991).Blood Urea Nitrogen is one of the important tools to know the renal function status. The values of BUN (6.5 to 48.2, 27.9, ± 13.7 mg /dl) was observed in free range tigers is commonly seen in malnutrition and hepatic insufficiencies, however, increased BUN is generally associated with renal disease congestive heart failure, shock, hypertension etc. Shrivastav et. al. (2011) observed the high rise might be also due to adlib intake of meat as the Royal Bengal Tiger can consume 35-40 kg meat of pray animal at a time (Prater, 2005).

4.14. Hepatic enzymes

The serum enzymes used routinely in clinical diagnosis are synthesized in liver (Schaffner, and Schaffner, 1991). In hepatocellular or in cholestatic forms of liver injury these hepatic enzymes are released in to the serum. The serum enzyme activities that are elevated in hepato cellulardamage are Alanine Aminotransferase (ALT) Aspertate Aminotransferase (AST) Ornithine Carbamoyltransferase (OCT), Glutamic Dehydrogenase (GD) Sorbitol Dehydrogenase (SDH) and arginase. The elevated serum activities that suggest cholestasis (intra hepatic or extrahepatic) are Alkaline phosphotase (AP), Gamma glutamyl transpeptidase (GGT) and 5′ nucleotidase (5′ND). The pathogenesis of the hepatic disease in carnivores especially in Felids are associated with viral hepatitis, parasitic infections or mechanical injuries (Rao and Acharjyo, 2002). The liver has great functional reserves and signs of hepatic failure often do not develop until 70% or more of the functional capacity of the liver is lost (Tennant, 1997).

4.15. Alanine aminotransferase (ALT)

Alanine Aminotransferase (ALT) was also termed as SGPT and used by many estimations and large number are found in Hepatocytes in cats, dogs and promates (Benjamin, 1979).The ALT was estimated 21.2 to 109.0, 67.9, 27.84 ± IU /L in free range healthy tigers (Shrivastav et. al, 2011).

4.16. Aspertate aminotransferase (AST)

Apart from liver, AST (Aspertate Aminotransferase) is also present in muscles and cardiac muscles. The higher value of AST though is not an organ specific but used as an indicator of liver dysfunctions. Shrivastav, et. al. (2011) reported 14.4 to 84.0, 57.9 17.27± IU /L in the free range tigers.

The haemato-biochemical profile of the Bengal tigers reported by Shrivastav et. al. (2011) was compared with the values of captive Bengal tigers (Seal et al. 1987), and no major differences were noticed except in ALT, AST and BUN. The mean values (BUN (27.90 ± 13.77 mg/dl), ALT (67.80 ± 27.84 IU/L) and AST (57.9. ± 17.27 IU/L) in free range tigers (Table1)) are comparatively higher with the values of BUN (23.4 ± 0.70 mg/dl), and AST (26.5 ± 4.7 IU/L) as recorded by Seal et al. (1987).The higher values in free range tigers might be associated with beasts of prey, its variety and intake of flesh in natural habits and habitat while zoo tigers are locally dependent on monitored diet in captivity.

Comprehensive information on haemato-biochemical parameters of free range tigers would be helpful for health monitoring and assessment of health status and prognosis of Bengal Tigers (Panthera *tigris tigris*) during treatment.

Author details

A.B. Shrivastav and K.P. Singh
Centre for Wildlife Forensic and Health,
M.P. Pashu Chikitsa Vigyan Vishwavidyalaya, Jabalpur, India

Acknowledgement

The Authors are highly thankful to Dr. H. S. Pabla, PCCF and Dr. Suhas Kumar APCCF (Wildlife) Govt. of M.P. for their interest and constant inspiration to support wildlife activities organized by the Centre for Wildlife Forensic and Health, MPPCVV, Jabalpur-482001, India.

5. References

[1] Benjamin, M.M. (1979) Outline of Veterinary Clinical Pathology, 3rd Edn the state University Press Ames, Iowa, USA., -108-109 pp.

[2] Chandranaik, B.M. Billarey,S.D. Das D; Renukaprasad, C and Krishnappa G (2006) Studies on haematological values in Tigers (*Panthera tigris*) Zoos Print Journal , 21(7) 2321.

[3] Crawford, J. M.; Hauser, S.C and Gollan, J.L. (1988) Formation of hepatic metabolism and transport of bile pigment.A status report semin. Liver Disease 8:105.

[4] Currier, M.J. P. and Russell K.R. 1982. Haematology and Blood Chemistry of the mountain Lion (*Felis concolor*) Journal of Wildlife Diseases, 18:99.

[5] Davidsohn L. and and Henry, J.B. (1969) Clinical Diagnosis by Laboratory Methods Saunders, Philadelphia, Pennsylvania.

[6] Douglas,A and Nelson,M.D.(1991)Basic Examination of Blood, Haematopoiesis Erythrocytic and Leukocytic Disorders. *In* Clinical Diagnosis and Management by Laboratory Methods 18th Edn. HBJ International Edition W. B.Saunders.
[7] Fowler, ME (1986) Hematological data for some exotic species of Falidae: zoo and wild animal medicine, 2nd Edn. Saunders, London, p 840.
[8] Gopal, R. (1993) Fundamentals of Wildlife Management 2nd Edn JH publication Allahabad.
[9] Galli, S. J. et. al. (1984).Basophils and Mast Cells: morphologic insights into their biology, secretary pattern and functions, Prog. Allergy, 34:1.
[10] Gallin et. al.(1982) Human neutrophils specific granules deficiencies: a model to assess the role of neutrophils specific granules in the evolution of inflammatory response, Blood, 59:1317 pp.
[11] Haden, R. L. Qualitative changes in neutrophilic leukocytes, Amer. Journal of Clinical Pathology, 5: 354-1935.
[12] Harvey, J.W (1997). The Erythrocyte: Physiology, Metabolism and Biochemical Disorders *In* Clinical Biochemistry of Domestic Animals Ed. Kaneko et. al. 5th Edn Harcourt Brace Academic Press, Asia Pp 157-203.
[13] Jain NC (1986) Materials and Methods for the study of the blood. Veterinary hematology, 3rd Edn. Lea & Fibiger, Philadelphia.
[14] Jain, N.C. and Kno, C.S (1975). Erythrocyte Sedimentation rate in dog cat. Comparison of two methods and influence of Packed Cell Volume, Temperature and storage of blood. Journal of Small Animal Practices 16:671.
[15] Karanth K.U and Gopal, R. (2005) An Ecology based policy framework for human –tiger coexistence in India. *In* People and Wildlife: Conict or co-existence 373-387. Woodruffe, R. Thirgood, S. and Rabinowitz, A. *Edn* Cambridge, Cambridge University Press.
[16] Mc Pherson, R. A. (1991) Specific Proteins: *In* Clinical Diagnosis and Management by Laboratory Methods 18th Edn. HBJ International Edition W. B.Saunders pp 215.
[17] Meyers-Wallen V.N et al. (1984) Hematologic Values in Healthy Neonatal, Weanling and Juvenile Kittens American Journal of Veterinary Research, 45: 1322.
[18] Prater S. M. (2005) Indian wild animals, 7th Edn Bombay natural history society, Bombay -37-45 pp.
[19] Pennington,R.J.(1971).Biochemical aspects of muscles disease. Adv.clin.Chem.14:409.
[20] Peters, T. (1977) Serum albumin: Recent progress in the understanding of its structure and biosynthesis.Clinical Chemistry., 23:5.
[21] Prasse K.W. et. al. (1973) Blood Neutrophilic Granulocyte kinetics in cats American Journal of Veterinary Research, 34:1021.
[22] Rao A. T., and Acharyjo, L.N (2002) Disease of Wild Felids, Reproprint Publisher, Bhubaneswar
[23] Richard A.M. (1991) Specific Proteins: *In* Clinical Diagnosis and Management by Laboratory Methods 18th Edn. HBJ International Edition W. B. Saunders pp 215.
[24] Schaffner, J.A. and Schaffner F (1991) Assessment of the Status of the Liver *In* Clinical Diagnosis and Management by Laboratory Methods 18th Edn. HBJ International Edition W. B. Saunders pp 229.

[25] Seal US, Armstrong DL, Simmons LG (1987) Yohimbine hydrochloride reversal of ketamine hydrochloride and xylazine hydrochloride immobilization of Bengal tigers and effects on haematology and serum chemistries. Journal of Wildlife Diseases 23(2):296–300.

[26] Shah, H.L. (1987) An integrated approach to the study of Zoonosis, Journal of Veterinary Parasitology, 1(1&2):7-12.

[27] Shrivastav, A. B. (2001) Wildlife health: A new discipline: Essential for Tiger Conservation Programme, Intas Polivet 2: (2) 134-136.

[28] Shrivastav, A. B. and Sharma, R. K.(2000) A Manual of Wildlife Health and Management in Protected Areas, College of of Veterinary Science and Animal Husbandry.

[29] Shrivastav A .B. and Sharma R .K (2005). Health Management of Tiger: A new discipline: Journal of Polyvet 2: 4-16.

[30] Shrivastav, A. B. Singh K. P, Mittal, S. K. and Malik P.K. (2011) Hematology and Biochemical Studies in Tigers, European Journal of Wildlife Research.

[31] Singh, K. P. (2004) Serum Biochemistry on Prognosis of animal diseases, In Training Manual for Field Veterinarians Published by JNKVV, 36-36.

[32] Taketa F, et.al. (1967). Studies on cat haemoglobin and hybrids with Human Haemoglobin A. Biochemistry 6: 3809.

[33] Tennant B.C. (1997) Hepatic Function *In* Clinical Biochemistry of Domestic Animals Ed. Kaneko et. al. 5th Edn Harcourt Brace Academic Press, Asia - 327.

[34] WII (1985) A Guide for the Chemical Restraint of Wild animals, Technical Report II, Wild Life Institute of India.

[35] Woo, J and Cannon, D. C. (1991) Metabolic intermediates and inorganic ions. *In* Clinical Diagnosis and Management by Laboratory Methods 18th Edn.HBJ International Edition W. B. Saunders pp141.

Chapter 13

Ascites Syndrome in Broiler Chickens – A Physiological Syndrome Affected by Red Blood Cells

S. Druyan

Additional information is available at the end of the chapter

http://dx.doi.org/10.5772/48307

1. Introduction

Reduced oxygen availability to the tissues (hypoxia) poses numerous challenges to animal life. Hypoxia occurs as a result of diminished partial pressure of oxygen, such as occurs with increasing altitude, or reduced oxygen percentage in the air capillaries of the lung. The oxygen partial pressure drops by approximately 7 mm Hg, i.e, approximately 2.5% in the case of atmospheric oxygen, for each 1,000 m increase in altitude, and thereby reduces the amount of oxygen available to the hemoglobin in red blood cells as blood passes through the lung.

The hypoxia tolerance of birds has been suggested to be greater than that of mammals. Early studies found that lowland house sparrows (*Passer domesticus*) in a wind tunnel at a simulated altitude of 6100 m behaved normally and flew for short periods [1]. Such findings support the anatomical and physiological evidence that the O_2 transport pathway of birds has several unique characteristics that help support energetic activity and aerobic metabolism during hypoxia.

The O_2 cascade from inspired air to the tissue mitochondria includes several convective and diffusive steps at which physiological adjustments can preserve the rate of O_2 flux in spite of hypoxia, thereby ensuring an uninterrupted supply of O_2 to the energy-producing machinery of the cells [2]. These steps include ventilatory convection, diffusion across the blood–gas interface, circulatory convection, diffusion across the blood–tissue interface (including myoglobin-facilitated diffusion), and O_2 utilization by the tissue mitochondria.

Breathing (ventilation) is stimulated when a decline in arterial PO_2 is sensed by chemoreceptors in the carotid bodies. However, this hypoxic ventilatory response increases respiratory CO_2 loss, causing a secondary hypocapnia (low partial pressure of CO_2 in the blood) and alkalosis (high pH) in the blood [3]. Hypocapnia reflexively inhibits breathing and causes an acid–base disturbance. It has been suggested that birds have a higher tolerance of hypocapnia than mammals [4], possibly because of an ability to rapidly restore blood pH in the face of CO_2 challenges [5]. The significance of this tolerance is that it would enable birds to ventilate more deeply before depletion of CO_2 in the blood impairs normal function, and thereby to enhance O_2 transport to the gas-exchange surface. It seems that every step in the O_2 transport pathway can be influential, and that the relative benefit of each step changes with the level of O_2 availability.

The acclimatization response to hypoxia generally involves increases in hematocrit (Hct) and in hemoglobin (Hb) concentration, but this adaptive erythropoietic response is complicated [6-9]. It is reasonable to expect that an increased Hct could confer a physiological advantage under hypoxia, by enhancing O_2-carrying capacity, but experimental results do not support this [10,11]. A moderately increased Hct enhances arterial O_2 content and therefore increases aerobic capacity [12-14], but the highest attainable Hct is not necessarily associated with the highest possible aerobic power output [15,16]. This is because the associated increase in blood viscosity increases the peripheral vascular resistance, and this might compromise cardiac output (Q), thereby reducing the O_2 consumption rate (VO_2) [17,18].

Another mechanism that can sustain/enhance O_2 transport under hypoxia is alteration in the O_2-binding properties of Hb in the blood. These alterations could be mediated by changes in the intrinsic Hb–O_2 affinity, changes in the sensitivity of Hb to allosteric cofactors that modulate Hb–O_2 affinity, and/or changes in the concentration of allosteric cofactors within the erythrocytes [19-22].

Numerous high-altitude birds, such as the bar-headed goose, the Andean goose [23], and the Tibetan chicken (*Gallus gallus*) [24], possess Hb with an increased O_2 affinity. This can dramatically increase O_2 delivery and pulmonary O_2 loading in hypoxia by increasing the saturation of Hb and, consequently, the O_2 content of the blood at a given O_2 partial pressure. Thus it can greatly improve the O_2 transport pathway [25].

Contrary to the hematological changes that are typically associated with the acclimatization response to hypoxia, genetically based changes in Hb structure that increase intrinsic O_2 affinity or that suppress sensitivity to allosteric cofactors are more important to hypoxia tolerance in naturally high-altitude birds [21,22,26], because in lowland birds an increased Hb–O_2 affinity may hinder O_2 unloading in the tissue capillaries.

Although these distinctive characteristics of birds should enhance hypoxia tolerance by improving the overall capacity for O_2 transport, being avian is not in itself sufficient for coping with hypoxia. Domesticated meat-type chickens (broilers) exhibit high O_2 requirements because of their very fast growth and, consequently, they may have a reduced blood O_2 level, i.e., hypoxemia [27-31] resulting from vigorous digestion and metabolism which have high O_2 requirements. When O_2 demand increases, heart rate and cardiac output increase, thereby increasing the flow of blood through the lung and the pressure required to force blood through the arterioles and capillaries of the lung. The increased flow rate and increased transit time may not allow the red blood cells to pick up a full load of O_2, so that hemoglobin O_2 saturation is not complete, which causes hypoxemia [32].

Hypoxia/hypoxemia directly stimulates the endothelial and smooth muscle cells in pulmonary blood vessels, causing vasoconstriction throughout the lungs and an increase in pulmonary blood pressure that can persist for a long time at high altitude [33,34]. This global vasoconstriction impairs O_2 diffusion because it can divert blood flow away from the gas-exchange surface to pulmonary shunt vessels [35], and the resultant pulmonary hypertension can cause fluid leakage into the air spaces, which, in turn, causes a thickening of the O_2 diffusion barrier [36,37]. Hypoxic pulmonary hypertension can also overburden the right ventricle of the heart and can contribute to pathophysiological conditions, such as chronic mountain sickness or ascites in broilers [9,38].

Ascites in fast-growing broilers:

The commercial broiler of today represents the culmination of dramatic changes over the past 60 years. These changes were caused by genetic selection processes that focused mainly on production traits [39,40]; it has been reported that 85-90% of the changes in commercial broilers were directly related to genetic aspects [39-42]. Commercial broilers of 1991 were compared with the Athens-Canadian Random Bred Control Population, which represents the commercial broilers of 1957 [39,40]. Average daily weight gain of the 1957 and 1991 broilers were 10 and 31 g/d, respectively, from hatch to 3 weeks of age, and 19 and 68 g/d, respectively, from 3 to 6 weeks. The higher growth rate (GR) is driven by a higher feed intake per unit time and higher metabolic rate and, consequently, a higher demand for O_2, from the embryonic stage onward [43-45]. However, it appears that the increase in growth rate occurred without concomitant development in the efficiency of the cardiovascular and the respiratory systems [41,46].

Thus, the increase in metabolic rate, coupled with exposure to environmental conditions such as temperature, lighting and ventilation, and nutritional factors such as feed form or content, all seem to promote the development of ascites [47]. The primary cause of the ascites syndrome, however, is believed to be hypoxia/hypoxemia [48,49], when the bird's demand for O_2 exceeds its cardiopulmonary capacity and causes pulmonary hypertension [50], which results in development of the ascites syndrome (AS) [51-53].

The etiology of the syndrome was well documented previously [52,54,55], and is characterized phenotypically by increased pulmonary hypertension, right-ventricle hypertrophy, fluid accumulation in the pericardium and abdominal cavity, increased hematocrit that results from increased red blood cell production (erythropoiesis), and a decline in arterial blood O_2 saturation [41,52,56,57].

An international survey in commercial broiler flocks showed that AS affected 4.7% of broilers worldwide [58]. Likewise, it was found that over 25% of overall broiler loss in the United Kingdom was a result of AS [59]. It is, therefore, apparent that this syndrome is a serious economic concern in the broiler industry. As the syndrome appears mainly at ages greater than 4 weeks, even 1% of mortality from AS causes significant economic losses, because it occurs toward the end of the growing period [58] and, therefore, affects heavy birds which have absorbed a considerable investment of labor and feed [60,61]. Two management approaches have been applied in order to minimize the actual AS mortality in commercial flocks: (1) increasing the broiler house temperature by means of heating and insulation, which are costly; and (2) reducing the actual growth rate and, therefore, the metabolic rate and demand for oxygen, by providing fewer hours of light so as to reduce the quantity of feed consumed, and using low-energy mash feeds to reduce intake of dietary energy [47,62]. Thus, while the genetic potential for rapid growth of commercial broilers has been continuously improved by breeding companies [41], its full expression is not allowed at the farm level, specifically to avoid morbidity and mortality of AS-susceptible birds. Consequently production costs are increased because of the longer period of rearing to marketing body weight.

There are two alternative hypotheses regarding the association between GR of contemporary broilers and their susceptibility or resistance to AS. Many studies showed that AS does not develop in slow-growing chickens, egg-type Leghorns [see, e.g., 63,64], or slow-growing broilers [see, e.g., 65,66]. It has been suggested that high GR is the direct cause of AS, because of the consequent high demand for oxygen by tissues and organs of these birds. According to this hypothesis, alleles or genotypes that increase GR of broilers also increase their tendency to develop AS. Such a situation should be manifested in a symmetrical genetic correlation between GR and AS: genetic differences in GR – whether between lines or families, or between individuals within lines – should be associated with corresponding differences in %AS. Symmetrically, individuals that develop AS, or families with higher %AS, should have a genetic potential for a higher GR than their counterparts that remain healthy under the same rearing conditions.

The second hypothesis asserts that broilers do not have to be the fastest growing birds in a flock in order to develop AS, but simply need to have their weight-gain rate exceed the growth rate of their pulmonary vascular capacity [67-71]. According to this hypothesis, there should be high-GR broilers that do not develop AS despite their high O_2 demand, because they are genetically resistant. Similarly, there should be broilers with genetically low GR that, nevertheless, are susceptible to AS, although they require special environmental conditions to express this susceptibility.

The hypotheses regarding an inherent association between AS and the genetic potential for high GR were tested by examining contemporary commercial broilers in 2002 and 2006, and an experimental low-GR slow-growing line [71]. All the lines were tested under the same experimental protocol, that allowed measurement of GR under standard brooding conditions (SBCs) up to d 19, and then efficiently distinguished between AS-susceptible and AS-resistant individuals, the latter being those that remained healthy under the same high-challenge, ascites-inducing conditions (AICs) – conditions based on exposure to low ambient temperatures while receiving different forms of diet [72]. Ascites syndrome incidence was 31 and 47% in the 2002 and 2006 birds respectively, and 32% in the 1986 slow-growing line (Table 1). Most broilers that remained healthy under the high-challenge AICs exhibited the same early GR and BW as those that later developed AS. These results, and the relatively high incidence of AS in the slow-growing line, indicated that there is very little, if any, direct genetic association between AS and genetic differences in potential GR, which suggests that AS-resistant broilers can be selected for higher GR and remain healthy, even under AICs

	2002 experiment				2006 experiment			
Age (d)	1986 broiler line		2002 broiler line		1986 broiler line		2002 broiler line	
Cumulative Mortality	n[1] ($N = 91$)	%	n[1] ($N = 42$)	%	n[1] ($N = 78$)	%	n[1] ($N = 97$)	%
28	0	0.0	1	2.4	0	0[a]	2	2.1[a]
35	5	5.5	2	4.8	3	3.8[b]	10	10.3[a]
42	10	11.0[b]	9	21.4[a]	12	15.4[b]	26	26.8[a]
54[2]	22	24.2	--	--	15	19.2	--	--
Morbidity[3] 42 or 54	7	7.6	4	9.5	11	14.1	20	20.6
Total AS incidence	29	31.8	13	31.0	26	33.3	46	47.4

[a, b] Mortality or morbidity percentages per line within rows (ages), within experimental year, without common superscript differ significantly (χ^2 test, $P < 0.05$)
[1] n = number of birds with AS; N = total number of birds in the line.
[2] The birds from the 1986 broiler line were kept under AIC through 54 d of age.
[3] Birds that survived to the end of trial (Day 54 for the 1986 broiler line; Day 42 for the 2002 and 2006 broiler lines) but were diagnosed with AS.

Table 1. Cumulative mortality and morbidity due to the ascites syndrome (AS) at various ages in broiler lines of the years 1986, 2002 and 2006, all reared together under high-challenge ascites-inducing conditions (AICs) from Day 19 to end of trial (According to [71]).

These results, supported by several previous studies [68,70-78], suggest that there is no "true" genetic correlation between the potential GR of broilers and their propensity to develop AS. It seems that AS is not caused by the increased O_2 requirement of a fast growth rate, but by an impairment of the O_2 supply needed to sustain the fast growth rate.

Thus, a better solution would be to select against AS susceptibility, because if all broilers were resistant to AS, management-induced reduction of growth rate would no longer be needed. Breeding against AS susceptibility should aim at identifying and eliminating all the AS-susceptible individuals in the selected population and selecting for high GR among the AS-resistant ones.

The questions raised by the last hypothesis concern what might cause broilers to be susceptible to ascites, and whether it is related to physiological disorders of the cardiovascular system.

This chapter will introduce readers to the physiological Ascites Syndrome and the complexity of the problems that highly productive broiler chickens face in coping with high-oxygen-demand conditions such as cold stress and high altitude. It will focus on: a. the ascites syndrome – its causes and etiology in broiler chickens; b. cardiovascular functioning and responsiveness in ascitic broilers; and c. genetic and physiological aspects of coping with the syndrome.

2. The Ascites syndrome: Its causes and etiology in broiler chickens

Ascites physiology and etiology:

The AS involves accumulation of fluids in the abdominal cavity [79], which prompted the common name of "water belly" to describe the syndrome; it occurs when broilers fail to supply sufficient oxygen to support their metabolic demands [80]. In the late 1970s AS was observed only at high altitudes [81], but since then it has been found also at low altitudes [82], mainly in broilers reared at low ambient temperatures and/or fed pelleted feed with high energy content.

The general pathogenesis of AS has been well documented [52,54,83,84]. Rapid growth requires a high resting metabolic rate, which requires adequate O_2 supply and utilization. The broiler chicken probably has more genetic potential for growth than it has potential to provide O_2 to sustain that growth, and in some broilers the demand for O_2 might exceed the cardiopulmonary capacity to supply sufficient O_2, ultimately leading to an O_2 deficit [85]. The heart responds by increasing its output of (deoxygenated) blood to the lungs for oxygenation. This increased blood flow causes an increase in the blood pressure required to push the blood through the capillaries in the lung which, in turn, causes pulmonary hypertension. This increase in work load results in an enhanced pressure load on the right ventricular muscle wall, to which the muscle cells respond by adding parallel sarcomeres, causing thickening (hypertrophy) of the right ventricular wall. The muscular right ventricular wall increases the pressure in the pulmonary arteries, arterioles and capillaries of the lung. This process continues, causing additional hypertrophy. Meanwhile, the right atrio-ventricular valve thickens and starts to leak, partly because the thicker valve is now less effective and partly because of the increasing back pressure from the pulmonary arteries and right ventricular chamber [86]. The leaking valve aggravates the excess pressure problem by admitting excess volume, the right ventricle dilates, and the wall-muscle cells lengthen by producing longitudinally arranged sarcomeres.

The increased blood volume raises the pressure overload until valve deficiency occurs, causing a drop in cardiac output and pulmonary hypertension, but marked pressure increases in the right atrium, sinus venosus, vena cava and portal vein. This increased pressure in the sinusoids of the liver causes leakage of plasma from the liver into the hepato-peritoneal spaces, i.e., ascites. The leaking valve and increased venous pressure result in hypoxemia and tissue hypoxia, and the kidney responds by producing erythropoietin in an attempt to increase the blood's O_2 carrying capacity by intensively producing more red blood cells.

Domestication had introduced several other insufficiencies into the cardiovascular system; among them is a thicker respiratory membrane than that in other birds, i.e., broilers have a thicker respiratory membrane than Leghorn-type laying fowl. This leads to: a. lower efficiency of O_2 transfer through the respiratory membrane; and b. lower hemoglobin oxygenation capability [62]. Research focusing on hemoglobin O_2 saturationin meat-type chickens indicated that fast-growing broilers have lower saturation than slow-growing broilers [30,87]. These results suggested that some meat-type chickens were not fully oxygenating their hemoglobin, even at low altitude. This might have been the result of increased blood flow rate through the lung capillary bed, which would reduce the time available for hemoglobin to be oxygenated in the lung interface [32,88], or to presence of immature red blood cells in the system [89]. In order to overcome this situation an increase in erythropoiesis takes place. However, such an increase, if not coupled to plasma volume expansion would increase blood viscosity, followed by increased blood-flow resistance [90]. The back pressure in the veins causes venous congestion, dilation and prominent vessels [50]. The lack of O_2 in the heart muscle results in hypoxic damage and, finally, right-ventricular hypertrophy. As cardiac output is reduced and tissue hypoxia becomes worse, the left ventricle loses muscle mass, the wall thins (because of hypoxia and disuse atrophy), the valves thicken and the chamber enlarges. Heart muscle damage is caused by the excess workload and by the tissue hypoxia associated with circulatory failure, not by the tissue hypoxia that increases cardiac output and triggers pulmonary hypertension.

Environmental causes of ascites syndrome:

Altitude: The partial pressure of oxygen becomes lower with increasing altitude. The ability of chickens to oxygenate their hemoglobin fully as the erythrocytes pass through the lung depends on the transit time in the lung, hemoglobin- O_2 affinity, the thickness of the air–hemoglobin barrier and, especially, the partial pressure of O_2 in the air [62]. The effects of high altitude or hypoxia on ascites and heart disorders in broilers were reported as early as the 1950s and 1960s [91-97]. Those reports indicated that birds raised at high altitudes died because of right ventricular hypertrophy, congested and edematous lungs, and accumulation of fluid in the abdominal cavity. Significant microscopic damage to the heart, lungs and kidneys was also found in birds reared at high altitude [95,97], as well as in 1-week-old broilers raised at high altitude [98] and in birds exposed to simulated high altitude [99-101].

Because AS was first noticed in birds raised at high altitude, the use of natural or simulated high-altitude conditions was one of the first experimental protocols to be used [see, e.g., 47,97]. The hypobaric chamber has been shown to be an effective tool for simulating high altitude and consistently inducing AS [102-106]; it simulates high altitude conditions by generating a partial vacuum, thereby reducing the partial pressure of O_2. Anthony and Balog [106], by simulating an altitude of 2,900 m above sea level, successfully induced 66% AS in a commercial sire line. In six lines of commercial broilers that were reared in the same hypobaric chamber, 47% of the birds developed AS [107].

When birds are exposed to low atmospheric O_2 levels pulmonary blood vessels constrict and pulmonary vascular resistance increases [108]. This immediate increase in pulmonary arterial pressure can, over time, cause right ventricular hypertrophy and eventually result in the ascites syndrome [81,89,109-111]. Additionally, hypoxemia leads to an increase in hematocrit, which, in turn, increases blood viscosity and results in increased resistance to blood flow through the pulmonary blood vessels [90,112-116].

Low temperature: Temperature is the most-studied environmental cause of ascites [see, e.g., 117-125]. In endothermic animals (mammals and birds) body temperature (Tb) is the most physiologically protected parameter of the body; therefore, the thermoregulatory system in these animals operates at a very high gain, in order to hold Tb within a relatively narrow range, despite moderate to extreme changes in environmental conditions [126]. The ability to maintain a stable Tb springs from the mechanisms that control heat production and heat loss; mechanisms that changed in the course of evolution, to enable endothermia to replace ectothermia [127,128]. Birds mostly respond to acute or chronic cold exposure by increasing their metabolic rate and oxygen requirement [129,130]. It was reported that a drop in environmental temperature from 20 to 2°C almost doubled the oxygen requirement of White Leghorn hens [131], and in another study there was a 32.7% increase in oxygen requirement in response to low temperatures [132].

Low temperatures were found to increase ascites by increasing both metabolic O_2 requirements and pulmonary hypertension [122,133]. This increase in pulmonary arterial pressure was attributed to a cold-induced increase in cardiac output, rather than to hypoxemic pulmonary vasoconstriction [134]. As a result, low ambient temperature has been widely used to induce AS in broilers [60,66,73,115,122,134-140]. Various protocols were developed, ranging from exposure to constant low temperatures [60,73,122,135,136,140], through gradual stepping down of ambient temperature [66,122,137,139], to episodic protocols under which the birds were exposed to natural fluctuations of winter temperatures [115,138]. The efficacy of a cold-exposure protocol depends upon its timing, duration and magnitude, as well as husbandry and the birds' genetic tendency to develop AS.

The effect of the timing of a cold-stress application on ascites development in broilers indicates that exposure to low temperatures during brooding has a long-lasting effect on ascites susceptibility [62,120,125,137,141,142]. The consensus appears to be that cold stress during the first two weeks of life affects the birds' metabolic rate for several weeks, and increases their susceptibility to ascites [62,120,125,137,141,142]. A novel AIC protocol for AS [72] involved rearing the tested birds in individual cages from 19 d of age, so that they could not escape the challenge of the environmental conditions, which comprised fan-induced air movement at about 2 m/s and moderately low ambient temperatures (18 to 20°C). The effects of the environmental conditions were augmented by early use of high-energy pelleted feed to enhance rapid growth and by lighting for 23 h/d. Under this combination of conditions, %AS among the broilers was 44% – much higher than those reported for cold-stressed broilers on litter, and similar to or slightly lower than that among broilers challenged by hypobaric chamber.

The birds that developed ascites as a result of exposure to low temperatures exhibited the same pathological symptoms as those that developed it under low O_2 partial pressure – symptoms including increased hematocrit, hemoglobin, heart weight, and right-ventricle:total-ventricle ratios [70-72,122,124,143-147].

3. Cardiovascular functioning and responsiveness in ascitic broilers

Blood O_2 transport, erythropoiesis and ascites

The blood system provides the main systemic response to environmental changes and metabolic demands, either through the cardiovascular system or through alteration in O_2-carrying capacity.

Reduced O_2 availability in the blood (hypoxemia), reduces the O_2 partial pressure (PO_2) of the arterial blood (PaO_2). In such a situation the blood system must maintain an adequate delivery of O_2 to the peripheral tissues, while maintaining an adequate PO_2 at the vascular supply source,, in order to permit O_2 diffusion to the tissue mitochondria.

Oxygen delivery can be enhanced by increasing the total cardiac output (Q) and by increasing the blood O_2 capacitance coefficient (βbO_2). The latter parameter is defined as the ratio $(CaO_2 - CvO_2)/(PaO_2 - PvO_2)$, where $CaO_2 - CvO_2$ is the arterial–venous difference in O_2 concentration and $PaO_2 - PvO_2$ is the arterial–venous difference in PO_2.

With regard to maintaining an adequate PO_2 at the vascular supply source, the lower critical PO_2 can be expressed as $PvO_2 = PaO_2 - [\beta bO_2 \times (Q/VO_2)] - 1$, in which VO_2 is the rate of O_2 consumption by the tissues and the product $\beta bO_2 \times (Q/VO_2)$ is the specific blood O_2 conductance [148,149]. Because PaO_2 is determined by ventilation and O_2 equilibration at the blood–gas interface, this equation shows that an increase in specific blood-O_2 conductance minimizes the decline in PvO_2 under hypoxia, thereby maintaining an adequate pressure head for O_2 diffusion to the tissue mitochondria [2].

Under severe hypoxia, an increased blood-O_2 affinity will tend to maximize βbO_2. The resultant increase in the specific blood O_2 conductance helps meet challenges of both delivery and supply: it minimizes the expected PO_2 decrement in the tissue capillaries while preserving a constant $CaO_2 - CvO_2$ difference. Likewise, an increased hemoglobin concentration increases CaO_2, thereby increasing blood O_2 conductance if PaO_2, Q and VO_2 all remain constant. With excessive polycythemia, however, potential advantages of an increased Hb concentration for O_2-carrying capacity might be more than offset by a corresponding reduction in Q.

Several significant alterations to the blood system in AS broilers were well documented: increased red blood cell numbers, through increased erythropoietin production [96,100,150-153]; elevation of hematocrit values and blood viscosity [54,72,154], and central venous blood congestion [50,155]. These findings raised the question of the association between the plasma and the fluid that accumulated in the abdominal cavity, and whether the increase in hematocrit resulted from a decline in plasma volume caused by plasma leakage out of the blood vessels, or from increased erythropoiesis that occurred as a compensatory reaction to the lack of oxygen in the tissue. In ascitic broilers the composition of the abdominal cavity fluid was fairly similar to that of the plasma, with regard to osmolality, and total protein and albumin concentrations, which suggests a deficiency in the selective permeability of the blood vessels [89]. These findings resemble those in cirrhotic human patients with ascites

[156-158]. The escape of plasma fluid out of the blood vessels was probably due to increased pulmonary hypertension and central venous congestion – symptoms found both in humans [158] and in broilers [56]. As in the case of human ascitic patients [159], AS broilers exhibited conservation of plasma volume similar to that of the healthy ones. However, the PCV in the AS broilers increased significantly, by up to 80%, as a result of a significant increase in the number of erythrocytes, which also contributed to a significant elevation in blood volume. Thus, enhanced erythropoiesis, and not plasma volume reduction, was found to be involved in the hemodynamics of the ascitic broilers [89]. This finding could also account for the blood congestion and the increased blood viscosity [90] that contribute to the enhanced cardiac workload [103,134], blood pressure [103], and blood-flow resistance [111] in AS chickens.

In AS birds, the high PCV, on the one hand, and the significant decline in blood oxygen saturation, on the other hand [30,57,66] raised the possibility of an impairment of blood O_2-carrying capacity. Increased erythrocyte rigidity appears to be another important factor in AS [54,62,113]: the nucleated erythrocytes will normally curl or fold to pass through lung capillaries [160], but hypoxemia and high hemoglobin concentrations decrease the deformability of erythrocytes [62]. Further calculations of hemoglobin content per 1,000 red blood cells revealed a significant reduction in the AS broilers compared with that in the healthy and control broilers [57,89]. These results suggest the possibility of inefficient enhancement of the erythropoiesis process.

Ascites-induction conditions elicited enhanced erythropoiesis, which resulted in an increased proportion of immature erythrocytes in the bloodstream. However, whereas in the healthy broilers only a moderate proportion (7.2%) of immature erythrocytes was observed, in the AS ones, immature erythrocytes contributed up to 23.5% to the total erythrocyte count [89]. The significant increase in immature erythrocytes, coupled with the significant decline in hemoglobin content, might provide the explanation for the decline of O_2 saturation in the blood of AS broilers [30,57,72,134].

The differences between healthy and AS chickens in their production of erythrocytes in general, and of immature erythrocytes in particular, suggest that erythropoiesis regulation in the ascitic birds is defective.

The heart

The avian heart is different from that of mammals in that the right atrio-ventricular valve is composed of a muscle loop made up mainly of muscle fibers from the right ventricle wall. The anatomy of this valve makes birds very susceptible to valve insufficiency [52,161,162]: when the right ventricle responds to an increased workload it becomes hypertrophic and the valve hypertrophies along with the ventricle [161]. This thickening of the valve interferes with its effectiveness and may lead to rapidly developing valve failure and ascites [161]. Although litter oiling did not reduce the average ascites score, litter oiling improved air quality significantly in the pens and also improved heart morphology by reducing the right ventricle area from 0.44 to 0.36 cm^2 in ad libitum birds [163, 164].

Alterations in the electrocardiogram (ECG) are seen in conjunction with AS. Of most importance has been the finding that increased S-wave amplitude in standard limb lead II indicates increased susceptibility to AS [111]. However, there were no ECG readings indicative of primary pulmonary hypertension in most birds that developed ascites [165]. A slower heart rate (bradycardia) [55,116], as well as reduction in the pulse rate had been found in birds developing AS [55] and in acutely cold-exposed birds [116].

Heart rate on days 1 and 7 was found to be significantly higher in the AS-susceptible (AS-S) genetic broiler line than in the AS-resistant (AS-R) broiler line, with only the lowest quartile of individual heart rates in the AS-S line overlapping the highest quartile in the AS-R line [57]. These results were in agreement with those of Druyan et al. [166], who found that generation S3 chicks from their AS-S line had a significantly higher heart rate on day of hatch than that of generation S3 chicks from the AS-R line. It was reported [167] that heart rate began to increase shortly after hatch, and reached a peak close to 4 wk of age; thereafter, it declined slowly [168]. The AS-S selected line exhibited increased heart rate only between d 1 and d 7, with a decline thereafter toward d 17, while the birds were kept under standard brooding condition [57]. Mild hypoxia was found to elicit an increase in heart rate [169,170], which suggests that the AS-S birds in that study experienced O_2 shortage already at the time of hatch, even when kept under optimal conditions. A higher mean partial pressure of CO_2 in broilers' venous blood (a marker for lung ventilation rate) on d 11 was found to be associated with increased ascites susceptibility [171,172]. Those results indicate that AS-susceptible birds suffer O_2 shortage at an early age. However, it also suggests that as long as the susceptible birds are under SBC, higher heart rate can compensate for a mild hypoxemia, and no other physiological parameter would be affected.

Effect on heart and blood vessels

Birds with ascites induced by either low ventilation or cold temperatures exhibited hypertrophy of the medial layer of arteriols, which was probably a response to primary pulmonary hypertension [173]. In low, ventilation-induced ascites, the broilers had significant inflammation or osseous-nodule formation in the lungs [174,175], whereas in cold-stress-induced ascites, birds showed no inflammation [173]. Wideman et al. [50] suggested that increases in pulmonary vascular resistance initiate increases in venous pressure by challenging the capacity of the right ventricle to thrust all the returning venous blood through the lungs. An acute reversal of systemic hypoxemia was reported to have no effect on pulmonary hypertension – a finding that discounted the influence of hypoxic pulmonary vasoconstriction [176]. It was hypothesized that this reversal of systemic hypoxemia increased total peripheral resistance and normalized arterial pressure and cardiac output, but could not decrease pulmonary hypertension because of the overwhelming influence of sustained pulmonary vascular resistance [176]. Development of techniques to measure changes in pulmonary arterial pressure and changes in wedge pressure helped to clarify that changes in pulmonary arterial pressure contribute to the mismatch between pulmonary vascular capacity and cardiac output, and that pulmonary hypertension is initiated as a consequence of excessive pulmonary arterial or arteriolar resistance [177,178]. The difference between individual broilers' susceptibility to ascites may be related to an innate or acquired variability in their pulmonary vascular responsiveness to vasoactive mediators [179].

4. Genetic and physiological aspects of coping with the syndrome

The genetic control of susceptibility to AS

Recent reports [71,72,107] indicate that about 50% of the broilers in commercial stocks develop AS under experimental protocols of high-challenge AIC. The term "high challenge" is used for AICs that apparently induce AS in all AS-susceptible individuals, whereas "low-challenge" AICs induce lower rates of AS, probably only in the AS-S individuals whose higher growth rates necessitate higher O_2 demands. The rates of AS reported in recent years are similar to those found under high-challenge AIC in the 1990s [68,73]. In recent years, however, actual AS mortality in commercial flocks has been significantly reduced or even completely eliminated by management practices that reduce feed intake and growth rate and, consequently, reduce the physiological O_2 demand [47,62]. The problem with this approach is that it compromises the efficiency of broiler production.

A better solution would be to select against AS susceptibility: once all the broilers were resistant to AS, a managed reduction in growth rate would no longer be needed. However, breeding is feasible only if there is an inherent susceptibility to AS and if effective selection against it can be applied.

Several studies have found the tendency of broilers to develop AS to be under genetic control, with estimates of heritability ranging from 0.1 to 0.7 [72-74,180,181]. Significant heritability of 0.5 to 0.6 has also been found for the ratio of right ventricle weight to total ventricle weight (RV:TV) – a postmortem indicator for AS development and severity [72-74,182]. These data indicate the feasibility of selecting against susceptibility to AS, but only if all the genetically susceptible birds are identified at the phenotypic level. Mortality or morbidity caused by AS provides the ultimate identification of AS-S individuals.

However, actual development of AS in susceptible birds depends on environmental conditions that lead to hypoxemia, either by reducing O_2 supply or increasing the O_2 demand [62]. It was found that a hypobaric chamber with a reduced O_2 partial pressure, equivalent to that at 2,900 m above sea level, successfully induced 66% AS in a commercial sire line, suggesting full exposure of genetic variation in AS susceptibility [103]. Surgical inactivation of one lung induced AS in all or most of the susceptible individuals [32,68,183,184]. The AIC protocol for broilers housed in individual cages, where the tested broilers could not avoid the environmental conditions that were based on movement of cool air driven by a fan, combined with high-energy pelleted feed and 23 h of light per day, resulted in about 50% AS among commercial broilers [70-72], suggesting that all or, at least, most of the susceptible broilers developed AS.

The successful induction of AS by means of any of these approaches suggests that breeding for AS resistance can be achieved by keeping all selection candidates under high-challenge AIC and awaiting mortality of all susceptible individuals. However, this direct-selection approach has not been used by breeding companies, because it would force them to compromise the selection for more important traits, such as growth rate and meat yield, which are not fully expressed under AIC.

Indirect selection against susceptibility to AS, cardiovascular indicators:

Many studies focused on identifying reliable diagnostic indicators for AS in broilers. Hematocrit (HCT) is a marker for high rate of erythropoiesis in ascitic birds, therefore it is always significantly higher in AS broilers than in their healthy counterparts reared under the same conditions [30,54,60,115,124,125,139,154]. HCT values from broilers aged 35 and 44 d were used to screen one sire line and two dam lines for AS susceptibility [154]: they were used to select individuals that were considered the most (> 36%) and least (< 29%) AS susceptible, and the males and females with the highest and lowest HCT values, from the two dam lines, were selected and classified as high hematocrit (H) and low hematocrit (L) groups. These individuals were then reared under broiler breeder management conditions. Males and females within each group were mated, to create offspring that were HH, HM-no definition for HM, LM, and LL. The progeny underwent screening for hematocrit on days 6, 42, and 49, and from d 33 onward birds were subjected to cold stress. Differences in HCT values were seen at d 6: the HH chicks had significantly higher values than all other groups. On d 49 HCT values of the HH birds were significantly higher than those of the LL birds. Cold stress increased AS mortality in all combinations, but the HH birds had significantly higher AS mortality then the LL birds, which suggests that HCT value is heritable. It was also suggested that HCT screening and selection based on HCT values could be effective in developing resistant populations of broilers. However, later studies revealed that the variation in HCT was a secondary manifestation of developing AS, therefore it could not be used as an early indicator of AS sensitivity under normal conditions [57,72]. Heart rate (HR), measured by pulse oximetry or by encephalography, was found to be lower in broilers suffering from AS than in healthy ones [111,163,185]. At 35 days of age, HR in feed-restricted broilers was significantly higher than that in fast-growing broilers, and the HR of broilers suffering from congestive heart failure, which is associated with hypoxemia and AS, was significantly lower than that of feed-restricted, slow-growing broilers and healthy fast-growing broilers [64]. Broilers with AS were found to have a significantly lower SaO_2 than their healthy counterparts at the age of 6 weeks (62.1 and 86.0%, respectively) [30]. Broilers with AS induced by a pulmonary artery clamp had a significantly lower SaO_2 and higher right-ventricle:total-ventricle weight ratio (hypertrophy of the right ventricle RV:TV) than those of healthy, non-AS broilers [32]. Therefore, low SaO_2 was suggested to be a reliable genetic early indicator for AS susceptibility [186]. In recent years, some breeding companies have selected against broilers with low SaO2, as measured in selection candidates at 5 wk of age [187]. However, because of the low %AS in these unstressed flocks, high SaO_2 levels are expected in susceptible individuals that do not develop AS; also, low heritability (0.15) was reported for SaO_2 at 5 wk of age in commercial breeding lines [187]. Because of this low heritability and only moderate genetic correlation with actual manifestation of AS, the effectiveness of 5-wk SaO_2 as an indicator for selection against AS susceptibility must be limited. All the cited findings suggest that there is a genetic component for AS mortality and also for several parameters (e.g., RV:TV and HCT) that have been found to be associated with development of AS; however, the exact biochemical and physiological precursor factors related to the genetic propensity to develop AS are still not known. It is often difficult to determine whether a particular change is primary in nature, and therefore determinative, or is a subsequent secondary manifestation in the development of AS. If parameters to specifically predict AS susceptibility or resistance are sought, it is of paramount importance that the primary changes be determined and evaluated. Moreover, in order to assess their significance as criteria for selection, it is necessary to estimate the heritability of these parameters, and their genetic correlation with consequent AS development under AIC.

In order to conduct advanced physiological and genomic research on AS, and to find the primary cause of AS, identification of all AS-susceptible individuals is crucial. This identification depends solely on mortality or morbidity under AIC. Under low- or medium-challenge AIC, relatively slow-growing broilers or those that can better withstand cold stress, have a relatively lower demand for oxygen and, therefore, do not develop AS. Incorrect identification of AS-susceptible chicks as AS-resistant leads to biased findings regarding the true genetic association between the measured traits and the genetic difference in broilers' susceptibility to AS.

To effectively select against AS susceptibility without interfering with the normal expression of other selected traits, one has to identify the genes responsible for the primary cause of AS or measure their phenotypic expression. There is evidence that the primary cause of AS is manifested in the prenatal or very early postnatal phases, when the cardiovascular system is being developed and is starting to function [188-190]. Measurements of such a manifestation, especially at the embryonic stage, necessitate sacrificing the investigated individuals, rendering it impossible to later determine, under AIC, if these individuals were susceptible or resistant to AS. Therefore, to conduct advanced physiological and genomic research on AS, one needs a pair of selected lines in which all the individuals are either AS-S or AS-R. Comparisons of tissues or functions of individuals from the divergent lines can help to identify the primary cause of AS and thereby to provide an effective indicator for selection against susceptibility. Resource populations derived from crosses between such divergent lines might facilitate genomic research aimed at identifying the genes involved in susceptibility or resistance to AS.

Direct selection against susceptibility to AS

Successful selection against AS susceptibility was conducted in a fully pedigreed elite commercial broiler breeder line [68,184]. Only males and females that did not develop AS following AS-inducing surgery, i.e., unilateral pulmonary artery occlusion, were used for reproduction. After two cycles of such selection, %AS among males that were exposed to low temperatures (14ºC) from 17 to 49 d of age was reduced to 4%, from 31% in the base population and 15% after one cycle. That study demonstrated the feasibility of selection based on mortality of AS-susceptible individuals under a protocol of high-challenge AIC. Divergent selection for AS mortality was conducted by Anthony et al. [78]: the AS was induced in a hypobaric chamber where oxygen content was reduced to the level equivalent to 2,900 m above sea level. After 10 generations of divergent sire-family selection, %AS increased to about 90% in the AS-susceptible line and decreased to about 20% in the AS-resistant line, thus reaching a divergence of about 70% [78]. Similarly successful divergent selection was applied by Druyan et al. [70]: the 1st selection cycle was based on progeny testing for AS mortality under low-challenge AIC, and two further cycles of full-pedigree progeny testing were conducted under a high-challenge AIC protocol [70,72]. Two divergent lines were established: AS-susceptible (AS-S) and AS-resistant (AS-R), with, respectively, 95 and 5% AS incidence, i.e., a divergence of 90%, when reared together under the same high-challenge AIC [70].

Genomic selection against susceptibility to AS

The very rapid genetic divergence between the selected lines, along with pedigree analysis of %ASF within the AS-S- and AS-R-selected lines implies that a single or a few major genes were responsible for the difference in %AS between the lines [70]. It was concluded that one or more genes was/were involved in the response to a two-cycle selection against AS susceptibility [68]. Single-gene inheritance was also suggested after a complex segregation analysis of data on oxygen saturation of the hemoglobin in arterial blood (SaO_2) [188], a trait known to be closely related to the AS [30,72]. Data on SaO_2 from 12,000 males in fully pedigreed populations of a male line that had been closed for 30 to 40 generations were available for that study. The results suggested that a single diallelic dominant locus was responsible for 90% of the genetic variation in SaO_2, with high levels of SaO_2 indicating AS resistance and low levels indicating AS susceptibility. Data from test-crosses between fully divergent AS-S and AS-R lines suggested a model of complementary interaction between the dominant alleles of two unlinked major genes [77].

If, indeed, only a few genes are involved in genetic control of susceptibility to AS, and in light of the current rapid development and application of genomic tools, the AS genes seem likely to be detected and mapped in the near future. Once mapped, with the help of current and future genomic methodologies, the causative SNPs (or closely linked ones, used as markers) in these genes will be identified. High-throughput genomic assays may soon facilitate efficient genotyping of these marker SNPs, and their routine utilization in commercial breeding programs. With availability of such markers, high-challenge AIC will not be needed to effectively select against susceptibility to AS, because breeders will be able to easily detect and cull individual birds, within the elite lines, that carry the alleles for AS susceptibility. All major broiler-breeding companies have been heavily involved in R&D efforts aimed at achieving this goal.

5. Overall conclusions

Broilers, being highly productive birds, have difficulties in maintaining a dynamic steady-state balance between higher metabolic rate, on the one hand, and, on the other hand, the consequently higher demand for O_2 – a demand that might exceed the cardiovascular system's capacity to satisfy the O_2 needs. This non-steady-state situation leads to the development of the physiological syndrome – ascites.

Following exposure to AIC of birds from various backgrounds, birds that manifested AS were found to differ significantly from their healthy counterparts, in traits that were measured after initiation of the various AIC protocols, e.g., RV:TV ratio, hematocrit, erythrocyte counts, SaO_2, heart rate, weight gain (WG). These differences are consistent with findings of numerous reports; they represent changes in secondary manifestations of AS and, therefore, could be useful in diagnosis of birds that are developing AS, but not in prediction of AS susceptibility.

Only Druyan's lines that were divergently selected for AS were found to differ significantly in heart rate during the first week of life, when reared under standard brooding conditions (SBCs). Heart rate was significantly higher in the AS-S line than the AS-R line, but before the manifestation of the syndrome no such differences were found between the sick and healthy birds from commercial flocks that were kept under SBCs. Therefore, it appears that higher heart rate cannot be used as a general indicator to identify AS-susceptible broiler chicks.

It is expected that the problem of AS will be solved by genetic eradication of the alleles for AS susceptibility. However, manifestation of AS by genetically susceptible individuals depends on environmental conditions as well as genetic variation in growth rate. Therefore genomic information is required for effective integration of selection against AS susceptibility into breeding programs of commercial broiler stocks.

Author details

S. Druyan
Department of Poultry and Aquaculture Science, ARO, the Volcani Center, Bet-Dagan, Israel

6. References

[1] Tucker VA (1968) Respiratory physiology of house sparrows in relation to high altitude flight. J. Exp. Biol. 48: 55-66.
[2] Storz JF, Scott GR, Cheviron ZA (2010) Phenotypic plasticity and genetic adaptation to high-altitude hypoxia in vertebrates. J. Exp. Biol. 213: 4125-4136.
[3] Scott GR, Milsom WK (2009) Control of Breathing in Birds: Implications for High Altitude Flight. In: Glass ML, Wood SC, editors. Cardio-Respiratory Control in Vertebrates: Comparative and Evolutionary Aspects. Berlin: Springer-Verlag. pp. 429-448
[4] Scheid P (1990) Avian Respiratory System and Gas Exchange. In: Sutton JR, Coates G, Remmers JE, editors. Hypoxia: the Adaptations. Toronto: B.C. Decker. pp. 4-7.
[5] Dodd GAA, Scott GR, Milsom WK (2007) Ventilatory roll off during sustained hypercapnia is gender specific in Pekin ducks. Respir. Physiol. Neurobiol. 156: 47-60.
[6] Bullard RW (1972) Vertebrates at Altitude. In: Yousef MK, Horvath SM, Bullard RW, editors. Physiological Adaptations. New York: Academic Press. pp. 209-225.

[7] Monge C, Whittembury J (1976) High Altitude Adaptation in the Whole Animal. In: Blight J, Cloudsey-Thompson J, MacDonald A, editors. Environmental Physiology of Animals. New York: Wiley.

[8] Winslow R, Monge C (1987) Hypoxia, Polycythemia, and Chronic Mountain Sickness. Baltimore, MD: Johns Hopkins University Press.

[9] Monge C, León-Velarde F (1991) Physiological adaptation to high altitude: oxygen transport in mammals and birds. Physiol. Rev. 71: 1135-1172.

[10] McGrath RL, Weil JV (1978) Adverse effects of normovolemic polycythemia and hypoxia on hemodynamics in the dog. Circ. Res. 43: 793-798.

[11] Winslow R, Monge C, Brown E, Klein H, Sarnquist F, Winslow N, McNeally S (1985) Effects of hemodilution on O_2 transport in high-altitude polycythemia. J. Appl. Physiol. 59: 1495-1502.

[12] Ekblom B, Hermansen L (1968) Cardiac output in athletes. J. Appl. Physiol. 25: 619-625.

[13] Kanstrup IL, Ekblom B (1984) Blood volume and hemoglobin concentration as determinants of maximal aerobic power. Med. Sci. Sports. Exerc. 16: 256-262.

[14] Ekblom B, Bergland B (1991) Effect of erythropoietin administration on mammal aerobic power. Scand. J. Med. Sci. Sports 1: 88-93.

[15] Villafuerte FC, Cárdenas R, Monge CC (2004) Optimal hemoglobin concentration and high altitude: a theoretical approach for Andean men at rest. J. Appl. Physiol. 96: 1581-1588.

[16] Schuler B, Arras M, Keller S, Rettich A, Lundby C, Vogel J, Gassmann M (2010) Optimal hematocrit for maximal exercise performance in acute and chronic erythropoietin-treated mice. Proc. Natl. Acad. Sci. USA 107: 419-423.

[17] Guyton AC, Richardson TQ (1961) Effect of hematocrit on venous return. Circ. Res. 9: 157-164.

[18] Connes P, Yalcin O, Baskert O, Brun JF, Hardeman M (2006) In health and in a normoxic environment, VO2 max is/is not limited primarily by cardiac output and locomotor muscle blood flow. J. Appl. Physiol. 100: 2099.

[19] Nikinmaa M (2001) Haemoglobin function in vertebrates: evolutionary changes in cellular regulation in hypoxia. Respir. Physiol. 128:17-329.

[20] Weber RE, Fago A (2004) Functional adaptation and its molecular basis in vertebrate hemoglobins, neuroglobins and cytoglobins. Respir. Physiol. Neurobiol. 144: 141-159.

[21] Weber RE (2007) High-altitude adaptations in vertebrate hemoglobins. Respir. Physiol. Neurobiol. 158: 132-142.

[22] Storz JF, Moriyama H (2008) Mechanisms of hemoglobin adaptation to high-altitude hypoxia. High Alt. Med. Biol. 9: 148-157.

[23] Black CP, Tenney SM (1980) Oxygen transport during progressive hypoxia in high altitude and sea level waterfowl. Respir. Physiol. 39: 217-239.

[24] Gou X, Li N, Lian L, Yan D, Zhang H, Wei Z, Wu C (2007) Hypoxic adaptations of hemoglobin in Tibetan chick embryo: high oxygen-affinity mutation and selective expression. Comp. Biochem. Physiol. 147B: 147-155.

[25] Scott GR, Milsom WK (2006) Flying high: a theoretical analysis of the factors limiting exercise performance in birds at altitude. Respir. Physiol. Neurobiol. 154: 284-301.

[26] Storz JF (2007) Hemoglobin function and physiological adaptation to hypoxia in high-altitude mammals. J. Mammal. 88: 24-31.

[27] Julian RJ, Wilson JB (1986) Right ventricular failure as a cause of ascites in broiler and roaster chickens. Proceedings of the IVth International Symposium of Veterinary Laboratory Diagnosticians, Amsterdam, the Netherlands. ed Borst G. H. A. (Iowa State University Press, Ames, Iowa) pp. 608-611.

[28] Peacock AJ, Pickett C, Morris K, Reeves JT (1989) The relationship between rapid growth and pulmonary hemodynamics in the fast-growing broiler chicken. Am. Rev. Respir. Dis. 139: 1524-1530.

[29] Peacock AJ, Pickett C, Morris K, Reeves JT (1990) Spontaneous hypoxemia and right ventricular hypertrophy in fast-growing broiler chickens reared at sea level. Comp. Biochem. Physiol. 97A: 537-541.

[30] Julian RJ, Mirsalimi SM (1992) Blood oxygen concentration of fast-growing and slow-growing broiler chickens, and chickens with ascites from right ventricular failure. Avian Dis. 36: 730-732.

[31] Mirsalimi SM, Julian RJ, Squires EJ (1993) Effect of hypobaric hypoxia on slow- and fast-growing chickens fed diets with high and low protein levels. Avian Dis. 37: 660-667.

[32] Wideman RF Jr, Kirby YK (1995). A pulmonary artery clamp model for inducing pulmonary hypertension syndrome (ascites) in broilers. Poult. Sci. 74: 805-812.

[33] Reeves JT, Grover RF (1975) High-altitude pulmonary hypertension and pulmonary edema. Prog. Cardiol. 4: 99-118.

[34] Gurney AM (2002) Multiple sites of oxygen sensing and their contributions to hypoxic pulmonary vasoconstriction. Respir. Physiol. Neurobiol. 132: 43-53.

[35] Lovering AT, Romer LM, Haverkamp HC, Pegelow DF, Hokanson JS, Eldridge MW (2008) Intrapulmonary shunting and pulmonary gas exchange during normoxic and hypoxic exercise in healthy humans. J. Appl. Physiol. 104: 1418-1425.

[36] Maggiorini M, Melot C, Pierre S, Pfeiffer F, Greve I, Sartori C, Lepori M, Hauser M, Scherrer U, Naeije R (2001) High-altitude pulmonary edema is initially caused by an increase in capillary pressure. Circulation 103: 2078-2083.

[37] Eldridge MW, Braun RK, Yoneda KY, Walby WF (2006) Effects of altitude and exercise on pulmonary capillary integrity: evidence for subclinical high-altitude pulmonary edema. J. Appl. Physiol. 100: 972-980.

[38] León-Velarde F, Villafuerte FC, Richalet JP (2010) Chronic mountain sickness and the heart. Prog. Cardiovasc. Dis. 52: 540-549.

[39] Havenstein GB, Ferket PR, Scheideler SE, Larson BT (1994) Growth, livability, and feed conversion of 1957 vs. 1991 broilers when fed "typical" 1957 and 1991 broiler diets. Poult. Sci. 73: 1785-1794.

[40] Havenstein GB, Ferket PR, Scheideler SE, Rives DV (1994) Carcass composition and yield of 1991 vs. 1957 broilers when fed "typical" 1957 and 1991 broiler diets. Poult. Sci. 73: 1795-1804.

[41] Havenstein GB, Ferket PR, Qureshi MA (2003) Growth, livability, and feed conversion of 1957 vs. 2001 broilers when fed representative 1957 and 2001 broiler diets. Poult. Sci. 82: 1500-1508.

[42] Havenstein GB, Ferket PR, Qureshi MA (2003) Carcass composition and yield of 1957 vs 2001 broilers when fed representative 1957 and 2001 broiler diets. Poult. Sci. 82: 1509-1518.
[43] Hulet RM, Meijerhof R (2001) Multi- or single-stage incubation for high-meat yielding broiler strains. In: Proc. Southern Poultry Science and Southern Conference of Avian Diseases, Atlanta, GA. p. 35.
[44] Tona K, Onagbesan OM, Jego Y, Kamers B, Decuypere E, Bruggeman V (2004) Comparison of embryo physiological parameters during incubation, chick quality, and growth performance of three lines of broiler breeders differing in genetic composition and growth rate. Poult. Sci. 83: 507–513.
[45] Druyan S (2010) The effects of genetic line (broilers vs. layers) on embryo development. Poult. Sci. 89: 1457–1467.
[46] Decuypere E, Buyse J, Buys N (2000) Ascites in broiler chickens: exogenous and endogenous structural and functional causal factors. World's Poult. Sci. 56: 367-377.
[47] Balog JM (2003) Ascites syndrome (pulmonary hypertension syndrome) in broiler chickens: are we seeing the light at the end of the tunnel? Avian Poult. Biol. Rev. 14: 99-126.
[48] Julian RJ (1987) The effect of increased sodium in the drinking water on right ventricular hypertrophy, right ventricular failure and ascites in broiler chickens. Avian Pathol. 16: 61-71.
[49] Julian RJ (1988) Pulmonary hypertension as a cause of right ventricular failure and ascites in broilers. Zootech. Internat. 11: 58-62.
[50] Wideman RFJ, Maynard P, Bottje WG (1999) Venous blood pressure in broilers during acute inhalation of five percent carbon dioxide or unilateral pulmonary artery occlusion. Poult. Sci. 78: 1443-1451.
[51] Bottje WG, Wideman RF Jr (1995) Potential role of free radicals in the pathogenesis of pulmonary hypertension syndrome. Poult. Avian Biol. Rev. 6: 211-231.
[52] Julian RJ (1993) Ascites in poultry. Avian Pathol. 22: 419-454.
[53] Wideman RF Jr, Kirby YK, Forman MF, Marson N, McNew RW, Owen RL (1998) The infusion rate-dependent influence of acute metabolic acidosis on pulmonary vascular resistance in broilers. Poult. Sci. 77: 309-321.
[54] Maxwell MH, Robertson GW, McCorquodale CC (1992) Whole blood and plasma viscosity values in normal and ascetic broiler chickens. Brit. Poult. Sci. 33: 871-877.
[55] Olkowski AA, Classen HL (1998) Progressive bradycardia, a possible factor in the pathogenesis of ascites in fast-growing broiler chickens raised at low altitude. Br. Poult. Sci. 39: 139-146.
[56] Wideman RF (2000) Cardio-pulmonary hemodynamics and ascites in broiler chickens. Avian Poult. Biol. Rev. 11: 21-43.
[57] Druyan S, Shinder D, Shlosberg A, Cahaner A, Yahav S (2009) Physiological parameters in broiler lines divergently selected for the incidence of ascites. Poult. Sci. 88: 1984-1990.
[58] Maxwell MH, Robertson GW (1997) World broiler ascites survey. Poult. Internat. 36: 16-30.

[59] Maxwell MH, Robertson GW (1998) UK survey of broiler ascites and sudden death syndromes in 1993. Br. Poult. Sci. 39: 203–215.

[60] Lubritz DL, McPherson BN (1994) Effect of genotype and cold stress on incidence of ascites in cockerels. J. Appl. Poult. Res. 3: 171-178.

[61] Anthony NP, Balog JM, Staudinger EB, Wall CW, Walker RD, Huff WE (1994) Effect of a urease inhibitor and ceiling fans on ascites in broilers. 1. Environmental variability and incidence of ascites. Poult. Sci. 73: 801–809.

[62] Julian RJ (2000) Physiological, management and environmental triggers of the ascites syndrome: a review. Avian Pathol. 29: 519-527.

[63] Olkowski AA, Classen HL (1999) Echocardiographic evaluation of heart function in normal chickens and chickens with heart failure and ascites. Poult. Sci. 78(Suppl. 1): Abstract 250.

[64] Olkowski AA, Abbott JA, Classen HL (2005) Pathogenesis of ascites in broilers raised at low altitude: aetiological considerations based on echocardiographic findings. J. Vet. Med. Ser. A 52: 4, 166-171,

[65] Gonzales E, Buyse J, Loddi MM, Takita TS, Buys N, Decuypere E (1998) Performance, incidence of metabolic disturbance and endocrine variables of food-restricted male broiler chickens. Brit. Poult. Sci. 39: 671-678.

[66] Buys N, Scheele CW, Kwakernaak C, Decuypere E (1999) Performance and physiological variables in broiler chicken lines differing in susceptibility to the ascites syndrome: 2. Effect of ambient temperature on partial efficiencies of protein and fat retention and plasma hormone concentrations. Brit. Poult. Sci. 40: 140-144.

[67] Wideman RF Jr (1998) Causes and control of ascites in broilers. In: Proc. National Meeting on Poultry Health and Processing, 33: 56-85.

[68] Wideman RF Jr, French H (2000). Ascites resistance of progeny from broiler breeders selected for two generations using chronic unilateral pulmonary artery occlusion. Poult. Sci. 79: 396-401.

[69] Decuypere E, Buyse J (2005) Further insights into the susceptibility of broilers to ascites. Vet. J. 169: 319–320.

[70] Druyan S, Ben-David A, Cahaner A (2007) Development of ascites-resistant and ascites-susceptible broiler lines. Poult. Sci. 86: 811-822.

[71] Druyan S, Hadad Y, Cahaner A (2008) Growth rate of ascites-resistant versus ascites-susceptible broilers in commercial and experimental lines. Poult. Sci. 87: 904-911.

[72] Druyan S, Shlosberg A, Cahaner A (2007) Evaluation of growth rate, body weight, heart rate, and blood parameters as potential indicators for selection against susceptibility to the ascites syndrome in young broilers. Poult. Sci. 86: 621-629.

[73] Lubritz DL, Smith JL, McPherson BN. (1995) Heritability of ascites and the ratio of right to total ventricle weight in broiler breeder male lines. Poult. Sci. 74: 1237-1241.

[74] de Greef K, Kwakernaak HC, Ducro BJ, Pit R, Gerritsen CL (2001) Evaluation of between-line variation for within-line selection against ascites in broilers. Poult. Sci. 80: 13-21.

[75] Deeb N, Shlosberg A, Cahaner A (2002) Genotype-by-environment interaction with broiler genotypes differing in growth rate. 4. Association between responses to heat stress and to cold-induced ascites. Poult. Sci. 81: 1454-1462.

[76] Pakdel A, van Arendonk JAM, Vereijken ALJ, Bovenhuis H (2005) Genetic parameters of ascites-related traits in broilers: effect of cold and normal temperature conditions. Br. Poult. Sci. 46: 35-42.

[77] Druyan S, Cahaner A (2007) Segregation among test-cross progeny suggests that two complementary dominant genes explain the difference between ascites-resistant and ascites-susceptible broiler lines. Poult. Sci. 86: 2295-2300.

[78] Pavlidis HO, Balog JM, Stamps LK, Hughes JD Jr, Huff WE, Anthony NB (2007) Divergent selection for ascites incidence in chickens. Poult. Sci. 86: 2517–2529.

[79] Riddell C (1991) Developmental, Metabolic, and Miscellaneous Disorders. In: Calnek BW, Barnes HJ, Beard CW, Reid WM, Yoder HW Jr, editors. Diseases of Poultry. 9th ed. Ames, IA: Iowa State University Press. pp. 839-841.

[80] Lister S (1997) Broiler ascites: a veterinary viewpoint. World's Poult. Sci. 53: 65-67.

[81] Cueva S, Sillau H, Vaplenzuela A, Ploog H (1974) High-altitude induced pulmonary hypertension and right heart failure in broiler chickens. Res. Vet. Sci. 16: 370-374.

[82] Albers G, Frankenhuis M (1990) Ascites, a high-altitude disease in the lowlands. Poultry (Misset). February March: 24-25.

[83] Currie RJW (1999) Ascites in poultry: Recent investigations. Avian Pathol. 28: 313-326.

[84] Wideman RF Jr (2001) Pathophysiology of heart/lung disorders: pulmonary hypertension syndrome in broiler chickens. World's Poult. Sci. J. 57: 289-307.

[85] Witzel DA, Huff WE, Kubena LF, Harvey RB, Elissalde MH (1990) Ascites in growing broilers: A research model. Poult. Sci. 69: 741-745.

[86] Olkowski AA, Classen HL, Kumor L (1998) Left atrio-ventricular valve degeneration, left ventricular dilation and right ventricular failure: a possible association with pulmonary hypertension and aetiology of ascites in broiler chickens. Avian Path. 27: 51-59.

[87] Reeves JT, Ballam G, Hofmeister S, Picket C, Morris K, Peacock A (1991) Improved arterial oxygenation with feed restriction in rapidly growing broiler chickens. Comp. Biochem. Physics 99A: 481-495.

[88] Wideman RF Jr, Kirby YK (1995) Evidence of a ventilation perfusion mismatch during acute unilateral pulmonary artery occlusion in broilers. Poult. Sci. 74: 1209-1217.

[89] Luger D, Shinder D, Wolfenson D, Yahav S (2003) Erythropoiesis regulation during the development of ascites syndrome in broiler chickens: a possible role of corticosterone. J. Anim. Sci. 81: 784-790.

[90] Fedde MR, Wideman RF Jr (1996) Blood viscosity in broilers: Influence on pulmonary hypertension syndrome. Poult. Sci. 75: 1261-1267.

[91] Smith AH, Wilson WO, Pace N (1954) The effect of high altitude on the growth of turkeys. Growth 18: 27-35.

[92] Smith AH, Wilson WO, Pace N (1955) Growth and reproduction in domestic birds at high altitudes. Poult. Sci. 35(Suppl.1): 1175.

[93] Smith AH, Abplanalp H, Harwood LM, Kelly CF (1959) Poultry at high altitudes. California Agriculture. November: 8-9.
[94] Siller WG, Hemsley LA (1966) The incidence of congenital heart disease in seven flocks of broiler chickens. Vet. Rec. 79: 451-454.
[95] Olander HJ, Burton RR, Adler HE. (1967) The pathophysiology of chronic hypoxia in chickens. Avian Dis. 11: 609-620.
[96] Burton RR, Smith AH (1967) Effect of polycythemia and chronic hypoxia on heart mass in the chicken. J. Appl. Physiol. 22: 782-785.
[97] Hall SA, Machicao N (1968) Myocarditis in broiler chickens reared at high altitude. Avian Dis. 12: 75-84.
[98] Maxwell MH, Spence S, Robertson GW, Mitchell MA (1990) Haematological and morphological responses of broiler chicks to hypoxia. Avian Pathol. 19: 23-40.
[99] Burton RR, Carlisle JC (1969) Acute hypoxia tolerance of the chick. Poult. Sci. 48: 1265-1269.
[100] Burton RR, Sahara R, Smith AH (1971) The haematology of domestic fowl native to high altitude. Environ. Physiol. 1: 155-163.
[101] Ploog HP (1973) Physiologic changes in broiler chickens (*Gallus domesticus*) exposed to a simulated altitude of 4267 m. (14000 ft). M.Sc. Thesis, Pennsylvania State University, University Park, PA, USA.
[102] Owen RL, Wideman RF Jr, Hattel AL, Cowen BS (1990) Use of a hypobaric chamber as a model system for investigating ascites in broilers. Avian Dis. 34: 754-758.
[103] Owen RL, Wideman RF Jr, Leach RM, Cowen BS, Dunn PA, Ford BC (1995) Physiologic and electrocardiographic changes occurring in broilers reared at simulated high altitude. Avian Dis. 39: 108-115.
[104] Owen RL, Wideman RF Jr, Barbato GF, Cowen BS, Ford BC, Hattel AL (1995) Morphometric and histologic changes in the pulmonary system of broilers raised at simulated high altitude. Avian Pathol. 24: 293-302.
[105] Anthony NB, Balog JM, Hughes JD, Stamp L, Cooper MA., Kidd BD, Liu X, Huff GR, Huff WE, Rath NC (2001) Genetic selection of broiler lines that differ in their ascites susceptibility. 1. Selection under hypobaric conditions. In: Proc. 13th Eur. Poult. Nutr. Symp., Blankenberge, Belgium. World Poultry Science Association, Belgium. pp. 327–328.
[106] Anthony NB, Balog JM (2003) Divergent selection for ascites: development of susceptible and resistant lines. In:Fifty-Second Annual National Breeders Roundtable Proceedings, St. Louis, Missouri, USA. pp. 39-58.
[107] Cisar CR, Balog JM, Anthony NB, Donoghue AM (2003) Sequence analysis of bone morphogenetic protein receptor type II mRNA from ascitic and nonascitic commercial broilers. Poult. Sci. 82: 1494-1499.
[108] Wideman RF Jr (1997) Understanding pulmonary hypertension syndrome (ascites). Hubbard Farms Technical Report, Walpole, NH, June. pp. 1-6.
[109] Sillau AH, Cueva S, Morales P (1980) Pulmonary arterial hypertension in male and female chickens at 3300 m. Pflugers Archiv. 386: 269-275.

[110] Owen RL, Wideman RF, Cowen BS (1995) Changes in pulmonary arterial and femoral arterial blood pressure upon acute exposure to hypobaric hypoxia in broiler chickens. Poult. Sci. 74: 708-715.

[111] Wideman RF Jr, Wing T, Kirby YK, Forman MF, Marson N, Tackett CD, Ruiz-Feria CA (1998) Evaluation of minimally invasive indices for predicting ascites susceptibility in three successive hatches of broilers exposed to cool temperatures. Poult. Sci. 77: 1565–1573.

[112] Maxwell MH, Spence S, Robertson GW, Mitchell MA (1990) Haematological and morphological responses of broiler chicks to hypoxia. Avian Pathol. 19: 23-40.

[113] Mirsalimi SM, Julian RJ. (1991) Reduced erythrocyte deformability as a possible contributing factor to pulmonary hypertension and ascites in broiler chickens. Avian Dis. 35: 374-379.

[114] Beker A, Vanhooser SL, Teeter RG (1995) Effect of oxygen level on ascites incidence and performance in broiler chicks. Avian Dis. 39: 285-291.

[115] Shlosberg A, Bellaiche M, Zeitlin G, Ya'acobi M, Cahaner A (1996) Hematocrit values and mortality from ascites in cold-stressed broilers from parents selected by hematocrit. Poult. Sci. 75: 1-5.

[116] Shlosberg A, Bellaiche M, Berman E, Perk S, Deeb N, Neumark E, Cahaner A (1998) Relationship between broiler chicken haematocrit-selected parents and their progeny, with regard to haematocrit, mortality from ascites and bodyweight. Res. Vet. Sci. 64: 105-109.

[117] May JD, Deaton JW (1974) Environmental temperature effect on heart weight of chickens. Int. J. Biometeorol. 15: 295-300.

[118] VillasenÄor J, Rivera-Cruz E (1980) Que estaÁ pasando on la ascitis? In: Proc. 29th Western Poultry Disease Conf., Acapulco, Mexico. pp. 89-92.

[119] Hernândez, A. (1984). Influencia de la temperatura en la incidencia de la ascitis de origen hipoxico en pollos de engorde. In: Memorias XIV Congreso Nacional de Medicina Veterinaria y Zootecnia, Cartagena, Colombia, p. 14.

[120] Acosta JM. (1986) Experimentos y observaciones de campo sobre ascites en el Ecuador. In: Proc. 35th Western Poultry Disease Conf., Puerto Vallarta, Mexico. pp. 1-3.

[121] Wideman RF Jr (1988) Ascites in poultry. Monsanto Nutr. Update. 6: 1-7.

[122] Julian RJ, McMillan I, Quinton M (1989) The effect of cold and dietary energy on right ventricular hypertrophy, right ventricular failure and ascites in meat-type chickens. Avian Pathol. 18: 675-684.

[123] Bendheim U, Berman E, Zadikov I, Shlosberg A (1992) The effect of poor ventilation, low temperatures, type of feed and sex of bird on the development of ascites in broilers. Production parameters. Avian Pathol. 21: 383-388.

[124] Shlosberg A, Pano G, Handji V, Berman E (1992) Prophylactic and therapeutic treatment of ascites in broiler chickens. Br. Poult. Sci. 33: 141-148.

[125] Shlosberg, A, Zadikov I, Bendheim U, Handji V, Berman E (1992) The effects of poor ventilation, low temperatures, type of feed and sex of bird on the development of ascites in broilers. Physiopathological factors. Avian Pathol. 21: 369-382.

[126] Silva JE (2006) Thermogenic mechanisms and their hormonal regulation. Physiol. Rev. 86: 435-464.

[127] Morrison, SF, Nakamura, K, Madden, CJ (2008) Central control of thermogenesis in mammals. Experimental Physiol., 93,773-797.

[128] Richards MP, Proszkowiec-Weglarz M (2007) Mechanisms regulating feed intake, energy expenditure, and body weight in poultry. Poult. Sci. 86: 1478-1490.

[129] Barott HG, Pringle EM (1946) Energy and gaseous metabolism of the chicken from hatch to maturity as affected by temperature. J. Nutr. 31: 35-50.

[130] Olson DW, Sunde ML, Bird HR (1972). The effect of temperature on metabolizable energy determination and utilization by the growing chick. Poult. Sci. 5: 1915-1922.

[131] Gleeson M (1986) Respiratory adjustments of the unanaesthetized chicken, *Gallus domesticus*, to elevated metabolism elicited by 2,4 dinitrophenol or cold exposure. Comp. Biochem. Physiol. 83A: 283-289.

[132] Huchzermeyer FW, Van der Colf WJ, Guinane PR (1989) Broiler ascites: increased oxygen demand with cold may explain high winter incidence. (SAPA) Poult. Bull.September, 474-483.

[133] Stolz JL, Rosenbaum LM, Jeong D, Odom TW (1992) Ascites syndrome, mortality and cardiological responses of broiler chickens subjected to cold exposure. Poult. Sci. 71(Suppl. 1): 4.

[134] Wideman RF Jr, Tackett CD (2000) Cardio-pulmonary function in broilers reared at warm or cool temperatures: effect of acute inhalation of 100% oxygen. Poult. Sci. 79: 257-264.

[135] Vanhooser SL, Beker A, Teeter RG (1995) Bronchodilator, oxygen level, and temperature effects on ascites incidence in broiler chickens. Poult. Sci. 74: 1586-1590.

[136] Wideman RF Jr, Ismail M, Kirby YK, Bottje WG, Moore RW, Vardeman RC (1995) Furosemide reduces the incidence of pulmonary hypertension syndrome (ascites) in broilers exposed to cool environmental temperatures. Poult. Sci. 74: 314-322.

[137] Deaton JW, Branton SL, Simmons JD, Lott BD (1996) The effect of brooding temperature on broiler performance. Poult. Sci. 75: 1217-1220.

[138] Shlosberg A, Bellaiche M (1996) Hematocrit values and mortality from ascites in cold-stressed broilers from parents selected by hematocrit. Poult. Sci. 75: 1-5.

[139] Luger D, Shinder D, Rzepakovsky V, Rusal M, Yahav S (2001) Association between weight gain, blood parameters, and thyroid hormones and the development of ascites syndrome in broiler chickens. Poult. Sci. 80: 965-971.

[140] Balog JM, Kidd BD, Anthony NB, Huff GR, Huff WE, Rath NC (2003) Effect of cold stress on broilers selected for resistance or susceptibility to ascites syndrome. Poult. Sci. 82: 1383-1388.

[141] Julian RJ, Squires EJ (1995) Suggestions for reducing ascites in meat-type chickens. In: Proc. 44th Western Poultry Disease Conf., Sacramento, CA. pp. 19-20.

[142] Groves PJ (2002) Environmental determinants of broiler ascites syndrome. In: Proc. Australian Poultry Sci. Symp., Sydney, Australia. 14: 83-88.

[143] Moye RJ, Washburn KW, Huston TM (1969) Effect of environmental temperature on erythrocyte number and size. Poult. Sci. 48: 1683-1686.

[144] Shlosberg A, Berman E, Bendheim U, Plavnik I (1991) Controlled early feed restriction as a potential means of reducing the incidence of ascites in broilers. Avian Dis. 35: 681-684.

[145] Scheele CW, De Wit W, Frankenhuis MT, Vereijken PFG (1991) Ascites in broilers. 1. Experimental factors evoking symptoms related to ascites. Poult. Sci. 70: 1069-1083.

[146] Vogelaere P, Savourey G, Daklunder G, Lecroat J, Braseur M, Bekaert S, Bittel J (1992) Reversal of cold induced haemoconcentration. Eur. J. Appl. Physiol. 64: 244-249.

[147] Kranen RW, Veerkamp CH, Lambooy E, Van Kuppevelt TH, Veerkamp JH (1998) The effect of thermal preslaughter stress on the susceptibility of broiler chickens differing with respect to growth rate, age at slaughter, blood parameters, and ascites mortality, to hemorrhages in muscles. Poult. Sci. 77: 737-744.

[148] Dejours P, Garey WF, Rahn H (1970) Comparison of ventilatory and circulatory flow rates between animals in various physiological conditions. Respir. Physiol. 9: 108-117.

[149] Bouverot P (1985) Adaptation to Altitude-Hypoxia in Vertebrates. Berlin: Springer-Verlag.

[150] Burton RR, Smith AH (1972) The effect of chronic erythrocytic polycythemia and high altitude upon plasma and blood volumes. Proc. Soc. Exp. Biol. Med. 140: 920-923.

[151] Julian RJ, Summers J, Wilson JB (1986) Right ventricular failure and ascites in broiler chickens caused by phosphorus-deficient diets. Avian Dis. 30: 453-459.

[152] Maxwell MH, Tullett SG, Burton FG (1987) Haematology and morphological changes in young broiler chicks with experimentally induced hypoxia. Res. Vet. Sci. 43: 331-338.

[153] Yersin AG, Huff WE, Kubena LF, Elissalde MH, Harvey RB, Witzel DA, Giroir LE (1992) Changes in hematological, blood gas, and serum biochemical variables in broilers during exposure to simulated high altitude. Avian Dis. 36: 189-196.

[154] Shlosberg A, Bellaiche M, Hanji V, Nyska A, Lublin A, Shemesh M, Shore L, Perk S, Berman E (1996) The effect of acetylsalicylic acid and cold stress on the susceptibility of broilers to the ascites syndrome. Avian Pathol. 25: 581-590.

[155] McGovern RH, Feddes JJR, Robinson FE, Hanson JA (1999) Growth performance, carcass characteristics, and the incidence of ascites in broilers in response to feed restriction and litter oiling. Poult. Sci. 78: 522-528.

[156] Parving HH, Jensen HA, Westrup M (1977) Increased transcapillary escape rate of albumin and IgG in essential hypertension. Scand. J. Clin. Lab. Invest. 37: 223–227.

[157] Parving H, Ranek HL, Lassen NA (1977) Increased transcapillary escape rate of albumin in patients with cirrhosis of the liver. Scand. J. Clin. Lab. Invest. 37: 643–648.

[158] Henriksen JH, Siemssen O, Krintel JJ, Malchow-Moller A, Bendsten F, Ring-Larsen H (2001) Dynamics of albumin in plasma and ascitic fluid in patients with cirrhosis. J. Hepatol. 34: 53–60.

[159] Salo J, Gines A, Gines P, Piera C, Jimenez W, Guevara M, Fernandez-Esparrach G, Sort P, Bataller R, Arroyo V, Rodes J (1997) Effect of therapeutic paracentesis on plasma volume and transvascular escape rate of albumin in patients with cirrhosis. J. Hepatol. 27: 645–653.

[160] Akester AR (1974) Deformation of red blood cells in avian lung capillaries. Proceedings of the Anatomical Society of Great Britain and Ireland. J. Anat. 117: 657–658.

[161] Julian RJ, Friars GW, French H, Quinton M (1987) The relationship of right ventricular hypertrophy, right ventricular failure, and ascites to weight gain in broiler and roaster chickens. Avian Dis. 31: 130-135.

[162] Julian RJ (1990) Cardiovascular disease. ed Jordan F. T. W. (Bailliere Tindall, London, United Kingdom), Poultry Diseases, 3rd ed. pp 345–353.

[163] McGovern RH, Feddes JJR. Robinson FE, Hanson JA (1999) Growth performance, carcass characteristics and the incidence of ascites in broilers in response to feed restriction and litter oiling. Poult. Sci. 78:522-528.

[164] McGovern RH, Feddes JJR. Robinson FE, Hanson JA (2000) Growth, carcass characteristics, and incidence of ascites in broilers exposed to environmental fluctuations and oiled litter. Poult. Sci. 79:324-330.

[165] Olkowski AA, Classen HL, Riddell C, Bennett CD (1997) A study of electrocardiographic patterns in a population of commercial broiler chickens. Vet. Res. Comm. 21: 51-62.

[166] Druyan S, Hadad Y, Yahav S, Cahaner A (2005) Ascites-resistant vs. ascites-susceptible broiler: physiological parameters and growth rate from hatch to 3 weeks of age. In: Abstracts 2nd Workshop on Fundamental Physiology of Perinatal Development in Poultry, (Berlin, Germany). Humboldt Univ. Berlin, Germany.

[167] Tazawa H, Takami M, Kobayashi K, Hasegawa J, Ar A (1992) Non-invasive determination of heart rate in newly hatched chicks. Br. Poult. Sci. 33: 1111–1118.

[168] Wideman RF Jr (1999) Cardiac output in four-, five- and six-week-old broilers, and hemodynamic responses to intravenous injections of epinephrine. Poult. Sci. 78: 392-403.

[169] Besch EL, Kadono H (1978) Cardiopulmonary responses to acute hypoxia in domestic fowl. In: Piiper J, editor. Respiratory Function in Birds Adult and Embryonic. New York: Springer-Verlag. pp. 71-78.

[170] Faraci FM (1986) Circulation during hypoxia in birds. Comp. Biochem. Physiol. 85A: 613-620.

[171] Scheele CW, Van Der Klis JD, Kwakernaak C, Buys N, Decuypere E (2003) Haematological characteristics predicting susceptibility for ascites. 1. High carbon dioxide tensions in juvenile chickens. Br. Poult. Sci. 44: 476–483.

[172] Scheele CW, Van Der Klis JD, Kwakernaak C, Dekker RA, Van Middelkoop JH, Buyse J, Decuypere E (2005) Ascites and venous carbon dioxide tensions in juvenile chickens of highly selected genotypes and native strains. World's Poult. Sci. J. 61: 113–129.

[173] Enkvetchakul B, Beasley J, Bottje W (1995) Pulmonary arteriole hypertrophy in broilers with pulmonary hypertension syndrome (ascites). Poult. Sci. 74: 1676-1682.

[174] Maxwell MH, Robertson GW, Spence S (1986) Studies on an ascitic syndrome in young broiler. 1. Haematology and pathology. Avian Pathol. 15: 511-524.

[175] Maxwell MH, Dick LA, Anderson IA, Mitchell MA (1989) Ectopic cartilagious and osseous lung nodules induced in the young broiler by inadequate ventilation. Avian Pathol. 18: 113-124.

[176] Wideman RF Jr, Fedde MR, Tackett CD, Weigle GE (2000) Cardio-pulmonary function in preascitic (hypoxemic) or normal broilers inhaling ambient air or 100% oxygen. Poult. Sci. 79: 415-425.

[177] Forman MF, Wideman RF Jr (2000) Measurements of pulmonary arterial pressure in anesthetized male broilers at two to seven weeks of age. Poult. Sci. 79: 1645- 1649.

[178] Chapman ME, Wideman RF Jr (2001) Pulmonary wedge pressures confirm pulmonary hypertension in broilers is initiated by an excessive pulmonary arterial (precapillary) resistance. Poult. Sci. 80: 468-473.

[179] Wideman RF Jr, Erf GF, Chapman ME (2001) Intravenous endotoxin triggers pulmonary vasoconstriction and pulmonary hypertension in broiler chickens. Poult. Sci. 80: 647-655.

[180] de Greef KH, Janss LLG, Vereijken ALJ, Pit R, Gerritsen CLM (2001) Disease-induced variability of genetic correlations: Ascites in broilers as a case study. J. Anim. Sci. 79: 1723–1733.

[181] Moghadam HK, McMillan I, Chambers JR, Julian RJ (2001) Estimation of genetic parameters for ascites syndrome in broiler chickens. Poult. Sci. 80: 844-848.

[182] Pakdel A, Van Arendonk JA, Vereijken AL, Bovenhuis H (2002) Direct maternal genetic effect for ascites related traits in broilers. Poult. Sci. 81: 1273–1279.

[183] Wideman RF Jr, Kirby YK, Owen RL, French H (1997) Chronic unilateral occlusion of an extrapulmonary primary bronchus induces pulmonary hypertension syndrome (ascites) in male and female broilers. Poult. Sci. 76: 400-404.

[184] Wideman RF Jr, French H (1999) Broiler breeder survivors of chronic unilateral pulmonary artery occlusion produce progeny resistant to pulmonary hypertension syndrome (ascites) induced by cool temperatures. Poult. Sci. 78: 404-411.

[185] Kirby YK, McNew RW, Kirby JD, Wideman RF Jr (1997) Evaluation of logistic versus linear regression models for predicting pulmonary hypertension syndrome (ascites) using cold exposure or pulmonary artery clamp models in broilers. Poult. Sci. 76: 392-399.

[186] Druyan S, Cahaner A, Bellaiche M, Rosner A, Shlosberg A (1999). Genetics of blood oxygenation, heart rate, and ECG waveforms, and their association with ascites in broilers. In: Proc. 1st European Poultry Genetics Symposium, Mariensee, Germany.. p. 112.

[187] Navarro P, Visscher, PM, Chatziplis D, Koerhuis AN, Haley CS (2006) Segregation analysis of blood oxygen saturation in broilers suggests a major gene influence on ascites. Br. Poult. Sci. 47: 671–684.

[188] Dewil E, Buys N, Albers GAA, Decuypere E (1996) Different characteristics in chick embryos of two broiler lines differing in susceptibility to ascites. Br. Poult. Sci. 37: 1003-1013.

[189] De Smit L, Tona K, Bruggeman V, Onagbesan O, Hassanzadeh M, Arckens L, Decuypere E (2005) Comparison of three lines of broilers differing in ascites

susceptibility or growth rate. 2. Egg weight loss, gas pressures, embryonic heat production, and physiological hormone levels. Poult. Sci. 84: 1446–1452.

[190] Tona K, Kemps B, Bruggeman V, Bamelis F, De Smit L, Onagbesan O, De Baerdemaeker J, Decuypere E (2005) Comparison of three lines of broiler breeders differing in ascites susceptibility or growth rate. 1. Relationship between acoustic resonance data and embryonic or hatching parameters. Poult. Sci. 84: 1439–1445.

Chapter 14

The Effects of the Far-Infrared Ray (FIR) Energy Radiation on Living Body

Kikuji Yamashita

Additional information is available at the end of the chapter

http://dx.doi.org/10.5772/36005

1. Introduction

1.1. A far infrared ray (FIR) energy

The power of the energy radiated from any material is dependent on the temperature. For example, the sun with the temperature of 6,000°C at the surface and ~15,000,000°C at the depths radiates the radio-magnetic ray with from the weak to the strong energy. The radio-magnetic ray with strong energy is absorbed before the arrives at the surface of the earth. But, if a human bathe in the ultraviolet ray even if it arrives only about 0.6% of whole ultraviolet ray radiated by the sun, the surface of skin is burned and strongly damaged. If the cell is poured the large quantities of ultraviolet ray, the DNA of nuclear is injured to induce a liver spot, freckles and aging of skin. Still more, it is thought that the immunity is inhibited and a cataract and a skin cancer can be induced by the ultraviolet ray. It was thought that the sunlight arrived at the surface of earth was finally composed of the ultraviolet ray (UVA, UVB) of 6%, the visible ray of 52% and the infrared ray of 42%. It was well known that the energy of these lights bring a lots of the good effects for living bodies. The other sides, the materials on the earth we are living radiated the narrow range of energy from 5 to 50μm in FIR under 30°C by getting the energy of sunlight.

In other words, thought the radiating energy on the earth creating a life was only FIR of 5~50μm by getting the energy of visual ray and FIR, the earth was filled with the energy of only FIR of narrow range. It was means that the energy of FIR may make contribution to the birth of a life. The National Aeronautics and Space Administration (NASA) reported which ray indispensable for the maintenance of the life was FIR of 4~20μm as the artificial sun in the space station. Therefore, it comes to a conclusion that the FIR is the raising ray for the living body (Fig.1). Recently, there have been many studies of the effects of FIR on health and food preservation. The available evidence indicates that whole-body FIR irradiation has biological effects [1-7]. Whole-body FIR irradiation is believed to improve human health and sleep by enhancing blood circulation in the skin [1, 2]. However, the effects of FIR on cells are not clearly understood. These thinking let me realize that there are a lot of natural materials radiating strongly the energy of FIR as a charcoal, stone, soil and tree. So, these natural materials were being used for our studies on the energy of FIR.

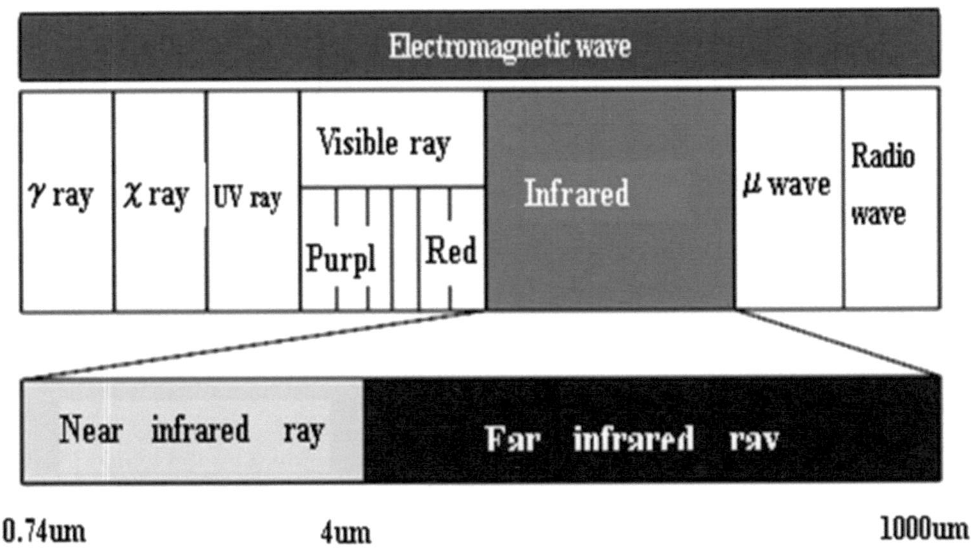

Figure 1. The classes of the electromagnetic wave by the wave length μm

2. The characteristics of rhyolite

In order to study strictly the effects of the energy of FIR in 4~20μm on the living body, the radiating machine of the energy of FIR should be developed. In order to develop it, the selection of a good FIR radiator were started at first. The most noticeable effect of FIR energy radiation was the activation of water molecules. The change of the weight of the ultrapure water on the FIR ceramics containing the five natural stones, 4 chemical products of mineral oxide and charcoal was exactly measured with time at 37°C. Though it was made clear that some natural stones activated the evaporation of pure water, the rhyolite especially strongly activated. Then, the rhyolite (MATERA Inc. Toon, Ehime, Japan) mined at Toon, Ehime in Shikoku Island was selected as the FIR radiation ceramics for the development of the radiating machine of the energy of FIR (Fig.2). The characteristic of rhyolite was the volcanic rock containing 70% over silicate dioxide with the flowing patterns formed by the phenocryst of magma (Fig.2). Though the components are the quartz, feldspar and biotite, the rhyolite is similar the granite. When the FIR energy radiated from the rhyolite was measured by Fourier transformed infrared spectrophotometer, it was made clear that the rhyolite was radiated 90% over the ideal black body at whole range of 5~20μm (Fig.3). It was proved that the rhyolite was the excellent radiator of FIR energy of 5~20μm.

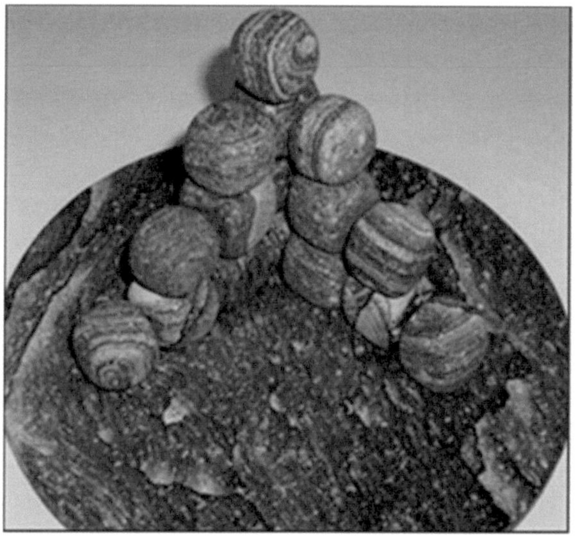

Figure 2. The photograph of the rhyolite

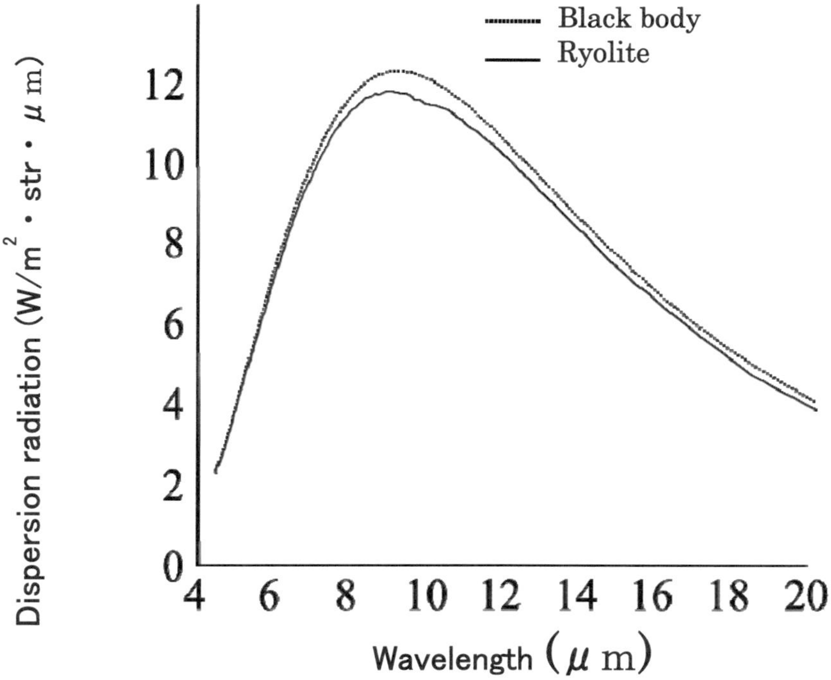

Figure 3. The radiation energy of the far infrared ray from the radiator

The powder of rhyolite showed the antibacterial action to the Staphylococcus aureus ATCC6538P at 1/5012. The adhesive sheet with the 15% powder of rhyolite showed at 1/1995. Still more, the paint containg the 10 % powder of rhyolite showed the antibacterial action to the Methicillin-Resistant Staphylococcus Aureus MRSAIID 1677 at 1/5012.

The values of antibacterial action of the materials containing rhyolite are respectively 3.7, 3.3 and 3.2. Though the values of antibacterial action over 2.0 was estimated as the antibacterial substance, the rhyolite was regarded to be the fairly mighty the antibacterial substance. Still more, the antibacterial action of rhyolite to the colon bacillus was verified in neutral condition at our laboratory also (Fig.4, Table 1). These results suggested that the antibacterial action of rhyolite did not depend on the change of pH. This graph showed the effects of rhyolite on the oxidation-reduction potential of water (Fig.5).

Item	The water treated with the powder of rhyolite	The water treated with the stone of rhyolite	Control
Biochemical oxygen demand mg/1	2.1	2.4	2.4
Chemical Oxygen Demand mg/1	3.4	3.9	3.9
Suspended solids	12	10	8
Dissolved Oxygen	9	8.9	9.1
Escherichia coli group number MPN/100ml	0	2200	14000
Conductivity	18.6	19.5	19

Table 1. The chemical analysis of the rhyolite treated water

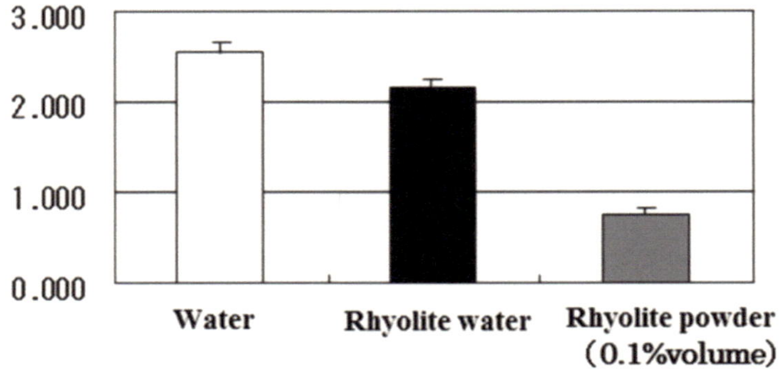

Figure 4. The effect of the rhyolite on Escherichia coli; Escherichia coli (DH50) were cultured for 16 hours in the sterilized pure water, the water containing the rhyolite and the water containing 0.1% rhyolite powder. The proliferation of the Escherichia coli inhibited at 15.6% in the water containing the rhyolite and 69.9% in the water containing 0.1% rhyolite powder.

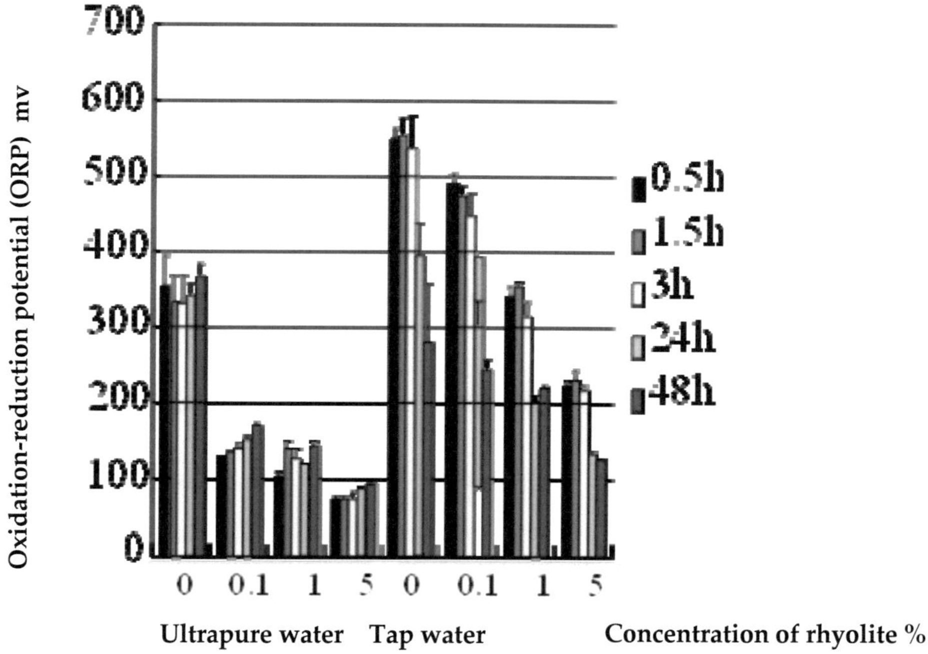

Figure 5. The change of the oxidation-reduction potential affected by the rhyolite. The oxidation-reduction potential (The longitudinal axis shows ORP, mv) decreased depending on the contents of the rhyolite(The transverse axis shows %) after 0.5-48h.

Though the oxidation-reduction potential of tap water is about 550, it decreased with time to be about 280 after 48 hours. When the powder of rhyolite was put into tap water at 0.1%, 1%, 5%, the oxidation-reduction potential of tap water decreased respectively up to 480, 340 and 220. Then, it decreased with time up to about 130 after 24 hours. It was thought that the high oxidation-reduction potential of the tap water caused by the residual chlorine. The reason why the oxidation-reduction potential of the tap decreased with time might be that the hypochlorous acid in tap water evaporated as the gas of chlorine with time. The oxidation-reduction potential decreased in the dependent upon the density of the rhyolite powder. It was thought that the reason was by the elution of any reducing agent from rhyolite. The small amounts of any elements with oxidative reaction were left in the ultrapure water. Therefore, the small amounts of rhyolite powder could reduce the most of oxidizers in the ultrapure water. The mighty oxidative powers of the residual chlorine attack the cell membrane of a microorganism and a virus to degenerate the inner protein and show the germicidal and disinfectant effects. It was thought that the reducer generally do not show a mighty antibacterial effect. Why the rhyolite shows the mighty antibacterial effects? Then, the 500g of rhyolite powder was put into 1l of ultrapure water. After keeping 18hours, the supernatant of the water was collected and filtrated with the filtering paper. Still more, the filtrate was centrifuged at

3000rpm for 10min. The supernatant of 600ml dried at 200°C for 5 hours up to get 13.4mg of white precipitates. The precipitates were analyzed by the x ray diffraction and the electron-micro analyzer. The results showed that the precipitates mainly consist of calcium and silicon (Fig.6). As the rhyolite contained 70% over silicate, the results suggested that the ceramics structure consist of silicate oxide should disintegrate. Then, the silicate radical molecule containing an additional electron could be formed. It was thought that the radical molecules are so active that the bacterium el.al was contacted to collapse the cell membrane with an antibacterial action. Though the mechanism to form the silicate radical molecule was not clear, the antibacterial effects of the rhyolite containing the 70% over silica were the experimental facts.

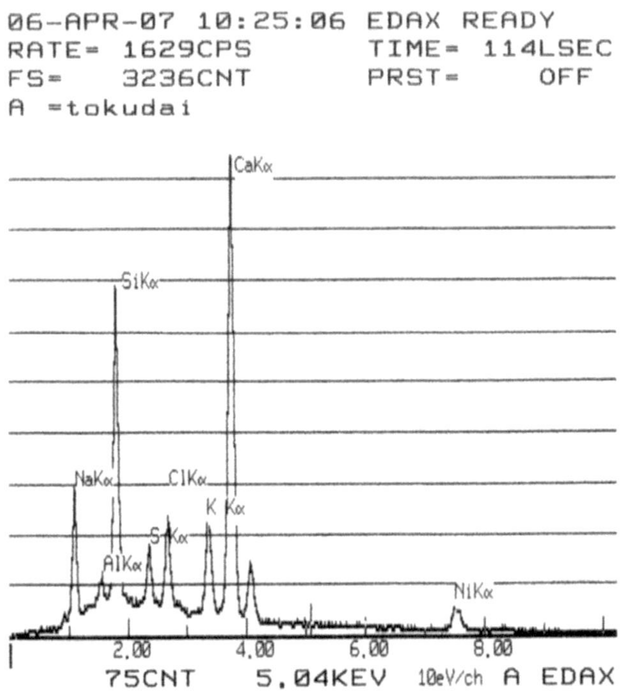

Figure 6. The analysis by the x ray diffraction of the components in the solution

3. The development of the FIR energy radiator

In order to clarify the effects of the FIR energy radiation on the living body at the rebel of a cell and animal, the FIR incubator for cell culture and animal raising apparatus was developed utilizing the valid ceramics as the rhyolite and the pureblack that the resemble effects as the ideal black body are well known.

The CO_2 incubator must be exactly controlled the temperature inside of the incubator at 37±0.5°C. Therefore, though the water jacket of about 40litter is equipped for the suppression of heat loss, the equipment of incubator becomes solid and heavy. Then, 0.5% CO_2 gas need be supply into the incubator to activate the culture cell breathing. Still more, the gas of 0.5% CO_2 in air must be supplied though the water layer in order to keep the humidity near 100%. So, we remodel the existing CO_2 incubator. The heating system was changed to FIR panel heater for keeping the temperature in the incubator at 37±0.5°C. The five face at up, down, both side and behind in the incubator except the front glass were coated with the valid ceramics as the rhyolite and the pureblack close to black body for raising the efficiency of FIR radiation. The all shelves were also coated with the same ceramics. Still more, the water jacket was change to the simple insulation, because the FIR energy directly and instantly heats the surface of objects even if the air and space lie between the surface of incubator and the objects. As a result, the light and compact CO_2 incubator that can continuously radiate the FIR energy for 24hours was developed with a great success (Fig.7) [8]. So, the strict comparative experiments on the effect of the FIR energy radiation on the culture cells become possible utilizing the same type of CO_2 incubator without remodeling as control.

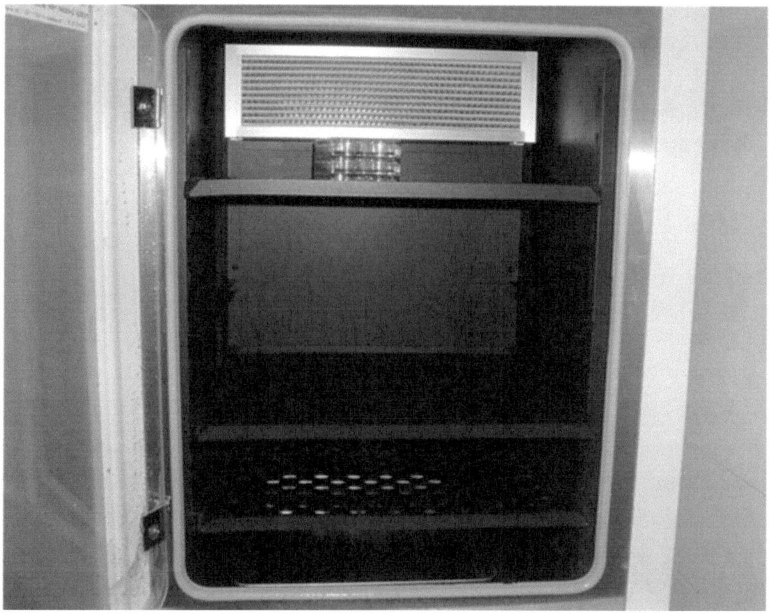

Figure 7. The FIR CO_2 incubator

Then, the FIR animal raising apparatus with same FIR radiating system of the FIR CO_2 incubator to control the temperature inside 20-40°C at will and break down any smell chemical products by photo-degradation with the light catalyst of TiO2 could be also developed (Fig.8). The FIR animal raising apparatus has the two chambers which the upper chamber is coated with the valid ceramics as the rhyolite and the lower chamber is no coating [9]. So, the strict comparative experiments on the effect of FIR energy radiation on animals become also possible by using the FIR animal raising apparatus.

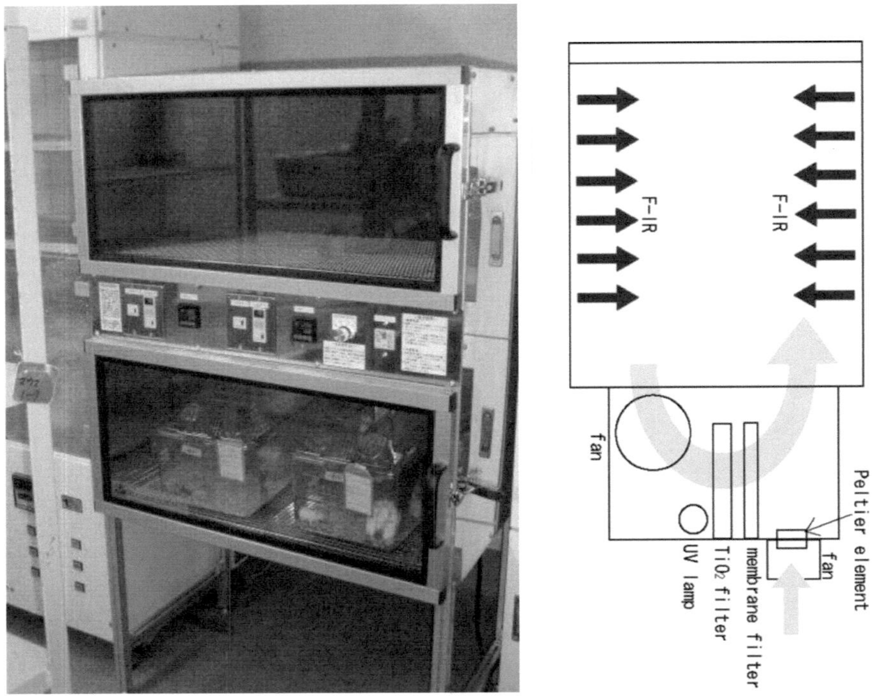

Figure 8. The FIR animal raising apparatus

4. The effects of FIR energy radiation on water

4.1. The volatility and fluidity of water

Water is indispensable for human life. As water is generally present surrounding us, the characteristics of water is hard to be considered as a strange matter. But, the truth that a boiling point of water is 100°C is peculiar comparing with the other elements with the similar molecular weight. For examples, though a sulfur is next of oxygen in the periodic table of the elements, the boiling point of hydrogen sulfate (H_2S) is -60.7°C. But, as the molecular weight of oxygen is smaller than that of sulfur, the boiling point must be smaller than -60.7°C. It is supposed that the boiling point of water should be theoretically at about -80°C. Then, the coagulating point of water is appropriate theoretically at about -110°C. Well, why the boiling and coagulating points are respectively at 100°C and 0°C? The reason is by the formation of cluster through the pulling against each other among the water molecules by a hydrogen bond et al. The imaginary molecular weight inferred from the boiling and coagulating points is about 100 by which 5, 6 water molecules gathered. Then, a water molecule has as much as four hydrogen bonds. Moreover, it was thought that the shapes of the cluster shows a straight chain, from a square to eleven-cornered shape, and the average shape is the pentagon. Moreover, it was thought that the cluster of water is not stable for long time, but it was formed and broken at the cycles of 10^{-12} seconds. But, this condition of cluster is only applied to the very pure water without any ion and impurity. The real water actually contained various impurities. Even if the very pure water is kept in air, the condition of water changes moment by moment by melting of a gas and molecules from air. Then, in order to estimate the present conditions of energy in the water, the change of the weight of water is exactly measured for the indicator of the volatility. When the difference of volatility between the tap water and the deionized water are compared, the deionized water is clearly volatilized more quickly than the tap water (Fig.9).

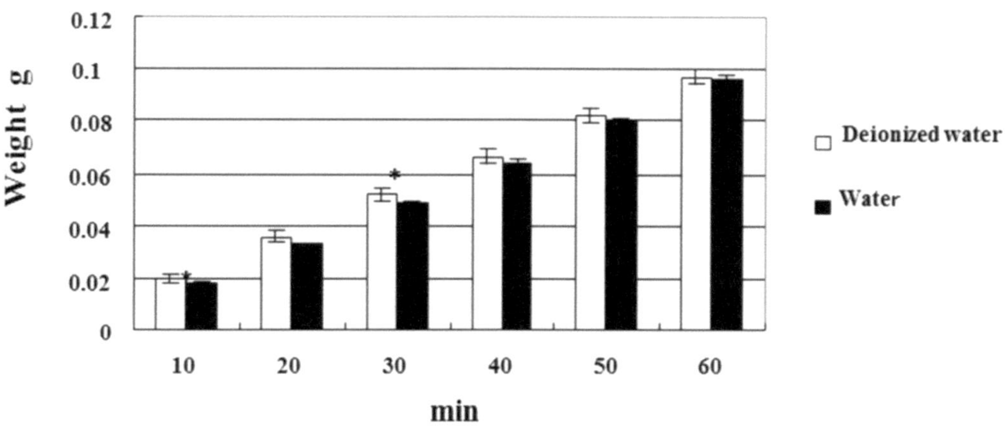

Figure 9. The change of the weight of the deionized water and the tap water

The high volatility means that a lot of water molecules spring out of the surface of water. Therefore, it is supposed that the energy of the water molecules is high and its cluster is small. This graph shows the change of weight of the deionized water radiated FIR energy through the grass layer by keeping in the FIR incubator for 12 hours and the untreated deionized water (Fig.10). Though the deionized water more quickly losses the weight than the tap water, the deionized water radiated FIR energy losses much bigger weight than the deionized water. In other words, it was made clear that the deionized water radiated FIR energy has high energy in the molecules to evaporate much easy. The results mean that the cluster of the water can become small by the FIR energy radiation. If that is the case, why the cluster formed by the water molecules changes by accepted the FIR energy? The water molecule consisting of two [O-H] bonds opening with 104°has three types of the vibration energies. One is the deformation vibration of 1594cm^{-1} and the others are the symmetrical and asymmetrical expansion and contraction energy of each 3656 cm^{-1} and 3756 cm^{-1}. When the energy were convert to the wave length, the deformation vibration is 6.27μm and the expansion and contraction energy are 2.74μm and 2.66μm [10]. If the FIR energy of 5~20μm radiated the water molecules, the deformation vibration of the water molecule was activated by the transmission of the energy through the resonance effect because the energy of deformation vibration was coincident with the radiating energy. Consequently, it was thought that the kinetic energy of the water molecule increased to rush out of a cluster. The cluster in the activated water by FIR energy radiation ought to raise the volatility. On the contrary, the strength of FIR energy radiation by any materials can be estimated by measuring the change of the volatility. Then, when the boiling points of water was measured, that of FIR radiated water was 97.4°C and that of control water was 98.9°C. The boiling point of water decreased clearly by FIR energy radiation. These results also suggested that the water molecules are at the condition to rush out easy from the surface of water. Still more, when the viscosity of water was measured, it was clarified that the viscosity clearly decreased by the FIR energy radiation (Fig.11). These results also suggest that the water become to flow easy by the same change of the cluster in water. It is thought that the water radiated FIR energy increases the volatility and fluidity at the same time. It is a very important finding. For example, it is thought that the blood and lymph flow in the human body become smoothly and activates by radiation of the FIR energy. It is only natural that the collection of lymph fluid into a lymph vessel rides the swelling in the body. Then, a tear, sweat and digestive juices become similarly to flow easy also. It is suggested that the activation of the secretion of a tear stimulate the para-sympathetic nerve system. Still more, the activation of the secretion of a sweat stimulates the various metabolisms in whole body. The activation of the secretion of the saliva and digestive juices stimulates the digestive function to make the body vigorously.

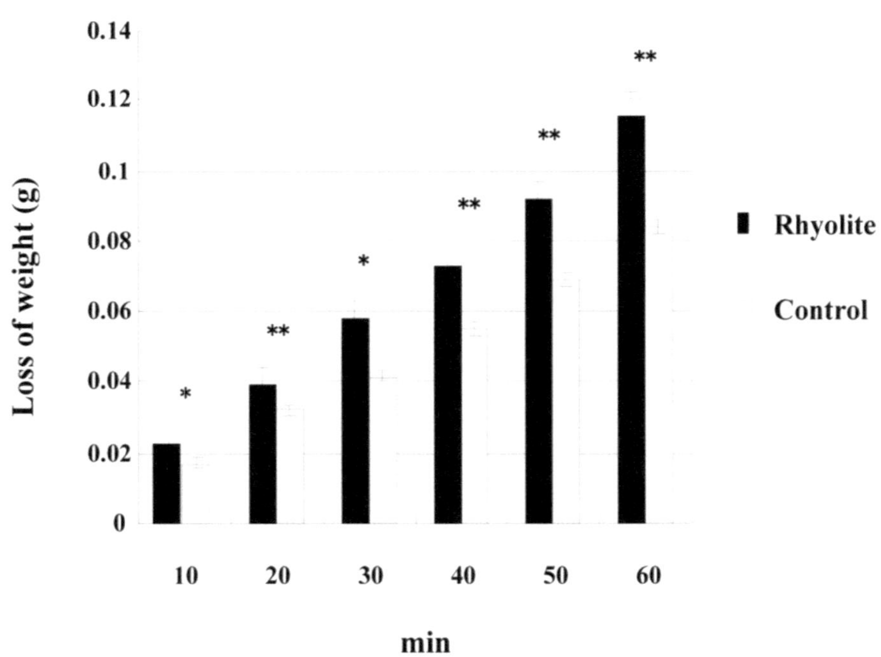

Figure 10. The change of the deionized water weight affected by the rhyolite as the FIR radiator

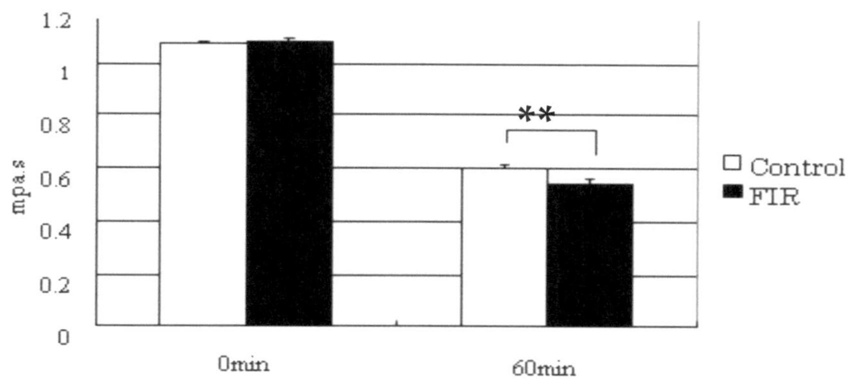

Figure 11. The change of the viscosity of water by the rhyolite as the FIR radiator

4.2. The solubility of water

It was found that the water radiated FIR energy by the rhyolite become to dissolve variable products. The plastic culture dish adhered proteins as bovine serum albumin (BSA) were prepared for the estimation of the solubility of water. The FIR energy radiated ultrapure water by the rhyolite and non-treated same water poured into the dish, and was collected for measurement of the UV absorbance for protein. The results showed that the FIR energy radiated ultrapure water could dissolve much more BSA than the non-treated same water (Fig.12). Not only protein but also sugar and sodium hydroxide were checked the solubility. The results showed that the FIR energy radiated ultrapure water could dissolve much more them. When the rhyolite powder was inserted into a fish tank at about 0.5%, the water in the tank became clear just after 4 days. These results were considered by which the deposited protein and other products in the tank dissolved in water to raise the degree of transparency by the FIR energy radiation from the rhyolite. It was confirmed that the fishes and shell fishes become live longer than usual and keep the freshness in the tank with the rhyolite. For the application of these effects of the FIR energy radiation on water, the development of the contact lens cleaner was tried. The force of cleaning in the FIR energy radiated ultrapure water were estimated to the contact lens attached the BSA on the surface. The results suggested that the force of cleaning of water was surely raised by FIR energy radiation from rhyolite. But, as the force of FIR was defeated to a detergent, the development of the contact lens cleaner was given up. However, it was expected that the effects of the FIR energy radiation from rhyolite, on which the force of solubilizing in water was activated, will be applied in various fields in future.

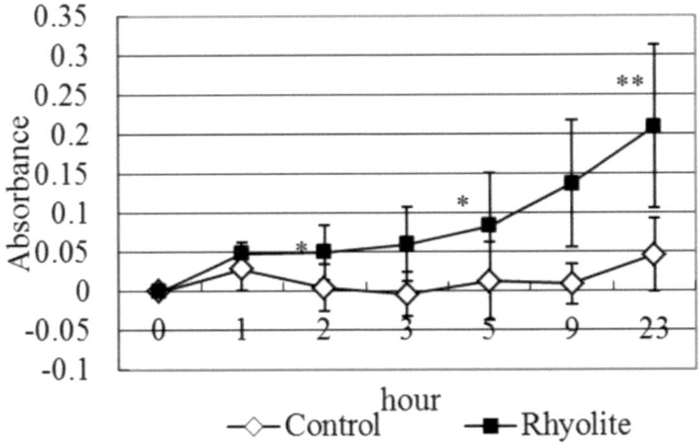

Figure 12. The solubility of BSA in the FIR energy radiated water

5. Experiment

5.1. The effects of the FIR energy radiation on an animal

5.1.1. The effect of the FIR energy radiation on the change of body weight of an animal

When the rats were raised by using the FIR animal raising equipment, the increase of the body weight of rats radiated FIR energy became gentler than that of control (Fig.13). Though the same experiments on the body weight of rats repeated five times, the results showed the same tendency that the FIR energy radiation inhibited the increase of the body weights. In some laboratories, the rats and the mice eat foods and drink water as much as wish. As a result, the rats and the mice naturally grow fat within a year. Therefore, it should be thought that the FIR energy radiation activates the exercise activity and keeps away the switchover to the obesity conditions.

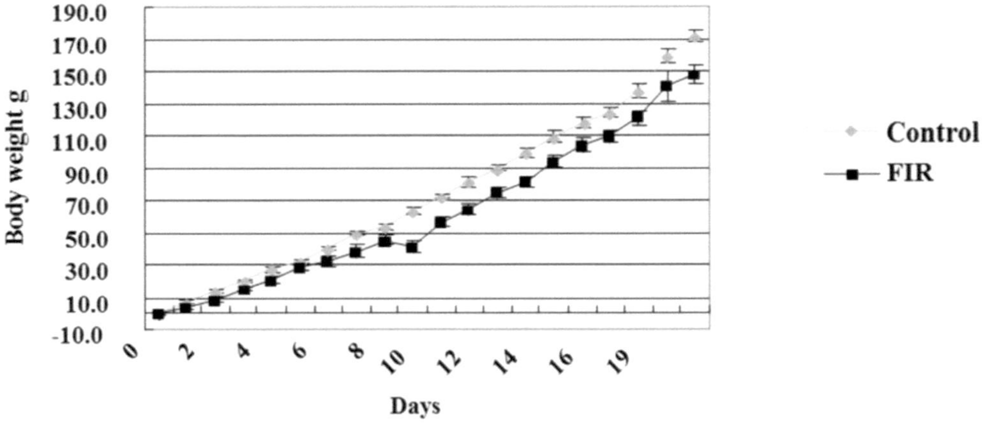

Figure 13. The change of the body weight affected by FIR. The growth of the rats was inhibited by the rhyolite as the FIR radiator.

5.1.2. The effect of the FIR energy radiation on the change of blood flow of an human

The Rhyolite powder with a peak diameter of about 10μm was printed to the blanket cloths made in Japan at 15%, like polka dots of about 2 cm (MATERA Inc. Toon, Ehime, Japan). The Rhyolite containing blanket and the control blanket were applied to the healthy volunteers for application of FIR energy of 20 min at room temperature 22°C and room humidity 50%, after acclimation of the condition in the room for 10 min. The velocity and the quantity of blood were continuously measured by the laser Doppler blood perfusion monitor and imagers in the same way for 20 min. The order of the application between the FIR and the control blankets was often changed at the condition of double blind. The velocity and the quantity of blood flow were accelerated 32.2% (Fig.14) and 19.1% (Fig.15) by the application of the Rhyolite containing cloths.

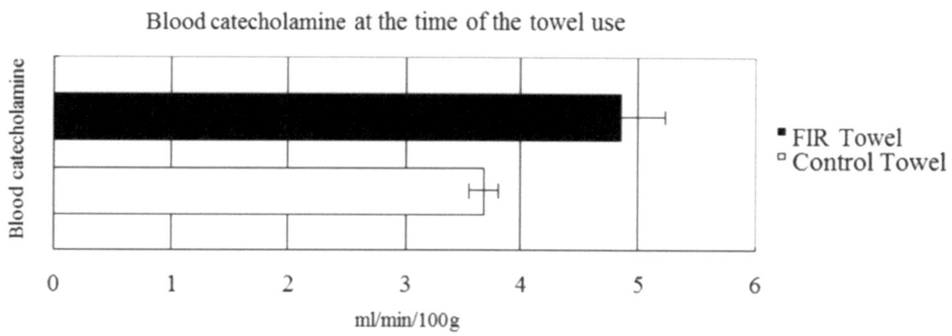

Figure 14. The change of the velocity of blood by the FIR blanket. This graph showed the velocity of the blood after 60 min of using the rhyolite containing blanket. The velocity of the blood increased 32.2% in the rhyolite containing blanket compared with the control blanket.

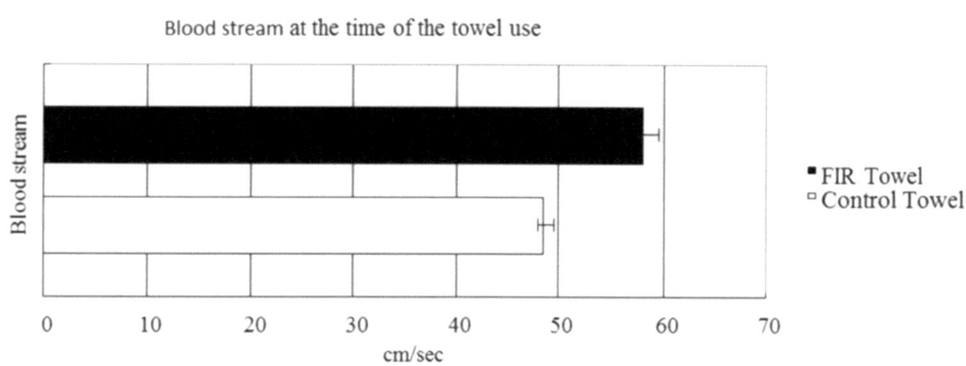

Figure 15. The change of the quantity of blood by the FIR blanket. This graph showed the quantity of the blood after 60 min of using the rhyolite containing blanket. The quantity of the blood increased19.1% in the rhyolite containing blanket compared with the control blanket.

5.1.3. The effect of the FIR energy radiation on the change of blood catecholamine

The amount of adrenaline, noradrenaline and dopamine in blood of the 40 mice keeping in the FIR and control animal raising apparatus for 40 days were measured at the blood center. It was shown that the amount of the dopamine in blood catecholamine significantly decreased, and the adrenaline and the noradrenaline in the blood catecholamine tend to decrease by radiated the FIR energy (Fig.16). These results suggested that the FIR energy radiation decreased the amount of the blood catecholamine in mice to inhibit the sympathetic nerve and activate the parasympathetic nerve. A mamma as a human body has the autonomous nervous system with the motor nervous and sensory nervous system. The autonomous nervous system distributes all internal organs to work in order to sustain a person's life independent of his mind.

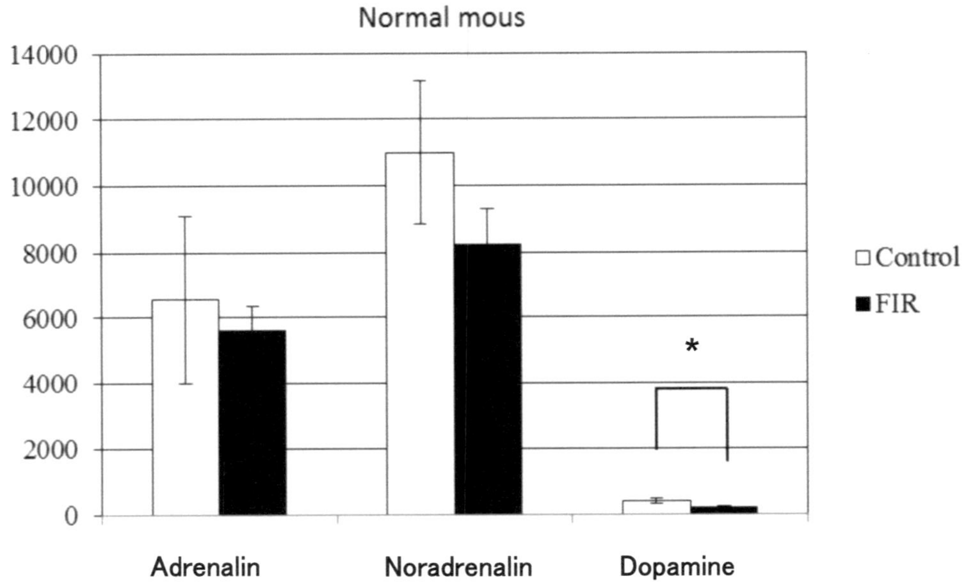

Figure 16. The change of the concentration of catecholamine in the blood affected by the FIR energy radiation. The concentration of the adrenaline, noradrenaline and dopamine in the FIR group were significantly lower 14.4%

There are the sympathetic nerves and the parasympathetic nerves in the autonomous nervous system which distribute every internal organ at the same times to control the function of each internal organ in spite of his mind. When the sympathetic nerves excited, the heart beat violently, the blood pressure increase, the breath become hard and the stress build up in the body. On the contrary, when the parasympathetic nerves excited, the feeling become confortable as at home to become feeling an appetite, sleep and sexual desire. It is thought that the rats and the mice radiate FIR energy become loss of the stress in the cage and lives the active and healthy life. In short, FIR energy radiation may avoid the stress and obesity.

5.1.4. *The effect of the FIR energy radiation on the biological macromolecules*

The effect of FIR energy radiation on the biological macromolecules is being made clear. The effects of FIR energy radiation on the activity of the enzyme can be estimated by using the FIR incubator developed by us. An enzyme is the special protein which has the various amino acids forming the three-dimensional structure with the various bonds to get a special role to a chemical reaction. In case that the activities of the 19 kinds of the enzymes appear in radiating FIR energy, it was made clear that the activity of some enzymes were accelerated or restrained. These results suggested that the efficiency of the enzyme activity changed because the various bond conforming the three-dimensional structure of the enzyme was affected by the FIR energy. In the enzymes measured by us, the results suggested that the activities of esterase, esterase lipase, lipase, leucin allylamidase, beta-glucuronidase were accelerated and that of alkaline-phosphatase, acid-phosphatase, naphtol-AS-BI-phospho hydrase were restrained. Especially, esterase, esterase lipase and lipase are the enzymes to decompose a fat. Though the experiments were preliminary study, it was made clear that the FIR energy radiation changed the three-dimensional structure of the various enzymes to accelerate or restrain the activities. Still more, it was possible from the results that the increase of body weight restrained because some decomposition enzyme of fat were restrained by FIR energy radiation. These results suggested that the FIR energy radiation has a diet effect.

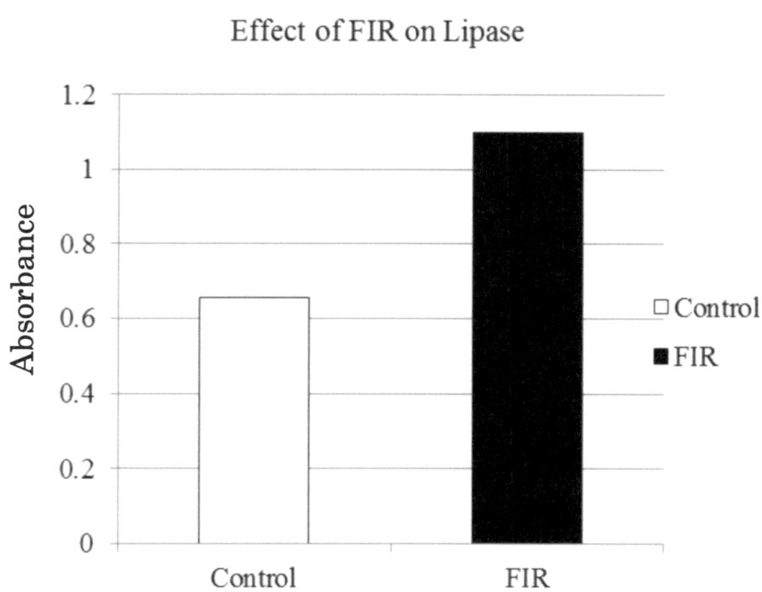

Figure 17. The change of activity of lipase by FIR energy radiation. The activity in the FIR radiation group was higher 40.5% than the control group at 530nm.

5.2. The effects of FIR energy radiation skin

5.2.1. The effect of FIR energy radiation on skin repair

The wound of circle with 8mm diameter was artificially made at the skin of rats keeping the FIR and the control animal raising apparatus. Then, the area of the wound was measured each several days. And the surface condition was observed. The results showed that though the surface of the wound in the FIR radiation group wet and soft, that of the control group was covered the hard scab (Fig.18).

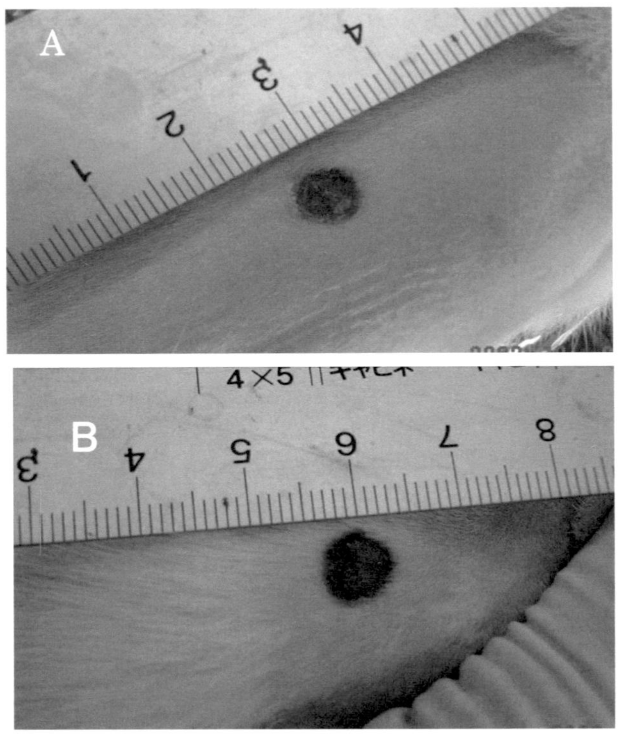

Figure 18. The surface of wound of skin affected by the FIR energy radiation. Control : (A) FIR energy radiation : (B)

The repair area of FIR radiation group increased each 30.54%, 28.27% and 14.22% after 5, 6 and 7days compared with control group (Fig.19). These results showed that the FIR energy radiation from out of body accelerated the wound healing at the surface of rat skin. Still more, the repair area of wound increased each 44.39% and 24.29% after 3 and 5 days by application of the ointment containing the 10% rhyolite as the FIR energy radiating ceramics. In other words, it was clarified that the FIR energy radiation promoted the wound hearing of skin, even if the radiation of FIR energy were by far from body or by contact with skin. If the blanket and sheet with FIR energy radiation effects were developed, the bedsore of the bedridden old persons or the sick persons in bed for a long time would be suppressed and restored to regenerate the skin and ease the pain of the patients. Now, though the rise in a fee for medical treatment becomes a social problem, if the bedsore could be suppressed to shorten the term of the admission to a hospital, the fee for the medical treatment would be reduced in the future. Still more, if the space of the residence was constructed with the FIR energy radiating building material as the rhyolite, the metabolism of skin would be promoted to hinder the aging of skin. Then, the FIR energy radiating ceramics as rhyolite may be tied together with a development of the creams and cosmetics to hinder the aging of skin.

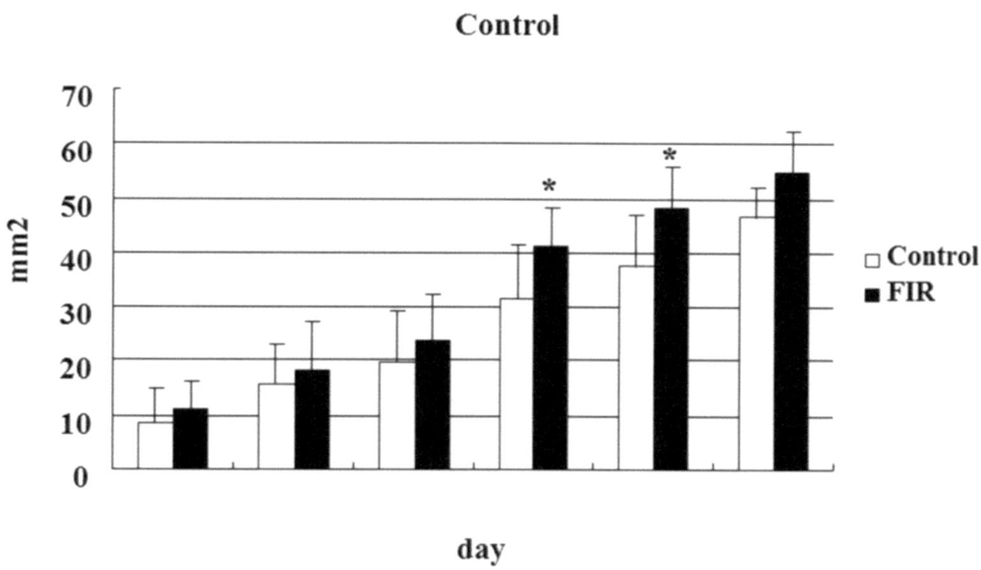

Figure 19. The repair area of wound hearing. The speed of repair was accelerated affected by the FIR energy radiation.

5.2.2. *Effect of the FIR energy radiation on a atopic dermatitis*

The mouse naturally induced a crisis of the inflammation of the skin as the atopic dermatitis with the application of a picric acid as the material raising the inflammation was imported from the United States. Then, the effects of the FIR energy radiation on the induction of the inflammation of the skin were analyzed by using the mouse. No an inflammation of skin in the mouse radiated FIR energy was detected after the application of a picric acid, though the atopic dermatitis of control mouse in the same condition were all induced without the FIR energy radiation (Fig.20). It was made clear that the area of the inflammation of skin and the number of the mast cells at the inflammation of skin as an atopic dermatitis clearly decreased by the FIR energy radiation (Fig.21).

These results suggested that the FIR energy radiation was effective for the prevention and the medical treatment to the inflammation of the skin as an atopic dermatitis. In the future, it is thought that the FIR ceramics as the rhyolite are tied together with the development of the medicine or the cure for the inflammation of the skin as an atopic dermatitis.

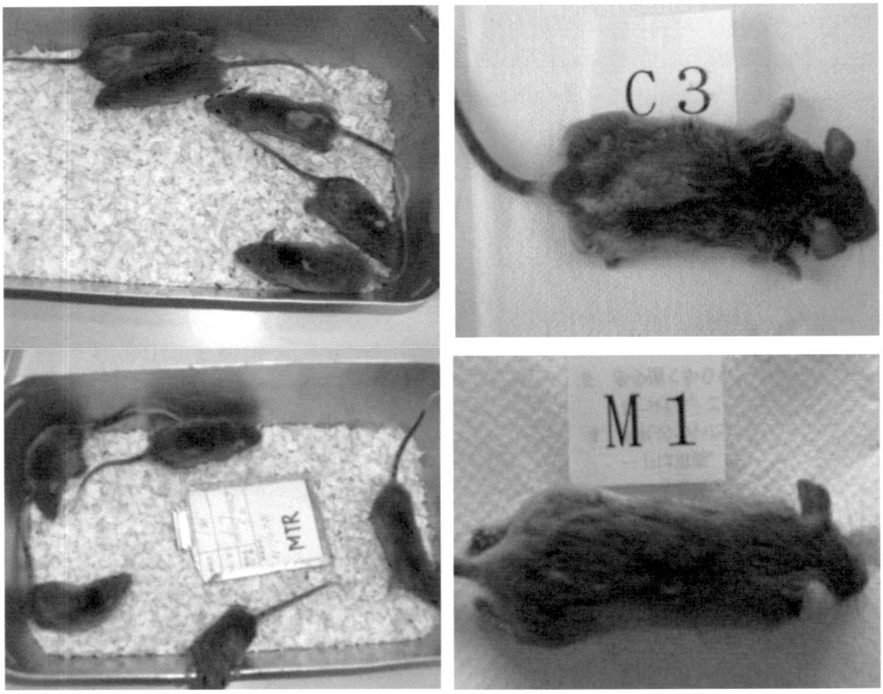

Figure 20. The change of the inflammation of the skin as the atopic dermatitis. The induction of the inflammation of the skin on all mice was suppressed by the FIR energy radiation

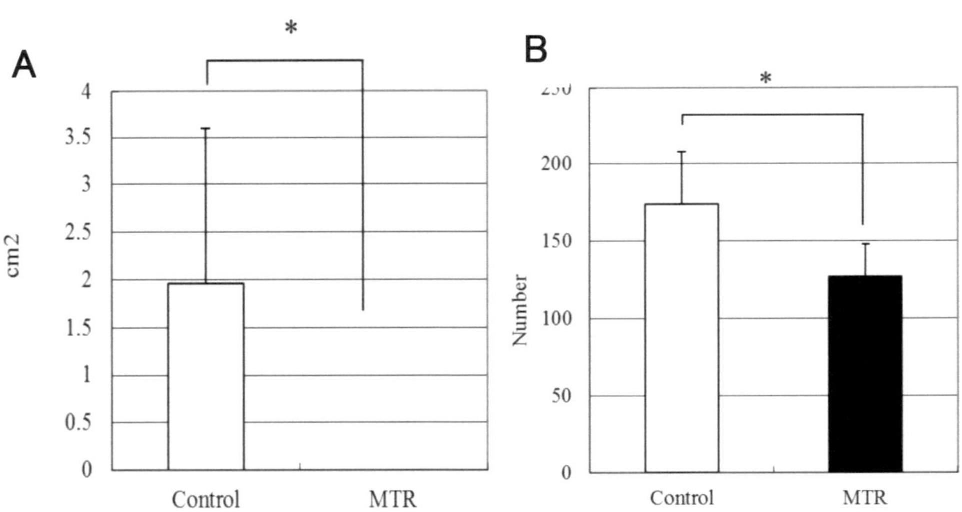

Figure 21. The area of the inflammation of skin and the number of the mast cells at the inflammation. Though the area of the inflammation in control group was 1.96cm^2, no inflammation was detected in the FIR energy radiation group (A). The number of must cells was smaller 26.9% in the FIR energy radiation group than the control group (B).

5.3. The effects of the FIR energy radiation on bone

5.3.1. The effect of the FIR energy radiation on the cultured osteoblast-like cells

The culturing osteoblast-like MC3T3-E1 cell (Riken Cell Banc, Tsukuba, Japan) were separated in the two groups in the FIR and the control CO_2 incubator. After 1, 3, 5, 7, 10 and 14days, the cell number of living cells in both groups were measured by a hematocytometer and observed by phase contrast microscope CK40 (Olympus, Tokyo, Japan). Still more, the gene expression of the 4 days culture cells in both groups was analyzed by the cluster analysis the microarray hybridization method (http://www.godatabase.org).

The proliferation of the osteoblast-like MC3T3-E1 cells in FIR group significantly inhibited each 19.08% and 12.24% after 3day and 10days culture compared with control group. But, it was considered that the formation of the calcified nodules in the FIR group was more than the control group by the observation of the culture cells stained with von kossa and with a phase-contrast microscope (Fig.22).

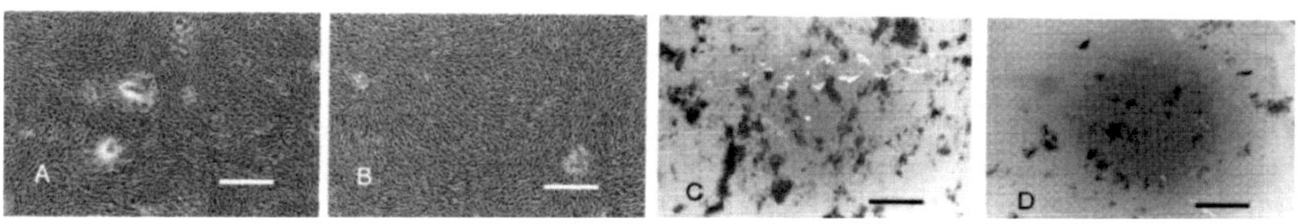

Figure 22. The effects of the FIR energy radiation on the bone nodules formed by MC3T3-E1 cells. The cultured MC3T3-E1 cells in FIR group (A) and control group (B) was observed by the phase contrast microscope CK40 (Olympus, Tokyo, Japan). Some samples after 4weeks culture were stained with Von Kossa method and observed by the same method. FIR group (C) Control group (D) Bar: 100μm

The results showed that the number and the area of the calcified nodules of the FIR group were 148.8 and 158.8 μm^2, though no calcified nodules was formed yet in control group after 2 weeks culture. Still more, that of FIR group increased each 2.92times and 4.91times compared with the control group after 4weeks (Fig.23). Consequently, the formation of the calcified nodules was clearly promoted by the FIR energy radiation. On the other hand, it was made clear by the results of cluster analysis after 4 day culture that the genes expression of Interferon activated gene 205, 203 and Interferon α-inducible protein 27 in the cell to cell signal field were reinforced and the gene expression of Interleukin 1 family member 6, Interleukin 17D, 17 receptor C, 17B, and Interleukin 3 related with inflammation were oppositely dropped (Table 2).

It was also made clear that the genes expression of Platelet-derived growth factor (PDGF) D polypeptide, Transforming growth factor β (TGFβ) induced and TGFβ inducible early growth response 1 in the cell proliferation field were reinforced, and the gene expression of PDGF B polypeptide and Fibroblast growth factor (FGF) 2, 21, 8 were oppositely dropped (Table 2). It was clarified by these data that the cell differentiation as the function of osteoblast estimated by the formation of calcified nodules were promoted by FIR energy radiation, though the proliferation was inhibited by it. In short, the FIR energy radiation shorts the term of cell proliferation and advances the timing of cell differentiation on the osteoblast. Finally, it was considered that the FIR energy radiation control these genes expression to inhibit the cell proliferation and promote the cell differentiation of osteoblast [8, 9]. It was made clear by these facts that the differentiation of cultured osteoblast-like cell as an osteoblast is promoted by the radiation of FIR energy.

Cell-cell signaling **Gene Name**	**Acc. No.**	**Fold change**
Interferon activated gene 205	NM_172648	1.597
Interleukin 15 receptor, alpha chain	NM_008358	1.422
Interferon alpha-inducible protein 27	AK010014	1.388
Mitogen activated protein 3K 7	BC006665	1.365
Interferon activated gene 203	NM_008328	1.328
Interleukin 1 family, member 6	NM_019450	-1.348
Interleukin 17D	NM_145837	-1.393
Heparin-binding EGF-like growth factor	NM_010415	-1.395
Interleukin 3	NM_010556	-1.471
Interleukin 17 receptor	NM_134159	-1.481
Interleukin 17B	NM_019508	-1.631
Growth **Gene Name**	Acc. No.	Fold change
Platelet-derived growth factor, D polypeptide	AK003359	1.555
Transforming growth factor, beta induced	NM_009369	1.505
TGFb Inducible early growth response 1	NM_013692	1.383
Mitogen activated protein kinase kinase kinase 7	BC006665	1.365
Growth differentiation factor 15	NM_011819	1.322
Fibroblast growth factor 8	D12483	-1.323
Fibroblast growth factor 21	NM_020013	-1.332
Epidermal growth factor receptor related gene	M99623	-1.337
Fibroblast growth factor 2	NM_008006	-1.342
Heparin-binding EGF-like growth factor	NM_010415	-1.395
Early growth response 3	NM_018781	-1.565
Growth factor receptor binding protein2-ap 1(Gab1)	NM_021356	-1.667
Platelet-derived growth factor, B polypeptide	NM_011057	-2.304

Table 2. The cluster analysis of the gene expression in MC3T3-E1 cells affected by FIR energy radiation by the microarray hybridigestion method These genes were reinforced and repressed at 1.3 over by the FIR energy radiation in the cluster of the Cell-to signaling and the growth.

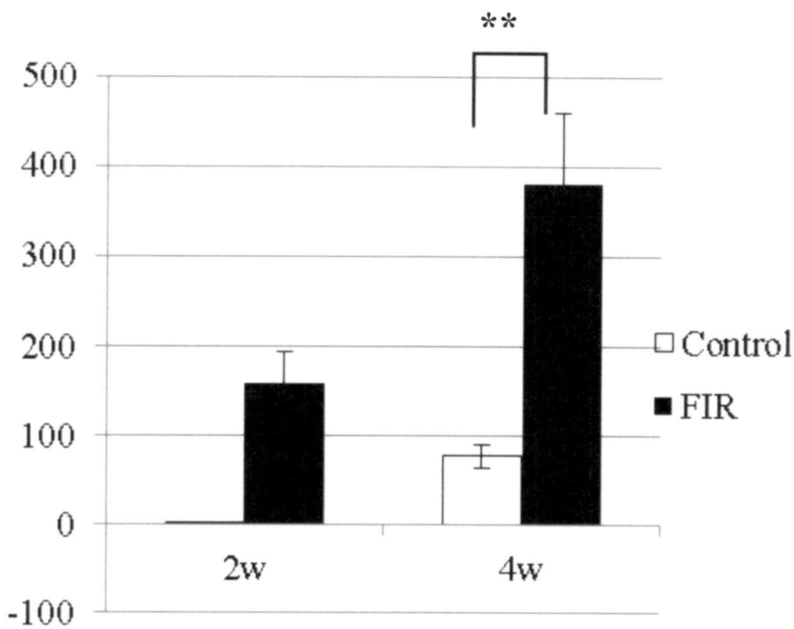

Figure 23. The effects of the FIR energy radiation on the number and the area of the bone nodules formed by MC3T3-E1 cells. Each five samples stained with Von Kossa method after 1, 2, 3 and 4 weeks in both groups were measured the nodules (A) and the number of the area (B) by Bio-system microscope BX-51. The measurement was analyzed by the average of five field of visions of each samples. Statistical analysis was carried out by t-test. *P<0.01

5.3.1.1. The effects of FIR energy radiation on the titanium implant

Pure titanium post (RTP post titanium #Ti, Dentech, Tokyo) were treated with the snowtech O solution (Nissan Chemical Industries, Tokyo) for 48 hours and immersed in MEM medium (Minimum Essential Medium Eagle, Sigma, St. Louis, MO, USA) for 5 days. Control group was only immersed in MEM medium at same condition. The 20 S.D. rats of 6 weeks old were implanted the titanium post into the central position of the femur. Left side was control group and Right side was the snowtech O solution treated group. These rats were separated two groups which the FIR energy radiating group kept in the FIR animal raising apparatus and the control group was kept in the normal animal raising apparatus. The femur with the titanium post was extracted and measured the intensity between the titanium and the bone by the tension test with the small omnipotent testing machine (Autograph, Shimadzu, Kyoto) after 1, 2 and 4 weeks raising. The same experiments were repeated twice. Though the data were easy affected by the damage of the surgical operation and the extent of the inflammation, the identical tendency was shown. The tension intensity of the implanted titanium post with the snowtech O solution in the FIR energy radiating group significantly reinforced 2.68 times as much as the same implant in the control group after 2 weeks (Fig.24).

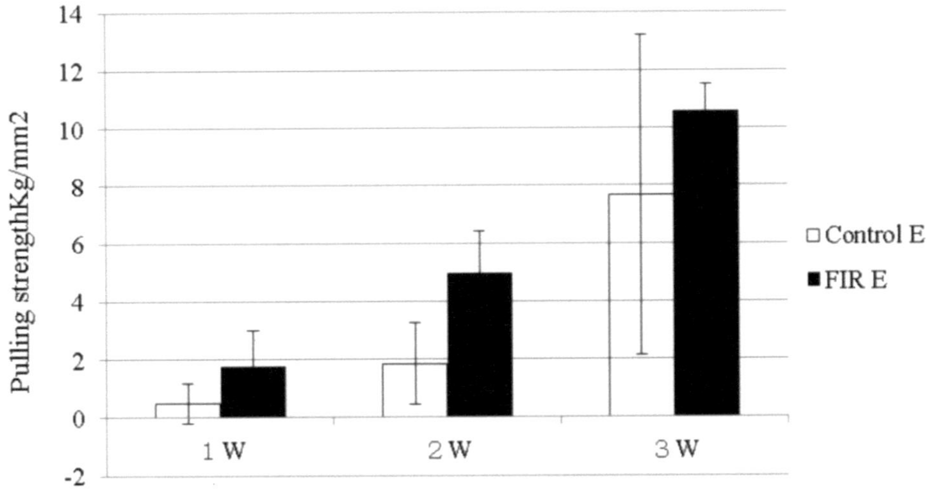

Figure 24. The effect of the FIR radiation on the strength of the bone bonding to titanium. The bone bonding to titanium was clearly promoted by the FIR energy radiation.

It was been thinking that FIR energy was too weak to permeate deep into the tissue of the living body. But, if the FIR energy radiation affects the water molecules in the blood as mentioned previously, the blood of the whole body was affected by FIR energy even if the deep position. The possibility is supported by the experimental results which the new bone formation inside of the femur was activated by the FIR energy radiation at the surface of the skin from outside of body.

It is suggested that the deformational vibration of the water molecules in the blood affected by the FIR energy radiation was activated by the transmission of the energy through the resonance effect because the energy of deformation vibration was coincident with the radiating energy. It was proved that the blood containing the activated water molecules become quickly flow into the bone to activate the new bone formation.

5.3.1.2. The effects of the feed containing the FIR ceramics on the growth of bone

The powder of the rhyolite mined at the vein of ore located on the Median Tectonic Line around Ehime prefecture was utilized for this experiment. The composition of the ingredient is SiO2 66.8%, Al2O3 13.52%, Fe2O3 6.98%, K2O 4.19%, Na2O 3.98%, CaO 2.55%. The 60 rats of SD strain at 4 weeks old were separated the three groups of 0.01% and 0.1%FIR treated and control. The each group was raised every 2 or 3 days with the standard feed containing 0.01% and 0.1% rhyolite and nothing for the each group in the measurement the amount of the eating feed. After 115days, all rats were killed by the over anesthesia and the femur and the tibia were measured at many parts of width and the length.

By the results of experiments, the amount of the eating feed of 0.01% FIR treated group increased up to 6.3%, that of 0. 1% FIR treated group decreased on the contrary compared with the control group. The width of the right femur at distal, central and postal position significantly grew each 3.2%, 21.4% and 12.3% and that of the right tibia at central position and the left femur at the distal position grew 1.3% also. The width of the right femur at central and distal position significantly grew each 3.7% and 6.1%, and that of the right tibia at central position and the left tibia at the distal position grew 11.8% also. Then, on the length of the long bone, the left tibia significantly grew 2.4% alone. The special affected parts were shown at Fig.25. It was clarified that the width of the femur and tibia quickly grew as shown in Fig.25.

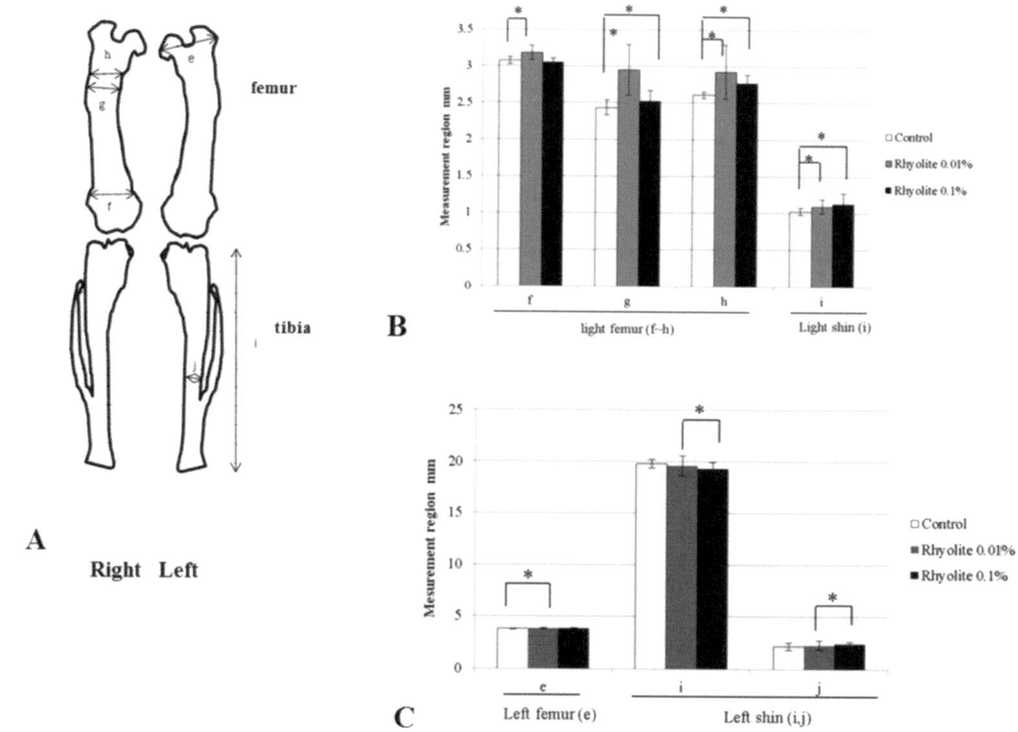

Figure 25. The effect of the eating the feed containing rhyolite on the growth of the bone. The measurement parts of the femur and the tibia were shown (A). The growth of the femur and the tibia of these three groups of 0.01% and 0.1%FIR treated and control were compared after 115days. Right : (B), Left : (C) It was clarified that the width of the femur and tibia quickly grew in the 0.01% FIR group.

It was made clear by these results that the bone formation was promoted by the inside radiation from the digestive organs by eating the feed containing the FIR energy radiating ceramics as same as the outside radiation of the FIR energy. These results suggest that the FIR energy radiation from the digestive organs arrives easy the deep posited bone of the living body. Still more, it was thought that the growth of length was a little inhibited and that of width was promoted. In other words, the FIR energy radiation does not promote the intrachondral ossification but the intra-membranous ossification that the osteoblast directly differentiates from the undifferentiated cells. As the effects of the bone affected more sensitive than the cartilage with the blood capillary, it was thought that the bone formation by the osteoblast is promoted by the FIR energy radiation. The results also prove that the

FIR energy radiation affected the living body though the blood containing many water molecules. It was clarified that the FIR energy radiation promotes the bone formation though the energy transmission to water molecules.

5.4. The Effects of the FIR energy radiation on the cancer

5.4.1. The Effects of the FIR energy radiation on the culture cancer cells

In order to clarify the effects of the FIR energy radiation on the culture cancer cells, A431 human epithelial vulva carcinoma cells, Sa3 human gingival squamous carcinoma cells, HSC3 human tongue squamous carcinoma cells, A549 human lung carcinoma cells, and MCF7 human breast carcinoma cells were cultured for the analysis of the effects on the proliferation, the shape of cells and the induction of apoptosis.

A431, A549, and MCF7 cells were cultured in Dulbecco's modified Eagle's medium/Ham's F-12 nutrient mixture (Sigma, St. Louis, MO, USA). HSC3 and Sa3 cells were cultured in Eagle's basal medium (Sigma). All culture medium was supplemented with 10% heat-inactivated fetal bovine serum. The cells (5×10^4) were plated and measured on days 8 using 0.2% trypan blue and the hemocytometer. Incorporation of 5-bromo-2'-deoxyuridine (BrdU) was used to determine the amount of DNA synthesis. Cells were observed with a CK40 phase contrast microscope (Olympus, Tokyo, Japan), fixed, and stained with hematoxylin and eosin. Still more, apoptotic cells were identified using an Apo-BrdU in situ DNA Fragmentation Assay Kit (Bio Vision, Mountain View, CA, USA).

Although the proliferation of A549, HSC3, and Sa3 cells was significantly suppressed from day 6 of culture (59.0%, 75.4%, and 76.2%, respectively) up to at least day 10, FIR irradiation had little effect on the growth of A431 or MCF7 cells. Measurement of BrdU incorporation on day 4 of culture also showed a significant suppression of growth by FIR irradiation in A549, HSC3, and Sa3 cells but not in A431 or MCF7 cells. Observation of the morphology by the phase contrast microscopy revealed that the cytoplasm and nucleus was enlarged in A549 cells. Some of the HSC3 cells also showed hypertrophy of the cytoplasm and nucleus and others tended to show atrophy. Finally, some of the Sa3 cells showed hypertrophy of the cytoplasm (to refer JEMAA 2010, 2, 382-394, Fig.1) [10]

To determine whether the inhibition of proliferation by FIR energy radiation was associated with apoptosis or necrosis, cancer cells were subjected to FIR irradiation of 48 h and analyzed on day 4 by staining with annexin V-FITC and PI and by TUNEL (TdT-mediated dUTP-biotin nick end labeling) (to refer JEMAA, 2010, 2, 382-394, Fig.3)[10]. These results indicated that FIR did not induce apoptosis in A431, HSC3, or Sa3 cells. A few of the Sa3 cells showed significant necrosis. These results indicate that the inhibition of proliferation by FIR in the cancer cells, particularly in HSC3 and Sa3 cells, was not due to apoptosis. Still more, in order to analyze all expressing genes induced by FIR energy radiation, the control and the FIR-irradiated samples after four days culture was monitored using a Qiagen RNeasy Mini Kit (Qiagen, Valencia, CA, USA) with elimination of low signal feature of background signal + 2.6 × SD, and P value < 0.01. Genes were further classified for process and function according to their

A431

Genbank	Description	Fold change
NM_014316	Calcium regulated heat stable protein 1, 24kDa	1.777
AJ131186	PRP19/PSO4 pre-mRNA processing factor 19 homolog	1.754
NM_007056	Splicing factor, arginine/serine-rich 16	1.706
NM_003824	Fas(TNFRSF6)-associated via death domin	1.518
NM_130469	Jun dimerization protein 2	1.493
NM_031209	queuine tRNA-ribosyltransferase 1(tRNA-guanine transglycosylase)	1.491
NM_003564	transgelin 2	1.482
NM_021826	FAST kinase domains 5(FASTKD5)	1.480
BT007321	general transcription facter IIH, polypeptide 4,52kDa	1.383
AF099011	EH-domin containing 1	1.382
NM_153361	Hypothetical protein MGC42105	-4.525
NM_009589	arylsulfatase D	-4.016
NM_000125	estrogen receptor 1	-3.891
NM_032726	phospholipase C, delta 4	-3.745
NM_006477	RAS-related on chromosome 22	-3.472
NM_004797	Adiponectin, C1Q and collagen domain containing	-2.513
NM_015555	zinc finger protein 451	-2.506
NM_002285	AF4/FMR2 family, member 3	-2.469
NM_012410	Seizure related 6 homolog(mouse)-like 2	-2.463
NM_005242	Coagulation factor II(thrombin) receptor-kike 1	-2.066

MCF7

Genbank	Description	Fold change
NM_006743	RNA binding motif(RNP1,RRM) protein 3	2.793
NM_012403	acidic(leucime-rich) nuclear phosphoprotein 32 family, member C	2.763
NM_012404	acidic(leucime-rich) nuclear phosphoprotein 32 family, member D	2.583
NM_014316	calcium regulated heat stable protein 1,24kDa	2.304
BC022779	v-akt murine thymoma viral oncogene homolog 2	1.846
NM_001719	bone morphogenetic protein 7(osteogenic protein 1)	1.817
NM_017590	zinc finger CCCH-type containing 7B	1.736
NM_052960	retinol binding protein 7, cellular	1.598
NM_005724	tetraspanin 3	1.577
NM_032129	pleckstrin homology domain containing, family N member 1	1.479
NM_020317	chromosome 1 open reading frame 63	-1.938
NM_005803	flotillin 1	-1.835
NM_001967	eukaryotic translation initiation factor 4A, isoform 2	-1.779
NM_005345	heat shock 70kDa protein 1A	-1.748
NM_015528	ring finger protein 167	-1.698
NM_032272	MAF1 homolog(S. cerevisiae)	-1.675
NM_024786	zinc finger, DHHC-type containing 11	-1.667
NM_005275	guanine nucleotide binding protein-like 1	-1.650
NM_003516	histone 2, H2aa	-1.645
NM_001964	early growth response 1	-1.623

Sa3

Genbank	Description	Fold change
NM_006743	RNA binding motif(RNP1,RRM) protein 3	3.046
NM_014563	trafficking protein particle complex 2	1.964
NM_014316	calcium regulated heat stable protein 1,24kDa	1.945
NM_001280	cold inducible RNA binding protein	1.825
NM_000475	nuclear receptor subfamily 0,group B, member 1	1.805
NM_145307	pleckstrin homology domain containing, family K member 1	1.788
NM_013962	neuregulin 1	1.731
NM_182687	protein kinase, membrane associated trysine/threonine 1	1.725
NM_024680	E2F transcription factor 8	1.710
NM_006123	iduronate 2-sulfatase(Hunter sysdrome)	1.688
NM_000508	fibrinogen alpha chain	-3.571
NM_005039	proline-rich protein BstNI subfamily 1	-3.185
NM_002113	complement factor H-related 1	-2.899
NM_001885	crystalline, alpha B	-2.801
NM_001964	eary growth response 1	-2.513
NM_004617	transmembrance 4 L six family member 4	-2.463
NM_006744	retinol binding protein 4, plasma	-2.410
NM_004543	nebulin	-2.353
NM_000204	I factor(complement)	-2.331
NM_021870	Fibrinogen gamma chain	-2.288

Genbank	Description	Fold change
NM_006121	keratin(epidermolytic hyperkeratosis)	2.383
NM_014316	calcium regulated heat stable protein 1,24kDa	1.934
NM_001946	dual specificity phosphatase 6	1.805
NM_005547	involucrin	1.756
BC006322	activating transcription factor 3	1.753
NM_005555	keratin 6B	1.750
NM_003125	small proline-rich protein 1B(cornifin)	1.656
NM_014604	Tax(human T-cell leukemia virus type I) binding protein 3	1.605
NM_003315	DnaJ(Hsp40)homolog, subfamily C, member 7	1.568
NM_002964	S100 calcium binding protein A8(calgranulin A)	1.564
NM_005359	SNAD, mothers against DDP homolog 4(Drosophila)	-1.976
NM_001348	death-associated protein kinase 3	-1.698
NM_130901	OTU domain containing 7	-1.695
NM_000524	5-hydroxytryptamine(serotonin)receptor 1A	-1.667
NM_006419	chemokine(C-X-C motif) ligand 13(B-cell chemoattractant)	-1.667
NM_032805	zinc finger protein 206	-1.623
NM_207370	G protein-coupled receptor 153	-1.618
NM_020999	neurogenin 3	-1.595
NM_005205	cytochrome c oxidase subunit Via polypeptide 2	-1.592
NM_004118	forkhead-like 18(Drosophila)	-1.590

Genbank	Description	Fold change
NM_014411	Nasopharyngeal carcinoma associated gene protein-8	4.253
NM_032972	protocadherin 11Y-linked	4.037
NM_005854	receptor(calcitonin)activity modifying protein 2	3.662
NM_001485	gastrulation brain homeobox 2	3.570
NM_015831	acetylcholinesterase (YT blood group)	3.528
NM_032237	hypothetical protein FLJ23356	3.478
NM_024867	KPL2 protein	3.472
NM_004132	hyaluronan binding protein 2	3.345
NM_002602	phosphodiesterase 6G, cGMP-specific, rod, gamma	3.205
NM_178536	lipocalcin 12	3.186
NM_002733	protein kinase, AMP-activated, gamma 1non-catalytic subunit	-2.309
NM_031266	heterogeneous nuclear ribonucleoprotein A/B	-2.212
NM_005556	keratin 7	-2.105
NM_006753	surfeit 6	-1.996
NM_006925	splicing factor, arginine/serine-rich 5	-1.988
NM_022044	stromal cell-derived factor 2-like 1	-1.984
NM_005694	COX17 homolog, cytochrome c oxidase assembly protein(yeast)	-1.828
NM_018645	Hairy and enhancer of split 6(Drosophila)	-1.821
NM_005954	matallothionein 3(growth inhibitory factor (neurotrophic))	-1.761

Table 3. The analysis of the extracted genes induced by the FIR energy radiation. The 10 most promoted genes and the 10 most inhibited genes in these changed genes showed

By the results that the significant changed genes of the 5 cancer cells by the FIR energy radiation were search, the cells inhibited the proliferation and showed that the many genes related the proliferation changed. The number of the inhibited genes by FIR energy radiation is more than that of the promoted gene except for the HSC3 cells. The 10 most promoted genes and the 10 most inhibited genes in these changed genes were shown at Table 3. There is no common gene in the expressed gene of 5 cells. These genes contained mainly the transcriptional factor and the control factor of the transcriptional factor.

5.4.2. The control system in the cancer cells for the FIR energy radiation

At the process of the analysis of the gene expression induced by the FIR energy radiation, it was made clear that the gene expression of HSP (Heat Shock Protein) 70 was reinforced by the FIR energy radiation. Therefore, the hyper expression cells and the knockdown cells of HSP70 were formed to analyze the effect on the proliferation.

In order to directly determine whether HSP70 can protect cells from FIR-induced cell death, we developed A431 and HSC3 cell lines stably expressing human HSP70A (A431-HSP70A and HSC3-HSP70A cells, respectively). Control cells were transfected with empty pcDNA3.1 (A431-Neo and HSC3-Neo). In our initial experiments, we found that the exposure of HSC3 and Sa3 cells but not A431 cells to the FIR energy radiation causes G2/M arrest and induces partial hypertrophy to the necrosis (data not shown) [12]. To determine whether the increased expression of HSP70A confers protection against the FIR energy radiation, the cell survival was examined in FIR-irradiated A431-HSP70, A431-Neo, A431-wt, and HSC3-HSP70, HSC3-Neo, and HSC3-wt cells. We found that over expression of HSP70A increased the cell proliferation in A431 and HSC3 cells. Furthermore, the proliferation of FIR-irradiated and control (unirradiated) A431-HSP70A cells was similar. The survival rate after 6 days of FIR irradiation was significantly higher in HSC3-HSP70A cells than in HSC3-Neo or HSC3-wt cells. In addition, the proliferation of FIR-treated HSC3-HSP70A cells was similar to that of control HSC3-HSP70A cells. The BrdU incorporation was significantly higher in FIR-irradiated or control A431-HSP70A cells than in A431-Neo or A431-wt cells. Although the BrdU incorporation of FIR-irradiated HSC3-wt and HSC3-Neo cells was lower than in unirradiated HSC3-wt and HSC3-Neo cells, it was similar in FIR-irradiated and unirradiated HSC3-HSP70A cells (to refer Med.Oncol 2008, 25, 229-237, Fig.3)[9].

HSP70 appears to be present in a variety of normal cell types and its expression may be induced by several stressors, such as hyperthermia, cardiac ischemia, infection, UV radiation, endotoxin, and nitric oxide to suppress or denature any foreign protein and restore an injured protein from lethal effects [13]. HSP70 seems particularly important for cancer cells. In human breast cancer, the expression of HSP70 correlates with increased cell proliferation, poor differentiation, lymph node metastases, and poor therapeutic outcome [14]. In vivo animal studies and clinical trials have revealed that hyperthermia may serve as a powerful tool in the treatment of prostate cancer [15-20]; at the cellular level, hyperthermic stress induces HSPs. Moreover, chemotherapeutic agents such as cisplatin, adriamycin, and bleomycin, as well as γ-radiation induce HSPs. HSP70 participates in cytoprotection and is associated with cellular resistance to lethal external effects [18-21]. However, in the present study, HSP70 was never induced by FIR. These results suggested that FIR has anti-tumor activity without inducing HSP70 as an anti-stress factor. This characteristic indicates that FIR may be suitable for medical treatment.

We next examined the effect of knocking down HSP70A and HSP70C mRNA and HSP70 protein expression using siRNA. Transfection with HSP70A/C siRNA effectively decreased HSP70A and HSP70C mRNA (Fig. 4A) and protein levels in both A431 and HSC3 cells without affecting the level of HSP70B mRNA or protein. HSP70A/C siRNA did not suppress BrdU incorporation in unirradiated A431 cells, but it suppressed BrdU incorporation in cells irradiated with FIR. Similarly, the HSP70A/C siRNA enhanced the suppression of BrdU incorporation by FIR irradiation. FIR irradiation also significantly suppressed BrdU incorporation in HSC3 cells transfected with the negative control siRNA. These results indicate that a decrease in HSP70 protein mediates the ability of limited FIR to inhibit the proliferation of A431 and HSC3 cells (to refer Med.Oncol 2008, 25, 229-237, Fig.4)[9].

5.4.3. *The effects of the FIR energy radiation on the implanted cancer cell to mice*

For experiments on body weight change, 10-week-old male skid mice (CB17/Icr-Prkdc) and 6- to 8-week-old male nude mice (Crlj:CD1-Foxn1) purchased from Charles River Japan (Yokohama, Japan) were housed with temperature control and a 12-h light-dark cycle. Male skid mice were weighed every 5 days, beginning at 10 weeks of age. FIR treatment by our developed animal raiser (FIR group), n=7 and control (control group), n=8.

The log-phase cancer cells cultured in 10% FBS and DMEM/HamF-12 medium (Sigma, St. Louis, USA) resuspended at a cell density of 1×10^7 ml in PBS containing 500 μg/ml of MatrigelTM basement membrane matrix (Becton Dickinson Labware, Two Oak Park, Bedford, MA). The tumor cells (1×10^6) were suspended in 0.1 ml of PBS containing 50 μg of MatrigelTM and were slowly hypodermically injected in the back using a 25-gauge needle. After injecting tumor cells, mice were separated two groups: FIR group and control group. During the experiments, the long and short diameters of the resulting tumor were measured in five-day intervals, and tumor volume was calculated by the following formula: tumor volume (mm3) =1/2× (long diameter) × (short diameter) 2.

For purpose of the ascertaining tumor organization change by the FIR energy radiation, the excised tumor was observed after stained with hematoxylin and eosin to detect tumor organization change after 30 days.

Then we carried out immunohistochemical analyses to detect matrix metalloproteinases (MMP) members MMP-1, MMP-9, MMP-10 and MMP-13 [9]. The increase in tumor volume after implantation was significantly suppressed by whole-body FIR starting from day 15, compared to the control group (to refer J Table1). The cDNA microarray analysis of tumor samples of control and FIR-treated showed that MMP-1, MMP-9, MMP-10, and MMP-13 in the MMP family were significantly down-regulated in the FIR group compared with control group (to refer ITEL 2005, 6(6), 597-601, Table1) [9]. The expression profiles obtained from cDNA microarray analyses as analyzed by quantitative real-time RT-PCR showed the control group to have highly significant overexpression of the genes for MMP-1, MMP-9, MMP-10, and MMP-13 compared to the FIR group (to refer ITEL 2005, 6(6), 597-601, Fig.4) [9].

These results suggest that suppression of tumor volume increase by in vivo FIR radiation was due to inhibition of MMPs by FIR radiation. In other words, FIR suppresses invasion and metastasis of tumor cells by inhibiting the expression of MMP-1, 9, 10 and 13.

As shown in (to refer ITEL 2005, 6(6), 597-601, Fig 5) [9], extensive portions of tumor tissue in the FIR group was encapsulated and necrotized in intra tumor division. On the other hand, in the control group tumor cells showed active proliferation and invasion into the surrounding muscular tissue. In addition, evaluation of the immunohistochemical expression of MMP-1, MMP-9, MMP-10 and MMP-13 using tumor tissues of control and FIR groups on day 30 after implantation showed MMP-1 and MMP-9 to be positively expressed in the tumor stroma of the control group, while MMP-10 and MMP-13 were strongly positive in tumor parenchyma (the part positively dyed at Cytokeratin10) (to refer ITEL 2005, 6(6), 597-601, Fig. 6) [9]. However, these MMPs in the FIR group were not significantly expressed. The result of immunohistological detection for these MMPs was concordant with the results of cDNA microarray and QRT-PCR. That is, FIR radiation seemed to suppress invasion of tumor cells by inhibiting the expression of MMP-1, MMP-9, MMP-10, and MMP-13.

The increased expression and activity of MMPs is associated with tumor invasion, metastasis, and angiogenesis [22]. The role of MMP-1 in tumor invasion and metastasis has only recently been determined [23]. MMP-1 has been shown to cleave entactin, thus contributing to the degradation of basement membranes and hence potentially contributing to the transitioning across epithelial barriers by tumor cells [24]. Immunohistochemical detection of MMP-1 expression is also associated with increased invasive potential and poor prognosis in colon and esophageal cancers [25, 26]. The first barrier to tumor invasion is the basement membrane, and because one of its principle constituents is type I collagen, the gelatinases (MMP-2 and MMP-9) are thought to play important roles in its degradation [27]. MMP-10 (stromelysin-2) is known to degrade various components of the extracellular matrix, and though it has been reported that MMP-10 (stromelysin-2) expression by lymphoma cells accelerates the growth of thymic lymphoma [28], the role of MMP-10 in other types of tumor growth is relatively unknown. MMP-13 (collagenase-3) is expressed in breast carcinoma and in articular cartilage of arthritic patients [29]. In addition, MMP-13 has high collagenolytic and gelatinolytic activity, and MMP-13 may be of importance in degradative processes involved in breast cancer progression [29]. In the present study, it was suggested that MMP-1, MMP-9, MMP-10, and MMP-13 are important for the invasion and metastasis of epithelial cancer of the human vulva A431 cell line in vivo and that the activities of MMP-1, MMP-9, MMP-10, and MMP-13 are selectively inhibited by FIR irradiation.

In conclusion, FIR irradiation can suppress tumor growth and invasion of epithelial cancer of the human vulva tumor by inhibiting the expression of MMP-1, MMP-9, MMP-10, and MMP-13 without critical side effects. Inhibition of MMP expression was considered to be one of the mechanisms by which multiplication of A431 tumor cells was suppressed in FIR irradiation.

6. Conclusion

It was made clear that the motion of the water molecules was surely and physically activated by the radiation of FIR with the CO_2 incubator and the animal raising apparatus. The analysis of the change of blood circulation conducted the conclusion that the FIR energy radiation activated not only the motion of water molecules but also the blood circulation in the living body. Still more, it was made clear that the activation effects on the water molecules developed the activation effects of the skin regeneration and the new bone formation. Moreover, the proliferation or metastasis of the various cancer cells were inhibited by the FIR energy radiation connected with the activation of blood circulation. It is expected that the present studies on the FIR energy radiation connect with the development of medical treatment for the regeneration of the tissue and organ as a skin and a bone, and the prevention medicine for cancer.

Author details

Kikuji Yamashita
Department of Oral and Maxillofacial Anatomy, Institute of Health Biosciences,
The University of Tokushima Graduate School, Tokushima, Japan

7. References

[1] Inoué S, Kabaya M. Biological activities caused by far-infrared radiation. Int J Biometeorol 1989;33(3) 145-150.
[2] Honda K, Inoué S. Sleep-enhancing effects of far-infrared radiation in rats. Int J Biometeorol 1988;32(2) 92-94.
[3] Udagawa Y, Nagasawa H. Effects of far-infrared ray on reproduction, growth, behaviour and some physiological parameters in mice. In Vivo 2000;14(2) 321-326.

[4] Udagawa Y, Nagasawa H,Kiyokawa S. Inhibition by whole- body hyperthermia with far-infrared rays of the growth of spontaneous mammary tumors in mice. Anticancer Res 1999;19(5B) 4125-4130.

[5] Toyokawa H, Matsui Y, Uhara J, Tsuchiya H, Teshima S, Nakanishi H, Kwon A-H, Azuma Y, Nagaoka T, Ogawa T, Kamiyama Y. Promotive effects of far-infrared ray on full-thickness skin wound healing in rats. Exp Biol Med (Maywood) 2003;228(6) 724-729.

[6] Udagawa Y, Inada K, Nagasawa H. Inhibition by Single Whole-Body Hyperthermia with Glucose Administration of the Growth of Spontaneous Mammary Tumors in Mice. Jpn J Hyperthermic Oncol 2000;16(4)229-236.

[7] Nagasawa H, Inada K, Ishigame H, Kusakawa S, Udagawa Y. Different Schedules of Whole-Body Hyperthermia with or without Glucose for the Inhibition of Mammary Tumors and Uterine Adenomyosis in SHN Mice. Bulletin of the School of Agriculture, Meiji University 2001；43-51.

[8] Yamashita K, Hosokawa H, Ishibashi J, Ishikawa N, Morimoto H, Ishikawa T, Nagayama M, Kitamura S. Development of CO2 Incubator with Limited Far-Infrared Radiation for Activation of Glucose Metabolism. ITE Letters BNTN 2005; 6(5) 53-57.

[9] Hosokawa H, Yamashita K, Ishibashi J, Ishikawa N, Morimoto H, Ishikawa T, Kitamura M, Nagayama M. A New Animal Raiser: Effect of Limited Infrared Radiation on Tumor Growth of A431 Cells. ITE Letters BNTM 2005; 6(6) 597-602.

[10] Egawa H, Takada K, Sasaki Y. (Eds) Far infrared ray. Ningentorekishisha Inc Tokyo 1999; 3.

[11] Ishibashi J, Yamashita K, Ishikawa T, Hosokawa H, Sumida K, Nagayama M, Kitamura S. The effects inhibiting the proliferation of cancer cells by far-infrared radiation (FIR) are controlled by the basal expression level of heat shock protein (HSP) 70A. Med Oncol (Northwood, London, England) 2008; 25(2）229–237.

[12] Yamashita K, Shine-Od Dalkhsuren, Ishikawa T, Sumida K, Ishibashi J, Hosokawa H, Ueno A, Nasu F, Kitamura S. Far-infrared ray radiation inhibits the proliferation of A549, HSC and Sa3 cancer cells through enhancing the expression of ATF3 gene. J Electromag Anal 2010; 4(2) 382-394.

[13] Wong H R, et al. Increased expression of heat shock protein-70 protects A549 cells against hyperoxia. Am J Physiol 1998;275(4 Pt 1) L836-41.

[14] Nylandsted J, Brand K, Jaattela M. Heat shock protein 70 is required for the survival of cancer cells. Ann N Y Acad Sci 2000; 926:122-125.

[15] Kaplan I, Kapp DS, Bagshaw MA. Secondary external-beam radiotherapy and hyperthermia for local recurrence after 125-iodine implantation in adenocarcinoma of the prostate. Int J Radiat Oncol Biol Phys 1991;20(3) 551-554.

[16] Kaver I, Ware JL, Koontz WW Jr.The effect of hyperthermia on human prostatic carcinoma cell lines: evaluation in vitro.Jr J Urol 1989;141(4) 1025-1027.

[17] Paulus JA, Tucker RD, Flanagan SW, Moseley PL, Loening SA, Park JB. et al. Heat shock protein response in a prostate tumor model to interstitial thermotherapy: implications for clinical treatment. Prostate 1993;23(3) 263-270.

[18] Roigas J, Wallen ES, Loening SA, Moseley PL. Effects of combined treatment of chemotherapeutics and hyperthermia on survival and the regulation of heat shock proteins in Dunning R3327 prostate carcinoma cells. Prostate 1998;34(3) 195-202.

[19] Servadio C, Leib Z. Local hyperthermia for prostate cancer. Urology 1991;38(4) 307-309.

[20] Yeushalmi A. Localized, non-invasive deep microwave hyperthermia for the treatment of prostatic tumors: the first 5 years. Recent Results Cancer Res 1988;107:141-146.

[21] Bellmann K, Jäättelä M, Wissing D, Burkart V, Kolb H. Heat shock protein hsp70 overexpression confers resistance against nitric oxide. FEBS Lett 1996;391(1-2) 185-188.

[22] Spiliotis ET, Kinoshita M, Nelson WJ. A mitotic septin scaffold required for Mammalian chromosome congression and segregation. Science 2005;307(5716) 1781-1785.

[23] Robinson CM, Stone AM, Shields JD, Huntley S, Paterson IC, Prime SS. Functional significance of MMP-2 and MMP-9 expression by human malignant oral keratinocyte cell lines. Arch Oral Biol 2003;48(11) 779-786.

[24] Sossey-Alaoui K, Ranalli TA, Li X, Bakin AV, Cowell JK. WAVE3 promotes cell motility and invasion through the regulation of MMP-1, MMP-3, and MMP-9 expression. Exp Cell Res 2005;308(1) 135-145

[25] Jia Y, Zeng ZZ, Markwart SM, Rockwood KF, Ignatoski KM, Ethier SP, Livant DL. Integrin fibronectin receptors in matrix metalloproteinase-1-dependent invasion by breast cancer and mammary epithelial cells. Cancer Res 2004;64(23) 8674-8681.

[26] Sires UI, Griffin GL, Broekelmann TJ, Mecham RP, Murphy G, Chung AE, Welgus HG, Senior RM. Degradation of entactin by matrix metalloproteinases. Susceptibility to matrilysin and identification of cleavage sites. J Biol Chem1993;268(3) 2069-2074.

[27] Hall C, Nelson DM, Ye X, Baker K, DeCaprio JA, Seeholzer S, Lipinski M, Adams PD. HIRA, the human homologue of yeast Hirlp and Hir2p, is a novel cyclin-cdk2 substrate whose expression blocks S-phase progression. Mol Cell Biol 2001;21(5) 1854-1865.

[28] Murray GI, Duncan ME, O'Neil P, Melvin WT, Fothergill JE. Matrix metalloproteinase-1 is associated with poor prognosis in colorectal cancer. Nat Med 1996;2(4) 461-462.

[29] Murray GI, Duncan ME, O'Neil P, McKay JA, Melvin WT, Fothergill JE. Matrix metalloproteinase-1 is associated with poor prognosis in oesophageal cancer. J Pathol 1998;185(3) 256-261.

Chapter 15

Laboratory Reference Intervals in Africa

Clement E. Zeh, Collins O. Odhiambo and Lisa A. Mills

Additional information is available at the end of the chapter

http://dx.doi.org/10.5772/48250

1. Introduction

Over the last decade, there has been a significant increase in the number of clinical trials taking place in sub-Saharan Africa in a concerted effort to identify safe and effective prevention and treatment strategies to combat the heavy burden of infectious diseases in this region [1-3]. This is because numerous viral, parasitic and bacterial diseases are endemic in this region, including: 66% of the global HIV/AIDS infections, 31% of tuberculosis infections, and 86% of malaria cases [3, 4]. Routine capacity for clinical laboratory testing is also increasing in Africa. Clinical trials and clinical care in sub-Saharan Africa require accurate laboratory reference intervals for appropriate assessment of patients/participants, monitoring disease progression, and reporting of possible toxicity and adverse events.

This is particularly important in phase I and II clinical trials. Phase I trials often enroll a small group of healthy participants in order to determine the metabolic and pharmacologic actions of drugs, side effects associated with increasing doses and early evidence of efficacy. Phase II trials on the other hand are controlled clinical studies conducted to evaluate efficacy of drug/vaccine for a particular indication in a larger group of participants and to further evaluate its safety. Many HIV vaccine trials are slated for Phase I–III trials in Africa. The inception of the US President's Emergency Plan for AIDS Relief in 2004, with a mandate to treat 2 million HIV infections with anti-retroviral therapy by 2008 has accelerated the implementation of lymphocyte immunophenotyping in urban and rural areas in Africa as initiation of therapy is often predicated on absolute CD4 T- lymphocyte counts. Central to any HIV vaccine and/or care and treatment program is the capability to measure absolute CD4 counts. CD4 counts are important in the context of breakthrough infections during HIV vaccine trials and informing treatment. Correct diagnosis in patient management often involves accurate interpretation of results from laboratory testing [5]. Hence it is critical for medical professionals to have access to an accurate management resource such as reference intervals.

Historically, clinical studies as well as routine clinical patient management in most African countries have relied on European-generated automated instrument values, US established reference intervals or the U.S. NIH division of AIDS (DAIDS) toxicity grading tables in assessing clinical parameters in study participants. The US-established reference intervals are obtained from the Massachusetts General Hospital reference values and serve as the standard reference interval comparison for most studies [6]. The DAIDS toxicity tables, also derived from a Caucasian population, are used for grading the severity of adult and pediatric adverse events, whether or not they are considered to be related to the study intervention [7]. DAIDS provides guidelines for estimating severity of adverse events using specific reference intervals (Table 1) as criteria for determining what is 'normal' and among abnormal values, how to grade the severity of the abnormality.

PARAMETER	GRADE 1 MILD	GRADE 2 MODERATE	GRADE 3 SEVERE	GRADE 4 POTENTIALLY LIFE-THREATENING
HEMOGLOBIN	10.0 – 10.9 g/dL	9.0 – 9.9 g/dL	7.0 – 8.9 g/dL	< 7.0 g/dL
NEUTROPHILS	1.0– 1.3 x 10^9 cells/L	0.75– 0.999 x 10^9cells/L	0.5– 0.749 x 10^9cells/L	< 0.5 x 10^9cells/L

Adult and pediatric values for age >57 days, HIV-negative from the DAIDS toxicity tables version 1.0, December 2004; clarification August 2009.

Table 1. Examples of DAIDS criteria of estimating severity grading based on laboratory parameters.

Reference values, in general, refer to the value or test result obtained by the observation or measurement of a particular type of quantity on an adequate number of persons (reference sample group) selected to represent the general population. Reference values are usually presented as reference intervals which refer to the interval between, and including two reference limits i.e., from the lower reference limit to the upper reference limit defined by a specific percentage (usually 95%). In certain parameters such as absolute counts of monocytes, eosinophils and basophils, only one reference limit (decision limit), more often the upper reference limit is of biological significance hence the lower reference limit assumes a value of zero.

Reference values go hand in hand with toxicity grading or decision limits, which can be defined as specific levels of the analyte that correspond to mild to life threatening clinical situations. Toxicity grading is particularly useful in the decision-making process of interpreting a measured value and assessing the health status of the subject being tested. For this reason reference values or toxicity grading are routinely used in clinical trials at enrollment to determine eligibility, establish baseline measures, and also during the course of the trial to monitor the participants' health. Moreover, several analytes are used either as markers for the possible presence of a disease or as direct evidence for that disease. Reference values, especially hematological and immunologic indices, are influenced by such factors as genetics, dietary patterns, pregnancy, gender, age, ethnic origin and prior exposure to environmental pathogens. Thus, it is important to consider these factors when applying reference intervals in diagnostics as well as in recruitment in clinical trials. According to the Clinical Laboratory and Standards Institute (CLSI) guidelines [8], it is recommended that laboratories establish their own reference intervals from the local population or validate the use of those obtained from a different setting. Despite this, clinicians and researchers in Africa have continued to use reference values of European or North American populations. Our group in Kenya has recently published reference intervals based on the CLSI guidelines and are currently assisting regional laboratories to establish their own reference intervals[9].

In this chapter, we give a brief background on the current status of participant recruitment in clinical trials and patient management in Africa. We will also describe how to select a reference population from which to derive the reference sample group. In addition, we describe various studies advocating the establishment of reference intervals performed in different regions of the African continent including our own. These studies show differences in hematological, biochemical and immunologic parameters between various African populations but these differences are statistically insignificant. However, most hematological, biochemical and immunologic parameters considered in the African studies are significantly different when compared to American and European derived values. This chapter will also discuss the proposed partitioning of adolescent males from adults given their increased recruitment into clinical trials. Adult males have significantly higher values for most hematological and biochemical parameters and we provide an explanation why this is so. While pregnant women and infants undergo physiological processes that alter their hematological and biochemical parameters, the partitioning of these cohorts has been slow. We discuss how pregnancy induces these changes and describe the particular parameters affected. We also highlight the dynamic changes in these parameters during infancy and how they differ from western-derived values. In this chapter, we also illustrate the downside of using inappropriate reference intervals in the recruitment of participants in clinical trials and patient management. We show how the use of such values results in exclusion of clinically healthy participants from clinical trials and may lead to inappropriate reporting of adverse events during the course of these studies. This potentially results in escalation of costs in the conduct of clinical trials. In this book chapter, we also propose the development of laboratory-derived African toxicity grades that, in addition to the already developed reference values, would be used for reporting adverse events in clinical trials and for determining critical values in routine health care.

2. Use of reference intervals, consequence of misclassification and selection of a reference population

2.1. The use of reference intervals

Reference intervals are useful both in the clinical and research environment. Medical laboratory reference intervals are primarily used for clinical purposes. They can be used as an indicator of good health. Alternatively, reference intervals/limits can be used to screen for physiological or pathological conditions hence important in routine health assessment, particularly for screening of anemia, blood disorders and diseases of the immune system. Reference intervals are important for accurate interpretation of laboratory data and provide assistance to the clinician in creating a more comprehensive clinical perspective for diagnosis and management of patients [10]. Of particular importance is the use of reference values as surrogate markers for monitoring disease progression and response to antiretroviral therapy in HIV-infected individuals [11]. For example, decisions to initiate, continue, or change antiretroviral therapy regimens are determined using CD4+ T-lymphocyte cell (CD4) counts, while drug toxicity is monitored using liver function tests, renal function tests, and full blood counts (FBC) [12, 13]. The hemoglobin concentration is used as a marker of anemia. As part of the management of anemia, the clinician conducts additional tests to identify a reversible etiology for anemia (eg, iron deficiency, infection) and if present treats it appropriately. However, in the clinical environment, the statistical definition of reference intervals may not allow certain clinical uses. Because these reference intervals have been derived statistically from a healthy population, they may not be used to rule in or rule out specific medical conditions. The statistically derived 95% reference interval would mean that 5% of normal subjects would have abnormal laboratory values. This is erroneously interpreted that 95% of diseased individuals would fall outside the derived reference interval. It is recommended that the number of diseased individuals who fall outside the defined 95% reference intervals be determined through a study of the distribution of such persons with the target condition [14]. Thus, it is necessary to confirm the validity of the proposed reference intervals with clinicians using a particular test to manage patients.

In the research environment, however, the aim is to define a reference population that is as similar as possible to that for which a particular test will be applied with the exception of the presence of the disease. During clinical trials, reference intervals relevant to the study of interest are required to interpret normal values of standard laboratory test results from the target population [15]. This is particularly important during phase I/II safety trials where healthy individuals are assessed without a control group [15-17]. Moreover, clinical reference intervals are necessary in order to accurately assess potential adverse events observed during the course of clinical trials.

2.2. Consequences of misclassification

A majority of clinically healthy participants have been excluded from several clinical trials in Africa because laboratory hematological and biochemical parameters are classified as abnormal [18-20]. Unnecessary exclusion of potential participants generally results in increased cost for study recruitment to achieve the target sample size. Accurate reference intervals are required for monitoring adverse events during vaccine and drug trials to limit misclassification that might otherwise lead to discontinuation of such trials or erroneous conclusions that the trial interventions are associated with adverse events. A study documented that the expense of adverse event investigation and reporting accounted for at least one-third of the study cost, irrespective of the adverse event grade [18]. To overcome these challenges, there is a need to establish accurate, locally derived reference intervals for the target population. Within the last decade, several studies in sub-Saharan Africa have attempted to establish hematological and biochemical reference intervals for use in clinical monitoring and patient management.

2.3. Selection of a reference population

The selection of a reference population is as per described in the Clinical Laboratory Standards Institute (CLSI, Wayne, PA, USA) guidelines [21]. The guidelines state that reference individuals selected for the determination of reference intervals should closely resemble the patient population undergoing medical examination and should be of similar age to be clinically significant [21]. The reference individuals should not be hospital or clinic patients unless absolutely necessary. The guidelines describe two selection methods for a reference population: *a priori* and *a posteriori*. *A priori* sampling method involves selection of reference individuals based on well-defined exclusion and partition criteria. The entire selection process takes place before any blood sample is drawn and a sufficient number of reference individuals are targeted to provide statistical validity. *A posteriori* sampling method involves selection of the reference population after the analyte has been tested. The CLSI guidelines recommend a minimum of 120 individuals to allow 90% confidence limits to be non-parametrically calculated for the reference limits [22]. Partitioning of reference intervals either by gender or age is recommended if clinically useful or physiologically well grounded. Even though 120 samples remains the recommended standard, an efficient laboratory, by considering the CLSI revised guideline strategies [8], can determine reference intervals using fewer samples [23]. Alternatively, a laboratory can adopt reference intervals established from another laboratory if the values are verified using the procedures set out in the guidelines.

In our study [9] of adolescents and adults living in rural western Kenya, all participants were screened by a review of medical history, a physical examination, tested for HIV and pregnancy (for females), and treated for any illnesses diagnosed. Participants were included if they were a permanent resident of the study area, between 13 and 34 years of age and able to provide informed consent or assent if a minor. Participants were excluded if they were HIV-seropositive, pregnant, exhibiting febrile symptoms or on any medication. Blood samples were therefore obtained from clinically healthy participants selected to generate hematologic and biochemical reference intervals. Data were partitioned by age (<18 years of age as adolescents and ≥18 as adults) and gender; median and 95th percentile intervals were calculated. The lower 95% reference limit was defined as the 2.5th percentile while the upper limit was defined as the 97.5th percentile. A Wilcoxon rank-sum test was used to test for age and gender differences. We compared our data against reference intervals from the Massachusetts General Hospital (MGH-USA) [6] and the U.S. NIH Division of AIDS (DAIDS) toxicity tables [7] to determine the number of study participants with values outside the MGH ranges or who had any adverse event as graded by the DAIDS criteria. However, while the CLSI guidelines recommend a description of the population from which reference intervals are derived, the DAIDS and Massachusetts General Hospital reference values do not provide such information.

3. Current status of reference values in Africa

Reference intervals for clinical laboratory parameters have traditionally been obtained from European and North American populations [2]. However, differences have been reported between these values when compared to healthy African population values [16]. These include lower hemoglobin, red blood cell counts, hematocrit, mean corpuscular volume, platelets and neutrophils, and higher monocyte and eosinophil levels for African population compared to their Western counterparts [16,24-26] and Africans of European decent [27, 28]. Moreover, variations in several indices have been reported between different African ethnic groups [26, 29-31]. These differences are postulated to occur due to factors such as genetics, dietary patterns, gender, age, ethnic origin and environmental pathogens which are known to influence hematological and immunologic indices [32-35].

While the differences observed in some laboratory parameters between African and Caucasian/Western populations may be attributed to nutritional differences, genetic polymorphisms, or more intense environmental exposure to endemic pathogens, it must be stressed that these reference values are being derived from population-based statistical analyses of norms among healthy persons. For example, healthy Africans tend to have lower white blood cell counts than Caucasians, but there is no evidence that they suffer any additional risk of developing severe infection or other sequelae. Also, African American populations, with environmental exposures more like their white American counterparts, tend to have lower 'normal values' in hematologic parameters than Caucasian Americans, suggesting a genetic basis for these population differences.

3.1 Variation in specific laboratory parameters

a. Hematologic parameters

The normal values of red cell counts and indices (i.e., hemoglobin concentration, hematocrit, mean corpuscular volume, red blood cell count), white cell counts and platelet counts are known to vary with age, sex and pregnancy [9, 16, 20, 31, 36]. In addition, genetic and environmental factors can also affect the reference intervals in certain populations [32-34, 37]. It is of particular importance that these differences in reference intervals be considered by clinicians in different settings.

i. Red blood cell (RBC) components

African RBC component values were significantly lower when compared to reference intervals obtained from the Massachusetts General Hospital [6] from a North American population, and thus a significant proportion are misclassified when the NIH DAIDS toxicity tables are applied [9, 34, 38]. Differences observed in the RBC components between African and Caucasian populations may be attributed to lower dietary iron intake, genetic polymorphisms such as thalassemia and sickle cell trait or chronic exposure to endemic parasites including helminths, malaria and schistosomiasis.

Statistically significant differences in median RBC, hemoglobin concentration (Hb) and hematocrit (Hct), mean corpuscular volume (MCV) and mean corpuscular hemoglobin

(MCH) by gender have been observed in several African studies, with adult males having higher values than adult females in East Africa [9, 16, 20, 31, 39, 40], Southern Africa [20, 36], West Africa [41] and Central Africa [42]. These gender differences in RBC parameters as illustrated in our findings (Table 2), are consistent with previously established evidence that males have higher values than females for these parameters and is partly attributed to the influence of the androgen hormone on erythropoiesis [43, 44] and to menstrual blood loss in women [16, 25, 39, 42, 45]. It has been reported that estrogens lower the Hb through hemodilution while testosterone increases the plasma volume but increases circulating RBC to an even greater extent [46].

		Age 13-17 years			Age 18-34 years			
Parameter	**Gender**	**n**	**Median (95th percentile)**	**p-value (gender)**	**n**	**Median (95th percentile)**	**p-value (gender)**	**p-value (age)**
Hemoglobin (g/dL)	**Female**	57	12.2 (8.1 - 14.2)	***<.0001***	83	12.1(8.0 – 14.2)	***<.0001***	*0.3243*
	Male	76	13.1 (10.6 - 15.6)		77	14.2 (11.4 - 16.9)		***<.0001***
Hematocrit (%)	**Female**	57	35.6 (24.8 - 43.1)	***<.0001***	83	35.8 (23.2 - 44.3)	***<.0001***	*0.8015*
	Male	76	38.8 (29.3 – 48.1)		77	41.7 (32.6- 51.5)		***<.0001***
RBC ($x10^{12}$/L)	**Female**	57	4.7 (3.3 - 5.4)	***0.0001***	83	4.5 (3.4 - 5.7)	***<.0001***	*0.2638*
	Male	76	4.9 (4.1 - 5.8)		77	5.3 (4.3 - 6.5)		***<.0001***
PLT($x10^{9}$/L)	**Female**	57	233 (134 – 439)	*0.2958*	83	220 (88 – 439)	***0.0222***	*0.4034*
	Male	76	224 (103 – 386)		77	201 (102 -307)		***0.0094***
WBC ($x10^{9}$/L)	**Female**	57	5.2 (3.9-10.2)	*0.6359*	83	5.6 (3.3-9.7)	***0.0189***	*0.2038*
	Male	76	5.6 (3.3-8.3)		77	5.3 (2.5-7.4)		*0.6382*
Lymphocytes ($x10^{9}$/L)	**Female**	57	2.2 (1.1 - 3.1)	*0.9820*	83	2.2 (1.3 - 3.8)	*0.6901*	*0.9388*
	Male	76	2.2 (1.0 - 4.2)		77	2.2 (1.0 – 3.5)		*0.585*
Ab Neutrophils ($x10^{9}$/L)	**Female**	57	2.0 (1.0-6.2)	*0.4991*	83	2.3 (1.3-5.4)	***0.0004***	*0.0576*
	Male	76	1.9 (0.8-5.0)		77	2.0 (0.8-3.9)		*0.6575*
CD4: Absolute	**Female**	58	934 (465- 1553)	*0.4074*	83	866 (440-1602)	***0.0141***	*0.509*
	Male	76	874 (367-1571)		77	811 (462-1306)		***0.0209***
CD8: Absolute	**Female**	58	506 (195-1068)	*0.4506*	83	472 (262 - 1167)	*0.8706*	*0.9213*
	Male	76	468 (195-988)		77	468 (201-1104)		*0.4194*
CD4/CD8 ratio	**Female**	58	1.8 (0.9-3.2)	*0.9215*	83	1.8 (0.8-3.0)	*0.0728*	*0.4879*
	Male	76	1.8 (0.8-2.8)		77	1.6 (0.8-2.8)		*0.0543*

Table 2. Test of difference in hematologic and immunologic parameters between gender and age-groups from healthy 13-34 year olds in a rural western Kenya cohort (2003-2005).

Age-related differences in the RBC component have also been observed among male participants, with adults (≥18 years) having higher levels of Hb, Hct and RBC compared to male adolescents (13-17 years) as shown here (Table 2) [9]. This age variation is similar to that reported in a study of Caucasian adolescents [34]. This difference could be attributed to higher levels of androgen hormones among older males. This explanation is further strengthened by the absence of age-related hematological difference among female participants. It has also been postulated that an increase in the size and mass of muscle fibers as occurs in males is associated with an increase in the number of circulating red blood cells [47].

There are limited data comparing reference intervals for hematologic values among African children compared to Caucasian children and also few studies on relevant local reference values for African infants. However, these studies, similar to the adult studies, have highlighted differences in RBC components compared to values obtained from Caucasian children [48]. The lower RBC parameters, as in the adolescent and adult groups, may be attributed to impaired hematopoiesis as a result of lower dietary iron intake, chronic blood loss due to hookworm infestation or chronic malaria infection [25]. Endemic sickle cell trait (HbS) and α-thalassemia may also play an important role [49].

ii. Platelets

In general, lower platelet counts are more common in African than in Western populations. While the lower platelet counts in African populations are consistent in several African studies [24, 25, 30, 31, 40], its etiology is unknown. Possibilities such as dietary, environmental and genetic factors have been proposed [24, 30, 31]. Nevertheless, the significant difference in the lower limit of the reference interval between African and Caucasian populations warrants consideration when interpreting platelet counts in patients or during clinical trial recruitment in African populations.

Among Africans males, significant age-related differences have been observed in platelet counts with adults having higher platelet counts compared to adolescents [9]. This variation is observed as a progressive increase with age from adolescence to young adulthood. In comparison, there is little age variation in platelet counts among females. However, females have higher platelet counts than males both in adolescence [9] and adulthood [9, 16]. These gender differences in platelet counts have been attributed to hormonal influences [50]. Platelet count have been observed to falls at the onset of menstruation while peak values are obtained in mid-cycle indicating that hormonal influences and/or menstrual blood loss may be involved [27]. While platelet levels remain stable during pregnancy, a decrease has been reported immediately after delivery, likely due to consumption during separation and delivery of the placenta.

iii. White Blood Cell (WBC) components

A high proportion of participants in the African studies have WBC counts below the lower range of the Massachusetts General Hospital US population-derived values [9, 20]. This phenomenon is consistent with a number of studies that have reported lower WBC counts in

African populations and those of African ancestry, including African Americans, than in Caucasian populations [24, 30, 51-53]. Because the reference interval for WBC counts is significantly different from that of Caucasian populations, it is advisable to use appropriate ethnic group intervals when interpreting blood counts [31].

Gender differences in the WBC counts exist in both African and Caucasian populations with females having higher values than males [9, 20, 54]. Age-related difference in WBC counts has been reported in several African studies [9, 25, 33]. Adolescents have higher WBC counts compared to adults as shown in our study (Table 2) [9].

1. Neutrophils

Within the U.S., lower neutrophil counts are more common among blacks compared to Caucasians [28]. Thus, it is not unsurprising to observe a higher proportion of African study participants (22.5-35%) having neutrophil counts below the lower range of Massachusetts General Hospital's population-derived reference interval [9]. It is estimated that about 25% to 50% of Africans have "benign ethnic neutropenia," maintaining consistently low absolute neutrophil counts with no evidence of increased susceptibility to infection or other adverse events [28]. Possibile explanations for the lower neutrophil count include diet, genetic or environmental influences [53, 55].

In general, there are significant differences in neutrophil counts between male and female adults, with the females having higher neutrophil counts than males. This increase in neutrophil counts observed in women may be related to estrogen since a decrease in counts has been reported after menopause [39]. Oral contraceptives have also been implicated in neutrophilia [56].

Additionally, several studies in southern Africa have documented high rates of neutropenia in infants of women receiving Prevention of Mother to Child Transmission interventions [57-591]. Evaluation of neutropenia in infants receiving antiretroviral prophylaxis or treatment (directly or indirectly through maternal exposure in utero or through breastfeeding) remains a challenge. Neutropenia is a known side effect of zidovudine [60] and trimethoprim/sulfamethoxazole, which is often prescribed for prevention of opportunistic infections in HIV-infected and/or HIV-exposed infants/children. This problem is further compounded by the paucity of normative data for hematologic values in African infants.

2. Basophils and eosinophils

Basophil and eosinophil counts in African populations are significantly elevated in both genders when compared to the US-based reference intervals [9, 20]. This may be due to a high prevalence of parasitic infections in the environment including schistosomiasis, helminthic infections, perennial malaria and exposure to a broader range of environmental antigens [25, 39]. However, the eosinophil counts do not vary significantly by gender or by age, as assessed between adolescent and adult African participants [9, 34].

3. Monocytes

Generally, no ethnic or age differences are observed between Caucasian and African populations [46]. Monocyte counts in Eastern and Southern Africa are comparable to the US derived valuesand thus there is no need for separate reference intervals [9, 20].

In the African studies, no differences are observed in absolute monocyte counts between adolescents and adults or by gender [9, 20]. Previous studies from Eastern and Southern African populations indicate an increase in monocyte counts in males compared with females but the difference is not significant [3, 24, 26, 29, 30].

4. Lymphocytes

Among healthy, HIV-uninfected persons, there are no significant differences in lymphocyte counts between Caucasian and African populations but females generally have higher lymphocyte counts than males [54]. This is corroborated by studies within Africa that indicated higher CD4 cell percentage and absolute CD4 counts in females compared to males [9, 26, 61].

However, geographical variation exists in lymphocyte counts with some populations in Southern African showing significantly lower reference values than other parts of Africa [62]. In assessing age-related variability, younger age is associated with higher CD4 cell counts and a higher CD4:CD8 ratio. However, the differences are not significantly except for CD4 cell counts between male adolescent and male adults [9]. These age and geographical variations need to be considered when interpreting lymphocyte counts.

b. Clinical chemistry parameters

Most African studies [9, 15, 16, 20] report reference intervals for most parameters (creatinine, direct bilirubin, amylase and albumin) that are in agreement with reference intervals published in the United States [6]. However, certain parameters such as Creatine Kinase (CK) and Lactose Dehydrogenase (LDH) have upper intervals that are substantially higher than those published in the Massachusetts General Hospital intervals [16, 20]. Other parameters with a similar trend include total bilirubin (T-bil) and blood urea nitrogen (BUN). The upper range for T-bil is about twice as high as that of the US-derived upper reference limit while the lower range for BUN is a about a third of the US-derived lower reference limit [9, 15, 20]. The etiology of high T-bil in the African population may arise from a number of factors including RBC hemolysis caused by malaria infection or sickle cell disease, malnutrition or physical exertion. Moreover, the presence of similar trends among other African populations is suggestive of a common environmental or genetic factor.

Our findings indicated gender and age variations in blood chemistry analytes of liver and renal function among African adolescents and adults. Male adolescents and adults had higher values for alanine aminotransferase (ALT), aspartate aminotransferase (AST), T-bil and creatinine than females adolescents and adults (Table 3). These gender differences were significantly greater for T-bil and creatinine in both adolescents and adults while for AST, the difference was significant only among the adolescents. However, these differences were not clinically significant. There were no gender differences in BUN and glucose levels for all age groups and no significant differences in T-bil, AST, ALT and glucose between the two age groups for both males and females. However adult men and women had higher values for creatinine and BUN compared to adolescent males and females, respectively.

			Age 13-17 years			Age 18-34 years		
Parameter	**Gender**	**n**	**Median (95th percentile)**		**n**	**Median (95th percentile)**	**p-value (gender)**	**p-value (age)**
AST/SGOT (μ/L)	**Female**	62	22.6 (12.0 – 43.1)	***0.0102***	82	22.2 (13.5 - 48.5)	*0.0822*	*0.5905*
	Male	77	26.9 (17.0 – 59.2)		77	26.7 (12.5-69.3)		*0.9147*
ALT/SGPT (μ/L)	**Female**	62	17.4 (4.2-65.3)	*0.6289*	82	18.9 (10.7-61.3)	*0.2247*	*0.1305*
	Male	77	20.5 (4.9-42.4)		77	22.4 (12.0-80.6)		*0.0901*
Total Bilirubin (μmol/L)	**Female**	62	9.7 (3.7-38.5)	***0.0331***	82	11.5 (5.8-36.1)	***0.0368***	*0.7132*
	Male	77	13.9 (5.7 – 62.6)		77	13.8 (5.3 - 50.7)		*0.6662*
Creatinine (μmol/L)	**Female**	62	64.5 (48.0-87.6)	***0.0229***	82	70.7 (52.4-96.8)	***<.0001***	***0.0013***
	Male	77	66.3 (49.6-103.7)		77	83.1(54.2-137.8)		***<.0001***

Table 3. Test of difference in clinical chemistry parameters between gender and age-groups from healthy 13-34 year olds in a rural western Kenya cohort (2003-2005).

4. Should establishing separate normal ranges for African adolescents and pregnant women be considered?

A number of studies similar to our published data [9], have reported age-related variation between male adolescents as compared to adults for Hb, Hct and RBC levels [25, 34, 45]. This observation is physiologically grounded on hormonal influence and as per the CLSI guidelines, partitioning reference intervals by age (or other subgroup considerations) may be appropriate. While these observations may not be of any medical significance, it should be taken into consideration whenever clinical trials target this population. To satisfy the statistical requirement for partitioning, there is need for further research on reference values among adolescents, as their participation in clinical trials increases.

Other than the RBC components mentioned above, no significant age differences have been observed in other laboratory parameters measured among males or in any parameters measured among females except for creatinine and BUN. Thus, for such parameters for which no differences are reported, adult values can be used in clinical trials involving adolescents.

With the advent of antiretroviral therapy for HIV and other interventions to improve maternal and child health, pregnant women and infants have become the focus of many health programs. However, few data exist regarding these important populations, despite increased clinical trials aimed at reducing mother-to-child HIV transmission. Although pregnancy-induced changes occur in hematological values including Hb, Hct and RBC count, very few laboratories provide specific reference ranges for pregnant women [63, 64].

In pregnancy, blood volume increases resulting in hemodilution. While the red cell mass increases during pregnancy, the plasma volume increases more resulting in a relative anemia. This leads to a lower Hb level, Hct and RBC. Hb is known to vary with gestational age with the highest values within the first and last trimesters and lowest during the second trimester. Similarly, the Hct and RBC decreases with gestational age. A stable higher upper reference limit for WBC count during pregnancy has been reported [65, 66]. WBC count is known to peak at delivery, thus limiting the use of this parameter as a marker for infection during delivery. This increase in WBC count results primarily from an increase in neutrophil counts and a slight increase in lymphocyte counts. Currently, there exists no African study designed to establish reference intervals during pregnancy and most laboratory information systems report reference values based on samples obtained from non–pregnant women which may not be useful for clinical decisions during pregnancy. Thus, there is an increased risk of overlooking important physiologic alterations resulting from pathological conditions and of misinterpreting normal changes as pathological events [64]. It is therefore important to develop reference intervals for women during pregnancy and the postpartum period for use in patient monitoring and management.

5. A case for African/ Region specific toxicity tables?

Under a research-based approach, applying the US Massachusetts General Hospital derived reference intervals to our reference population from western Kenya during screening for a clinical trial (Table 4), over 58% of the volunteers would have been excluded from the trial despite having laboratory results consistent with the general population from which they were derived. This erroneous screening out of otherwise healthy volunteers would have important implications on study costs, work load and time, as more volunteers would be need to be screened in order to meet the required target [15].

Similarly, applying the DAIDS toxicity tables to our population, some of our calculated reference intervals fall between the normal, and grade 1–2 toxicity grading in the DAIDS system (Table 4). Using the clinic based approach, 40% of our otherwise healthy study participants would have erroneously been considered to have at least one laboratory-based grade 1–4 toxicity adverse event. The lower range for Hb, neutrophil counts, as well as the upper range for eosinophil counts and bilirubin would be considered as grade 2 adverse events, for example. Even though studies have documented these findings, this information is not widely known and as a result, DAIDS has issued only 1 set of "standard" toxicity tables without considering racial or ethnic differences [57]. Thus, during international clinical trials, these tables are used as guidelines in the conduct of such trials. This may result in a situation where the results of a clinical trial cannot be generalized to the population in question since a majority of otherwise healthy participants are screened out. Moreover, given that the investigational product is intended for use within the same population being sampled, this may complicate post-market analysis or application of the product for the general population. Unfortunately, there are no comparable tables from Africa on which such clinical decisions can be based. It is therefore important that African countries carry out large studies in different regions of Africa for such parameters to establish African toxicity tables.

		MGH USA reference intervals (25th percentile)[6]			Division of AIDS (DAIDS) toxicity grading							
		out of range Comparison			Grade 1		Grade 2		Grade 3		Grade 4	
Parameter	n	95th percentile	n	%	n	%	n	%	n	%	n	%
Hemoglobin Males (g/dl)	140	13.5-17.5	65	46	2	1.3	0	0	2	1.3	0	0
Hemoglobin Females (g/dl)	153	12-16	61	40	11	7.9	8	5.7	14	10	0	0
Hct (females) (%)	140	36-46	74	53								
Hct (males) (%)	153	41-53	88	58								
RBC (males) (10^{12} cells/L)	140	4.5-5.9	29	19								
RBC (females) (10^{12} cells/L)	153	4.0-5.2	32	23								
MCV (fL)	293	80-100	157	54								
Platelets (10^9 cells/L)	293	150-350	53	18	6	2	6	2	0	0	0	0
WBC (10^9 cells/L)	293	4.5-11.0	66	23	2	0.7	0	0	0	0	0	0
Lymphocyte count (10^9 cells/L)	293	1.0-4.8	6	2	0	0	0	0	0	0	0	0
Neutrophil count (10^9 cells/L)	293	1.8-7.7	110	38	25	8.5	9	3.1	1	0.3	0	0
Eosinophil (10^9 cells/L)	293	0-0.5	130	44	60	20.5	12	4.1	0	0	0	0
Basophil count (10^9 cells/L)	293	0-0.2	5	2								
Monocyte count (10^9 cells/L)	293	0-0.8	0	0								
ALT (SGPT) (U/ L)	293	0-35	30	10	12	4.1	1	0.3	0	0	0	0
AST (SGOT) (U/ L)	293	0-35	40	13	9	3.1	3	1	0	0	0	0
Total Bilirubin (μmol/L)	293	5.1-17.0	90	30	37	12.7	27	9.2	4	1.4	1	0.3
Creatinine (μmol/L)	293	0-133	4	1	4	1.4	0	0	0	0	0	0
Glucose mmol/L	293	4.2-6.4	210	71								
BUN (mmol/L)	293	3.6-7.1	246	84								
***CD4** (Cells/ μl)	293	404-1612	6	2	3	1	1	0.3	0	0	0	0
***CD8** (Cells/ μl)	293	220-1129	13	4								

*Reference ranges provided by Becton-Dickinson with the MultiTEST IMK Kit Reagent package (12/2000;23-3602-02) - DAIDS- Division of AIDS tables for grading the severity of adult and pediatric adverse events [26] - MGH- Massachusetts General Hospital weekly case records [25]

Table 4. Frequency of adverse events and out of range values comparing western Kenyan cohort to DAIDS and North American derived MGH values

6. Conclusion

While it is desirable to generate reference intervals for different populations, the procedure remains a challenge due to the prohibitive cost involved in performing these studies and the limitation in identifying suitable healthy reference individuals. Thus, the CLSI recommendation that all diagnostic laboratories should determine and maintain their own reference interval for each laboratory parameter is impractical. The revised CLSI guidelines have recommended that if it is not possible to establish detailed reference studies, then validation of published reference intervals can be performed using methodology tailored for the population served by the laboratory. As few as 20 specimens can be used to validate reference values within each laboratory by performing a formal outlier test.

Given the number of clinical trials and persons receiving clinical services is expected to increase substantially in sub-Saharan Africa, there is a need for the establishment of locally derived clinical laboratory reference values to ensure appropriate general health assessment, treatment monitoring, and efficient implementation of clinical trials. Even more important is the need for the establishment of toxicity grading tables for application in clinical care among Africans based on the documented differences between laboratory reference values from African populations and Caucasians or Western populations of mixed ethnic origin.

Author details

Clement E. Zeh, Collins O. Odhiambo and Lisa A. Mills
U.S. Centers for Disease Control and Prevention (CDC-Kenya), Kisumu, Kenya,
Centre for Global Health Research, Kenya Medical Research Institute/U.S. CDC Research and Public Health, Kisumu, Kenya

Acknowledgement

The authors would like to acknowledge Kayla Laserson and Laurie Kamimoto and Professor Barbara Bains for their thorough review of this chapter. The authors would also like to appreciate vital contributions made by KEMRI/CDC Kisumu, HIV-Research Laboratory. This chapter is published with the approval of the Director of KEMRI.

Disclaimer: The findings and conclusions in this article are those of the authors and do not necessarily represent the views of the U.S. Centers for Disease Control and Prevention. Use of trade names is for identification purposes only and does not constitute endorsement by the U.S. Centers for Disease Control and Prevention or the Department of Health and Human Services.

7. References

[1] Esparza J, O.S., *HIV vaccines: a global perspective.* Current Molecular Medicine, 2003. 3: p. 183–193.

[2] Jaoko W, N.F., Anzala O, Manyonyi GO, Birungi J, Nanvubya A, Bashir F, Bhatt K, Ogutu H, Wakasiaka S, Matu L, Waruingi W, Odada J, Oyaro M, Indangasi J, Ndinya-Achola J, Konde C, Mugisha E, Fast P, Schmidt C, Gilmour J, Tarragona T, Smith C, Barin B, Dally L, Johnson B, Muluubya A, Nielsen L, Hayes P, Boaz M, Hughes P, Hanke T, McMichael A, Bwayo J, Kaleebu P, *Safety and immunogenicity of recombinant low-dosage HIV-1 A vaccine candidates vectored by plasmid pTHr DNA or modified vaccinia virus Ankara (MVA) in humans in East Africa.* Vaccine, 2008. 26(22): p. 2788–2795.

[3] UNAIDS, *Report on the global AIDS epidemic. Geneva, Switzerland, WHO press,* WHO, Editor. 2010, UNAIDS.

[4] TheGlobalFund, *The Global Fund to Fight AIDS, TB and Malaria;''Global FundARVFactSheet*. 2009.

[5] Bakerman S, B.P., Stausbauch P *ABC's of Interpretive Laboratory Data*. 2002, Scottsdale. AZ, USA: Interpretive Laboratory Data, Inc.

[6] Kratz A, F.M., Sluss PM, Lewandrowski KB, *Case records of the Massachusetts General Hospital. Weekly clinicopathological exercises. Laboratory reference values.* New England Journal of Medicine, 2004. 351(15): p. 1548-1563.

[7] DAIDS, *Division of AIDS Table for Grading the Severity of Adult and Pediatric Adverse Events*, DAIDS, Editor. 2004: Bethseda, MD, USA.

[8] CLSI, *Defining, Establishing, and Verifying Reference Intervals in the Clinical Laboratory; Approved Guideline*. 2008, Wayne, PA: Clinical and Laboratory Standards Institute.

[9] Zeh C, A.P., Inzaule S, Ondoa P, Oyaro B, Mwaengo DM, Vandenhoudt H, Gichangi A, Williamson J, Thomas T, DeCock KM, Hart C, Nkengasong J, Laserson K, *Population-based biochemistry, immunologic and hematological reference values for adolescents and young adults in a rural population in Western Kenya.* PLoS One, 2011. 6(6).

[10] Ritchie RF, P.G., *Selecting clinically relevant populations for reference intervals.* Clin Chem Lab Med, 2004. 42(7): p. 702-709.

[11] O'Brien WA, H.P., Daar ES, Simberkoff MS, Hamilton JD, *Changes in plasma HIV RNA levels and CD4+ lymphocyte counts predict both response to antiretroviral therapy and therapeutic failure.* Ann Intern Med, 1997. 126: p. 939–945.

[12] Cengiz C, P.J., Saraf N, Dieterich DT, *HIV and liver diseases: recent clinical advances.* Clinics in Liver Disease, 2005. 9: p. 647–666.

[13] Phillips AN, S.S., Weber R, Kirk O, Francioli P, Miller V, Vernazza P, Lundgren JD, Ledergerber B, *HIV viral load response to antiretroviral therapy according to the baseline CD4 cell count and viral load.* JAMA, 2001. 286: p. 2560–2567.

[14] Boyd, J.C., *Defining laboratory reference values and decision limits: populations, intervals, and interpretations.* Asian Journal of Andrology, 2010. 12: p. 83-90.

[15] Eller LA, E.M., Ouma B, Kataaha P, Kyabaggu D, Tumusiime R, Wandege J, Sanya R, Sateren WB, Wabwire-Mangen F, Kibuuka H, Robb ML, Michael NL, de Souza MS, *Reference intervals in healthy adult Ugandan blood donors and their impact on conducting international vaccine trials.* PLoS ONE, 2008. 3(12).

[16] Kibaya RS, B.C., Sawe FK, Shaffer DN, Sateren WB, Scott PT, Michael NL, Robb ML, Birx DL, de Souza MS, *Reference ranges for the clinical laboratory derived from a rural population in Kericho, Kenya.* PLoS One, 2008. 3(10).

[17] Omosa-Manyonyi GS, J.W., Anzala O, Ogutu H, Wakasiaka S, Malogo R, Nyange J, Njuguna P, Ndinya-Achola J, Bhatt K, Farah B, Oyaro M, Schmidt C, Priddy F, Fast P, *Reasons for ineligibility in in phase 1 and 2A HIV vaccine clinical trials at Kenya AIDS vaccine initiative (KAVI), Kenya.* PLoS One, 2011. 6(1).

[18] Chou VB, O.S., Hussain H, Mugasha C, Musisi M, Mmiro F, Musoke P, Jackson JB, Guay LA, *The costs associated with adverse event procedures for an International HIV Clinical Trial determined by activity-based costing.* Journal of Acquired Immune Deficiency Syndrome, 2007. 46: p. 426–432.

[19] Lubega IR, F.M., Musoke PM, Elbireer A, Bagenda D, Kafulafula G, Ko J, Mipando L, Mubiru M, Kumwenda N, Taha T Jackson, JB, Guay L, *Considerations in using US-based*

laboratory toxicity tables to evaluate laboratory toxicities among healthy malawian and Ugandan infants. J Acquir Immune Defic Syndr, 2010. 55(1): p. 58-64.

[20] Karita E, K.N., Price MA, Kayitenkore K, Kaleebu P, Nanvubya A, Anzala O, Jaoko W, Mutua G, Ruzagira E, Mulenga J, Sanders EJ, Mwangome M, Allen S, Bwanika A, Bahemuka U, Awuondo K, Omosa G, Farah B, Amornkul P, Birungi J, Yates S, Stoll-Johnson L, Gilmour J, Stevens G, Shutes E, Manigart O, Hughes P, Dally L, Scott J, Stevens W, Fast P, Kamali A, *CLSI derived hematology and biochemistry reference intervals for healthy adults in eastern and southern Africa.* PLoS One, 2009. 4(2).

[21] NCCLS, *How to define and determine reference intervals in the clinical laboratory; approved guideline.* 2000, National Committee for Clinical laboratory Standards

[22] Reed AH, H.R., Mason WB, *Influence of statistical methods used on the resulting estimate of normal range.* Clin. Chem, 1971. 17: p. 275-284.

[23] Horn PS, H.G., Pesce AJ, *Determining Laboratory Reference Intervals: CLSI Guideline Makes the Task Manageable.* Laboratory Medicine, 2009. 40(2): p. 75-76.

[24] Gill GV, E.A., Marshal C, *Low platelet counts in Zambians.* Transactions of the Royal Society of Tropical Medicine and Hygiene, 1979. 73(1): p. 111-112.

[25] Lugada ES, M.J., Kaharuza F, Ulvestad E, Were W, Langeland N, Asjo B, Malamba S, Downing R, *Population-based hematologic and immunologic reference values for a healthy Ugandan population.* Clin Diagn Lab Immunol, 2004. 11: p. 29-34.

[26] Tugume SB, P.E., Lutalo T, Mugyenyi PN, Grant RM, Mangeni FW, Pattishall K, Katongole-Mbidde E, *Hematological reference ranges among healthy Ugandans.* Clin Diagn Lab Immunol, 1995. 2: p. 233–235.

[27] Morley, A., *A platelet cycle in normal individuals.* Aust Ann Med, 1969. 18: p. 127-133.

[28] Haddy TB, R.S., Castro O, *Benign ethnic neutropenia: what is a normal absolute neutrophil count?* The Journal of Laboratory and Clinical Medicine, 1999. 133(1): p. 15-22.

[29] Abdulkadir J, B.G., *Haemoglobin and haematocrit levels in young adult Ethiopian males in Addis Ababa.* Ethiopian Medical Journal 1979. 17: p. 5–8.

[30] Bain B, S.M., Godsland I, *Normal values for peripheral blood white cell counts in women of four different ethnic origins.* Journal of Clinical Pathology, 1984. 37: p. 188-193.

[31] Ngowi BJ, M.S., Bruun JN, Morkve O . , . 9: p. 1., *Immunohaematological reference values in human immunodeficiency virus-negative adolescent and adults in rural northern Tanzania.* BMC Infect Dis, 2009. 9(1).

[32] Choong ML, T.S., Cheong SK, *Influence of race,age and sex on the lymphocyte sub-sets in peripheral blood of healthy Malaysian adults. .* Annals of clinical biochemistry, 1995. 32(6): p. 532–539.

[33] Lee BW, Y.H., Chew FT, Quah TC, Prabhakaran K, Chan GS, Wong SC, Seah CC, *Age- and sex-related changes in lymphocyte subpopulations of healthy Asian subjects: from birth to adulthood.* Cytometry, 1996. 26(1): p. 8-15.

[34] Romeo J, W.J., Gomez-Martinez S, Diaz LE, Moreno LA, Castillo MJ, Redondo C, Baraza JC, Sola R, Zamora S, Marcos A, . , . 83: p. . *Haematological reference values in Spanish adolescents: the AVENA study.* European Journal of haematology, 2009. 83: p. 586–594.

[35] Shahabuddin, S., *Quantitative differences in CD8+ lymphocytes, CD4/CD8 ratio, NK cells, and HLA-DR(+)-activated T cells of racially different male populations.* Clin Immunol Immunopathol 1995. 75: p. 168–170.

[36] Mwinga K, V.S., Chen YQ, Mwatha A, Read JS, Urassa W, Carpenetti N, Valentine M, Goldenberg R L, *Selected hematologic and biochemical measurements in African HIV-infected and uninfected pregnant women and their infants: the HIV Prevention Trials Network 024 protocol.* BMC Pediatr, 2009. 9.

[37] Shahabuddin, S., *Quantitative differences in CD8+ lymphocytes, CD4/CD8 ratio, NK cells, and HLA-DR(+)-activated T cells of racially different male populations.* Clin Immunol Immunopathol, 1995. 75: p. 168–170.

[38] Hsieh MM, E.J., Byrd-Holt DD, Tisdale JF, Rodgers GP, *Prevalence of Neutropenia in the U.S. Population: Age, Sex, Smoking Status, and Ethnic Differences.* Annals of Internal Medicine, 2007. 146(7): p. 486-492.

[39] Saathoff E, S.P., Kleinfeldt V, Geis S, Haule D, Maboko L, Samky E, de Souza M, Robb M, Hoelscher M, *Laboratory reference values for healthy adults from southern Tanzania.* Trop Med Int Health, 2008. 13: p. 612–625.

[40] Tsegaye A, M.T., Tilahun T, Hailu E, Sahlu T, Doorly R, Fontanet AL, Rinke de Wit TF, *Immunohematological reference ranges for adult Ethiopians.* Clin Diagn Lab Immunol 1999. 6: p. 410–414.

[41] Koram KA, A.M., Ocran JC, Adu-Amankwah S, Rogers WO, Nkrumah F K, *Population based reference intervals for common blood haematological and biochemical parameters in the Akuapem north district.* Ghana Medical Journal, 2007. 41(4): p. 160-166.

[42] Menard D, M.M., Tothy MB, Kelembho EK, Gresenguet G, Talarmin A, *Immunohematological reference ranges for adults from the Central African Republic.* Clin Diagn Lab Immunol, 2003. 10: p. 443–445.

[43] Gordon AS, M.E., Wenig J, Katz R, Zanjani ED, *Androgen actions on erythropoiesis.* Annals of the New York Academy of Sciences, 1968. 149: p. 318–335.

[44] Krabbe S, C.T., Worm J, Christiansen C, Transbol I *Relationship between haemoglobin and serum testosterone in normal children and adolescents and in boys with delayed puberty.* Acta Paediatr Scand, 1978. 67: p. 655–658.

[45] Hawkins WW, S.E., Leonard VG, *Variation of the hemoglobin level with age and sex.* Blood, 1954. 9(10): p. 999-1007.

[46] Gardener FH, N.D., Piomelli S, Cummins JF, *The erythrocythaemic effects of androgens.* British Journal of Haematology, 1968. 14(6): p. 611–615.

[47] Daniel, W., *Hematocrit: maturity relationship in adolescence.* . Pediatrics, 1973. 52(3): p. 388-394.

[48] Troy SB, R.-R.A., Le Dyner L, Musingwini G,. Shetty AK, Woelk G, Stranix-Chibanda L, Nathoo K. Maldonado YA, *Hematologic and Immunologic Parameters in Zimbabwean Infants: A Case for Using Local Reference Intervals to Monitor Toxicities in Clinical Trials.* J Trop Pediatr 2011. 58(1): p. 59-62.

[49] Saxena S, W.E., *Heterogeneity of common hematologic parameters among racial, ethnic, and gender subgroups.* Archives of Pathology and Laboratory Medicine, 1990. 114: p. 715–719.

[50] Tikly M, B.D., Solomons HD, Govender Y, Atkinson PM, *Normal haematological reference values in the adult black population of the Witwatersrand.* S Afr Med J, 1987. 72(2): p. 135-136.

[51] Ezeilo, G., *Non-genetic neutropenia in Africans.* . Lancet 1972. 300(7785): p. 1003-1005.

[52] Orfanakis NG, O.R., Bishop CR, Athens JW, *Normal blood leukocyte concentration values.* Am J Clin Pathol, 1970. 53: p. 647-651.

[53] Shaper AG, L.P., *Genetic neutropenia in people of African origin.* Lancet, 1971. 2: p. 1021–1023.

[54] Bain, B., *Ethnic and sex differences in the total and differential white cell count and platelet count.* Journal of Clinical Pathololoogy, 1996. 49: p. 664–666.

[55] Ezeilo, G., *The aetiology of neutropenia in healthy Africans.* East African Medical Journal, 1974. 51(12): p. 936-942.

[56] Cruickshank JM , A.M., *The Effect of Age, Sex, Parity, Haemoglobin Level, and Oral Contraceptive Preparations on the Normal Leucocyte Count* British Journal of Haematology, 1970. 18(5): p. 541–550.

[57] Kourtis AP, B.B., van der Horst C, Kazembe P, Ahmed Y, Chasela C, Knight R, Lugalia L, Tegha G, Joaki G, Jafali R, Jamieson D J, *Low Absolute Neutrophil Counts in African Infants.* Journal of the International Association of Physicians in AIDS Care, 2005. 4(3): p. 73-76.

[58] Shetty AK, C.H., Mirochnick MM, Maldonado Y, Mofenson LM, Eshleman SH, Fleming T, Emel L, George K, Katzenstein DA, Wells J, Maponga CC, Mwatha A, Jones SA, Abdool Karim SS, Bassett MT, *Safety and trough concentrations of nevirapine prophylaxis given daily, twice weekly, or weekly in breast-feeding infants from birth to 6 months.* journal of Acquired Immune Deficiency Syndrome, 2003. 34(5): p. 482-490.

[59] Wells J, S.A., Stranix L, Falkovitz-Halpern MS, Chipato T, Nyoni N, Mateta P, Maldonado Y, *Range of normal neutrophil counts in healthy zimbabwean infants: implications for monitoring antiretroviral drug toxicity.* J Acquir Immune Defic Syndr 2006. 42(4): p. 460-463.

[60] Englund JA, B.C., Raskino C, McKinney RE, Petrie B, Fowler MG, Pearson D, Gershon A, McSherry GD, Abrams EJ, Schliozberg J, Sullivan JL, *Zidovudine, didanosine, or both as the initial treatment for symptomatic HIV-infected children. AIDS Clinical Trials Group (ACTG) Study 152 Team.* New England Journal of Medicine, 1997. 336(24): p. 1704-1712.

[61] Urassa WK, M.E., Swai AB, Gaines H, Mhalu FS, Biberfeld G, *Lymphocyte subset enumeration in HIV seronegative and HIV-1 seropositive adults in Dar es Salaam, Tanzania: determination of reference values in males and females and comparison of two flow cytometric methods.* J Immunol Methods, 2003. 277: p. 65–74.

[62] Bussmann H, W.C., Masupu KV, Peter T, Gaolekwe SM, Kim S, Reich AM, Ahn S, Wu Y, Thior I, Essex M, Marlink R, *Low CD4+ T-lymphocyte values in human immunodeficiency virus-negative adults in Botswana.* Clin Diagn Lab Immunol, 2004. 11(5): p. 930-935.

[63] Abbassi-Ghanavati M, G.L., Cunningham FG, *Pregnancy and laboratory studies: A reference table for clinicians.* Obstetrics and gynecology, 2009. 114(6): p. 1326-1336.

[64] Larsson A, P.M., Hansson L-O, Axelsson O, *Reference values for clinical chemistry tests during normal pregnancy.* Obstretics and Gynaecology, 2008. 115(7): p. 874-881.

[65] Belo L, S.-S.A., Rocha S, Caslake M, Cooney J, Pereira-Leite L, Quintanilha A, Rebelo I, *Fluctuations in C-reactive protein concentration and neutrophil activation during normal pregnancy.* European Journal of Obstetrics & Gynecology and Reproductive Biology, 2005. 123: p. 46–51.

[66] Lurie S, R.E., Piper I, Golan A, Sadan O, *Total and differential leukocyte counts percentiles in normal pregnancy.* Eur J Obstet Gynecol Reprod Biol, 2008. 136: p. 16–19.

Chapter 16

Principles of Blood Transfusion

Nuri Mamak and İsmail Aytekin

Additional information is available at the end of the chapter

http://dx.doi.org/10.5772/48332

1. Introduction

The aim of this chapter is to present a revised overview of small and large animal transfusion medicine based on a review of the veterinary literature. Blood transfusion has become more performable in small and large animal practice. By donor selection and the availability of blood component substitutes, usage of the blood products improved. The use of blood component therapy safely needed knowledge of blood groups, antibody prevalence and the impact of blood groups on veterinary transfusion medicine. Animal blood transfusions antibodies against blood group antigens also play a role. In addition knowledge of the means to decrease the risk of adverse reactions by using proper donors and screening assays that simplify detection of serological incompatibility is important. The clinical significance of blood group antigens in veterinary medicine is generally in the areas of transfusion reactions and neonatal isoerythrolysis (NI). This chapter includes an update on canine and feline, horse, donkey, cattle, sheep, gaot, pig, llama and alpaca blood groups and known blood incompatibilities, donor selection and blood collection, storage of blood components, available equine blood products and indications for transfusion, whole blood (WB) and blood product transfusion in ruminants and camelids, blood component and blood substitute therapy, administration, and adverse reactions in small and large animal blood transfusion.

2. Blood types in dogs and cats

Blood types are classified according to specific antigens on the surface of erythrocytes. Platelets, leukocytes, and body tissues and fluids may also consists of erytrocyte antigens. [1]. In immunogenicity and clinical significance these antigens can differ. They can serve as markers of disease in some cases and taking part in recognition of self. The clinical significance of blood group antigens is generally noted in transfusion reactions and neonatal isoerythrolysis (NI) in veterinary medicine [2]. These antigens can characteristically trigger a reaction caused by circulating anti-erythrocyte antibodies in the opposite host or donor.

These antibodies can occur naturally. Also they can be induced by a previous transfusion. Interaction leads to the destruction by hemolysis of red blood cells (RBCs). This is one of the severe and potentially life-threatening situation. [3].

The dog erytrocyte antigen types or blood types are categorized by the DEA (Dog Erythrocyte Antigen) system. DEA 1.1, 1.2, and 1.3 are termed A system. There are also DEA 3, DEA 4, DEA 5, DEA 6, DEA 7 and DEA 8. [2]. In the United States the incidence of DEA 1.1 is approximately 45% and DEA 1.2 is 20% [4]. DEA 1.3 is common in German shepherd dogs and has been reported only in Australia [5]. Frequency of DEA 1.1 in Kangal Dog was found as 61.1% in Turkey [6]. In Croatia where the closest data studied the rate was 66.7% [7]. The rate was also 56.9% in Portugal [8] and 55% in Japan [9]. Approximately 60 % of the canine population is in DEAs 1.1 and 1.2 group. DEA 1.1 is the strongest antigen in the dog. Two membrane proteins of 50 and 200 kD has been identified by a monoclonal antibody to DEA 1.1 using immunoprecipitation techniques. [10]. Presenting in a single band DEA 1.2 has been found to be an 85-kD protein [11].

DEA 1.1 is the most antigenic group in respect to transfusion medicine. Little is investigated about DEA 3, 4, 5 and 7 in comparison to DEA 1.1. In literature, the frequency of DEA 3 is lower in comparison to DEA 1.1 blood type. In the United States it is determined that approximately 6% of the general dog population is DEA 3 positive [12]. This rate is reported as 13% in Brazil [13]. In Turkey, DEA 3 is most found blood type in the Kangal Dog [6]. In the canine blood groups DEA 4 is the most common type. In USA, it is indicated that overall 98% of the general dog population have DEA 4 blood [12]. In Brazil, all dogs blood type were positive for DEA 4 [13]. The molecular weight of DEA 4 present in a single band has been found to be 32 to 40 kD using immunoprecipitation techniques [11].

In the United States typing sera can be commercially obtained only for DEA 1.1, 1.2, 3, 4, 5, and 7 [4]. In Brazil a report studied on German shepherd dogs determined that 14% of the dogs were positive for DEA 5 and 8% were positive for DEA 7 [13]. The frequency of DEA 5 and 7 positive dogs was 55.5% and 71.7% respectively in Turkey [6]. Also, DEA 7 may cause an antibody response in dogs that lack it. A system of nomenclature about antigen Tr has described. The Tr antigen system is a 3-phenotype, 6-genotype system [14]. The molecular weight of DEA 7 present in 3 distinct bands has been found to be 53, 58, and 63 kD by using immunoprecipitation techniques [11].

An exact definition of a canine universal donor is not agreed among veterinary transfusion experts. Well excepted description of the universal donor is that a dog negative for DEA 1.1, 1.2, DEA 3, DEA 5, DEA 7, and positive for DEA 4. It is difficult to find DEA 4 negative dog because 98% of all dogs are positive for DEA 4. Thus there is a very little chance to influence donor selection. If the dog is DEA 7 positive, some other experts do not exclude it from the donor pool [15]. In most populations the incidence of DEA 4 blood type is more than 98% [16]. Because of this in transfusion medicine these dogs are the best candidate for being a donor. If other donors are known to be compatible with the recipient they can also be utilized [17]. DEA 3, 5 and 7 negative dogs have naturally occurring antibodies to DEA 3, 5 and 7 positive red cells. However during the first transfusion these blood groups do not possess a major transfusion reaction [4]. In Turkey, the most common blood types were DEA 1.1, 4 and 7. Because all Kangal dogs have DEA 4 positivity it does not seem to be important in respect to transfusion medicine. The prevalence and antigenic properties of DEA 1.1 and 7 are significantly important. If unmatched transfusion is performed in Turkish Kangal dogs they can constitute acute hemolytic transfusion reactions [6]. Dogs with DEA 1.1 or 1.2 are called group A positive. Adversely, dogs do not have DEA 1.1 or 1.2 are called group A negative [1].

A blood group system described as N-acetylneuraminic acid and N-glycolylneuraminic acid present on gangliosides (hematosides) of the RBC membrane in Japan [18]. It is referred as the D system. This system is consist of two antigens, D1 and D2, with phenotypes, D1, D2, and D1D2. The D1 and D2 antigens are codominanat factors. Anti-D1 is identical to anti-DEA3. The importance of this system in transfusion medicine pointed out by transfusion of D2 type blood into a D1 type patient, or of D1 type blood into a D2 type patient consistently cause severe acute transfusion reactions [19, 20]. RBCs of some dogs designated as type C at titre sup to 128 are aglutinated rather than lectin extracted from seeds of Clerodendron tricotomum. Type C is completely negative for other dogs. C system was compared to the DEA system and determined to be different [10, 19, 21]. Specific IgG alloantibodies in previously sensitized Dalmatian dog by blood transfusion is described as the Dal blood type. The frequency is not known. Typing sera for this antigen also is commercially not available [2, 22, 23].

Three blood types are described in the feline AB blood group system and mik group system. In cats a new blood group defined as Mik. It is named after the alloantibody identified in the first blood donor cat, Mike. In three cats that had not previously received transfusions Mik antibodies were detected. They are defined as a cause of incompatibilities between donor and recipient blood that are not related to the AB blood group system [24].

The phenotypes type A, type B, and type AB are occured. A null phenotype is not exist. The most common blood type is Type A. Type B is less common. Type AB is rare [2, 25]. Type B is indicated in Australia (26.3%), and Greece (20.3%) ([26] , [27]). In large studies of both pedigree and non-pedigree cats in the USA distribution of type AB cats is demonstrated to be rare (0.14%) ([28]). Type AB were 0.4% in Australia (([26]). In Scotland the incidence of AB cats is 4.4% ([29]).

Type B is indicated in Australia (26.3%), and Greece (20.3%) ([26, 27]. In large studies of both pedigree and non-pedigree cats in the USA distribution of type AB cats is demonstrated to be rare (0.14%) [28]. Type AB were 0.4% in Australia [26]. In Scotland the incidence of AB cats is 4.4% [29].

In Turkey, 60 % of Van cats and 46.4 % of Angora cats are type B [30]. And 220 (73.1%) nonpedigree domestic cats had type A blood, 74 (24.6%) had type B and seven (2.3%) had type AB [31] in Turkey. Except type AB group, cats have naturally occurring alloantibodies. It is known that cats have naturally occurring alloantibodies (isoantibodies) against the blood type they are lacking. Because of this to prevent blood incompatibility reactions in cats feline blood typing is important in clinical practice. Blood type incompatibility can especially result in two fatal reactions. The first is acute haemolytic transfusion reactions, occur particularly in cat transfused with type A blood [32]. Feline neonatal isoerythrolysis (NI) is the second incompatibility reaction. It occurs when type A or AB kittens born to type B queens are nursing. Naturally occurring anti-A alloantibodies result in blood incompatibility reaction in the type B queen's colostrum and milk [25, 30].

Cats constitute non-self antibodies in contrast to dogs. As a result of this non-self antibodies potentially fatal antibody-mediated reactions can occur towards non-self red blood cells. Nearly 20% of type A cats have anti-B antibodies. These antibodies are usually weak. All type B cats have strong anti-A antibodies. In contrast AB cats do not have alloantibodies [32]. In previously unsensitized cats naturally occuring isoantibodies are responsible for transfusion reactions. Nearly all type B cats have highly titered anti-A agglutinins and hemolysins. RBCs can be destructed rapidly in type B cats taking type A blood. In type B cats the high titres of naturally occurring anti-A antibodies cause rapid intravascular destruction of transfused type A red blood cells [33]. This can be mediated by IgM, complement fixation and the release of potent vasoactive compounds. As a result of this shock can develop usually due to possessed antibodies towards the transfused RBCs [3, 34]. This can cause severe transfusion reaction and death even if as little as 1 ml of type A blood is administered to a type B-cat [2, 35]. Because of their endotheliochorial placenta newborn kittens have no alloantibodies. Nevertheless colostral transfer of immunoglobulin (Ig) G and a small amount of IgM occurs. Neonatal isoerythrolysis develops in cats. It is one of the cause of the fading kitten syndrome. Kittens that are type A or AB and those that are born to type B queens are at risk. In affected kittens Clinical sings can range from unapparent, to severe hemolytic anemia with hemoglobinuria, icterus, and death [1, 36, 37, 38].

3. Transfusion therapy

Packed red blood cells (pRBCs) and fresh frozen plasma (FFP) are components generally provided for canine transfusions. If processed at once, 1-4 each unit (450 mL) of whole blood can be seperated into 1 unit of pRBCs and 1 unit of FFP. It is difficult to prepare components from a small volume of blood. Because of this cat blood transfusions are usually administered as fresh or stored whole blood. If patients requires specific components like pRBCs and FFP, in this case whole blood can be separated into them [39].

In veterinary medicine, red blood cell transfusions are used more frequent recently. They are the integral part of lifesaving. They are used in critically ill as advanced treatment. Situations required transfusions include life-threatening anemia from acute hemorrhage or surgical blood loss, hemolysis from drugs or toxins, immune-mediated diseases, severe nonregenerative conditions, and neonatal isoerythrolysis [40].

Indications of red blood cell transfusions are in the treatment of anemia caused by hemorrhage, hemolysis, or ineffective erythropoiesis. Oxygen is poorly soluble in plasma. Because of this oxygen in blood is mostly carried by hemoglobin (Hgb). In anemic patient, RBC transfusions increase the oxygen-carrying capacity. Therefore inadequate delivery of oxygen to tissues with consequent tissue hypoxia are prevented or treated [41].

The treatment of severe anemia caused by hemorrhage, hemolysis, ineffective erythropoiesis, auto-immune hemolytic anemia, or neoplasia is primary indication for blood transfusion. Lethargy and altered mentation, increased respiratory effort, pale mucous membranes and tachycardia are the clinical signs of anaemia. The body carry out a number of adaptive responses physiologically, to maintain carrying of oxygen to the tissues [42, 43]. The solution of oxygen in plasma is weak. Because of this hemoglobin (Hgb) carries approximately whole oxygen in blood [41]. The decision to conduct a RBC transfusion is generally based on a measurement of the patient's packed cell volume (PCV), hematocrit (Hct) or Hgb concentration (Hgb) and especially on clinical evaluation of the patient [41]. Clinically animals should be evaluated individually. Generally when the hematocrit is less than 10%, the treatment of anemia is transfusion. However, animals with acute-onset anemia usually require transfusion before their hematocrit decreases to 15%. This contrasts with the situation in animals with chronic anemia. Other indications for transfusion are hypovolemia, thrombocytopenia, clotting factor deficiency, and hypoproteinemia [1]. Electrocardiographic signs of myocardial ischaemia are similar to those identified in human patients with myocardial infarction. It can ocur with anemia [44].

The usage of administration of FFP are for the treatment of a single or multiple clotting factor deficiency, vitamin K deficiency or antagonism, surgical bleeding or where a massive transfusion is required [45]. Hypoalbuminaemia and coagulopathies especially due to liver disease are the main reported indications for FFP transfusions in cats [46].

Stored blood is more than 8 hours old. The length of storage depends on the anticoagulant/preservative solution used. It varies from 48 hours for 3.8% sodium citrate (no preservative) to 4 weeks for CPD-A1 (citrate, phosphate, dextrose, and adenine). Acid citrate dextrose (ACD), citrate phosphate dextrose (CPD and CP2D), and citrate phosphatedextrose-adenine (CPDA-1) are mostly used as preservatives. The viability of RBCs is provided by the added dextrose, phosphate, and adenine. Due to the preservative used, the storage can extend up to 3 to 5 week ([3, 41, 47].

In patients that are hypothermic or receiving large volumes of blood, refrigerated RBC products should be prewarmed to temperatures between 22°C and 37°C immediately before transfusion. In the routine practice of RBC products to normovolemic anemic patients, refrigerated blood components do not need warming before transfusion. Warming may accelerate the deterioration of stored RBCs and may cause rapid growth of contaminating microorganisms [48].

In clinical practice advances in safety of blood transfusion is important in preventing transfusion-transmitted infections (TTI). The most frequent severe infectious outcome of transfusion has been known as bacterial contamination of platelets, with resultant sepsis in the recipient recently. Using automated or semi-automated blood culture devices, apheresis platelets and prestorage pooled platelets are most often tested [49].

Generally, before a blood transfusion is given to animals, blood typing and/or cross-matching of the recipent and donor should be done to avoid the likelihood of a transfusion reaction. Also, ineffective therapy is caused by shortened survival of transfused mismatched red cells. In order to prevent primary sensitization and risk of developing hemolytic disease in breeding females, cross-matching and/or blood typing is important. In general veterinary practise, blood typing for canine DEA 1.1 and for feline types A and B is applied [1].

To decrease adverse reactions one sould pay attention to blood typing and crossmatching procedures as much as monitoring. There is always risk in blood transfusions. For this reason, they should be performed only when warranted. When taking history, previous transfusion therapy should be asked and in a history of previous transfusion therapy cross-matching is necessary [1, 50].

Depending on availability and indication for transfusion, whole-blood or blood-component therapy may be administered. RBCs, white blood cells (WBCs), platelets, all the coagulation factors, albumin and immunoglobulins constitute whole blood (WB) [51].

In cats, fresh whole blood is the most common product used recently. Stored whole blood, packed red blood cells and fresh frozen plasma (FFP) are also given as transfusions [45].

The heavier cellular elements from the supernatant plasma are sedimented by centrifugation of whole blood sediments. Due to separation of blood collection within 8 hours all protein activity and concentration are maintained in the plasma. The obtained supernatant usually frozen. For subsequent transfusion, it is stored as fresh frozen plasma (FFP). In addition it can also processed to provide cryoprecipitate and cryosupernatant. It can also be transfused immediately as fresh plasma [52, 53]. Fresh frozen plasma have to be stored frozen at -30°C before used. Also it should be identified with the donor blood type, name and collection date. Samples thawed and not used sould discarded or stored in a fridge and used within 12-24 h and should not be refrozen [43].

Recently an ultra-purified polymerised bovine haemoglobin solution is the only commercially available alternative to red cell transfusion (Oxyglobin). It is not licensed in cats but it has been used in treatment of anaemia in cats and also in therapy of carbon monoxide poisoning [54, 55].

Hemostatic protein deficiencies lead to hemorrhagic disorders and the treatment is done principally by plasma components [56]. In animals with von Willebrand disease (vWD) and hereditary coagulation factor deficiencies active hemorrhage is controlled by plasma components. Plasma components are also used for preoperative prophylaxis in these diseases [53].

For preparation of plasma components sterile plastic bags are used. After that they are stored and transferred as frozen in individual boxes. Products have to be stored at -20°C or lower. Just before transfusion they warmed to 37°C in a water bath or incubator. Preferred route of administration is the intravenous transfusion of plasma components. If attempts at vascular access have failed, intraosseous transfusion can be used in emergency situations. When acut allergic reactions occur transfusion is stopped and antihistamines and/or short-acting steroids are given [53, 57].

Cats have antibodies to non-self blood types within the plasma. Because of this only type-specific plasma should be administered to cats in contrast to dogs. Using one of the commercially available systems whole blood can be separated into FFP and packed red cells if it is taken aseptically. The blood spun at 3800 rpm at 10°C in a refrigerated centrifuge for 12 mins. Using a plasma extractor the plasma is extracted and stored at –20°C [57].

In hypoalbuminemic dogs and cats, human serum albumin has been used for therapeutic use [58].

3.1. Platelet transfusion

Correction of coagulation by fresh platelets are shown by in vitro coagulation studies. Freshly collected platelets correct thrombocytopenia, control associated hemorrhage, and prevent death from bleeding. Hemorrhagic diathesis are prevented by platelet replacement for thrombocytopenia [59].

Severe thrombocytopenia or thrombopathia result in bleeding. Platelet transfusion is used for the control of this bleeding. In veterinary medicine platelet transfusion has been used rarely compared to red blood cell (RBC) and plasma transfusion. In dogs, reports related to platelet transfusion are generally associated with experimental hematopoietic stem cell transplantation. Platelet-rich blood products consist of fresh whole blood (FWB), platelet-rich plasma (PRP) and platelet concentrate (PC). They are used for aggressive anticancer therapy and treating complex hematologic disorders. Centrifugation of whole blood constitute platelet-rich plasma (PRP) and centrifugation of platelet-rich plasma constitude platelet concentrates (PC). Platelet activation is induced by centrifugation so that the resuspension of the platelet pellet during PC preparation from dogs is difficult. The preparation efficiency of PC from dogs can be improved by addition of PGE1 in PRP before the centrifugation of PRP. Also therapeutic efficacy of the platelets are maintained. In 10-28 kg body weight dogs plateletpheresis has been used successfully. On the canine donor thrombocytopenia and hypocalcemia are the main adverse effects of plateletpheresis [60-62].

At room temperature (RT) (20-24°C), PRP and PC can be stored for 5-7 days with continuous or intermittent agitation. At RT FWB can be stored for up to 8 hours. The interest in freezed (4°C) storage of platelets is increasing because of the increased risk of bacterial proliferation at RT storage. Storage of human PRP and PC are limited to 5 days because of prevention of bacterial proliferation at room temperature [60- 63].

Platelet transfusions as with RBC and plasma components should be performed with 170 μm filters standard blood administration sets. Transfusion sets which can bind platelets should be exempt from latex [60].

The most common reaction to PC are febrile reactions. The frequency is decreased by pre-storage leukoreduction. In immunocompetent dogs receiving multiple transfusions, alloimmunization to platelet antigens occurs. Leukocyte reduction and ultraviolet B irradiation are recently accepted methods for preventing the development of platelet alloimmunization [64-66].

Recently platelet cryopreservation are used to provide long-term storage and immediate availability of platelet products for transfusion. When fresh platelets are unavailable cryopreserved platelets can be activated in vitro and provide therapeutic benefit [63].

3.2. Granulocyte transfusion

Granulocyte transfusion can be used as supportive therapy. It is used in patients with life-threatening neutropenia caused by bone marrow failure or in patients with neutrophil dysfunction. Granulocyte transfusions is shown to be useful in treatment of infections in patients after treatment with high-dose chemotherapy. It is helpful especially in the chemotherapy associated with conditioning for hematopoietic stem cell transplant. By using granulocyte colony-stimulated factors higher doses of granulocytes for transfusion are produced. Thus recently the use of therapeutic granulocyte transfusion has been increased. The outcome of transfusion are effected by the type of infection being treated, the likelihood of recipient marrow recovery, and recipient alloimmunization [67].

In small animals therapeutic granulocyte transfusions have been used especially in experimental models of myelosuppression and neonatal sepsis. In clinical veterinary medicine they have been used rarely. Granulocytes can be used to identify the site of inflammation. Beside leukapheresis, centrifugation of FWB, with or without colloid-facilitated sedimentation, may be used to isolate canine and feline buffy coats. Only sedimentation may also be used in the cat. At RT granulocytes are stored immobil for 24 hours. The dose for beginning is 1×10^{11} granulocytes/kg in a volume of 15mL/kg. It is used once to twice in a day [68-70].

4. Donor selection

To select permanent blood donors, blood typing have to be performed. Donors should be healthy young adults. They undergo routine physical check up and hematology and clinical chemistry evaluations are done. They should never taken a blood transfusion and should be free of blood parasites and other infectious diseases [1].

Nulliparous and spayed female dog and cat donors have to be chosen. Blood have be collected via jugular venipuncture aseptically. Acepromazine interferes with platelet function. Because of this donors should not be sedated with it [1].

Every 3 to 4 weeks, dogs can donate between 13 and 17 ml of blood per kilogram of body weight. Features of donors sould include well nourished, supplemented with oral iron, bled less than once per month to prevent iron deficiency, greater than 25 kg, and negative for antigens for DEAs 1.1, 1.2, 3, 5, and 7. Donors should not have heartworm disease, babesiosis, brucellosis, ehrlichiosis, and Rocky Mountain spotted fever. Donors have appropriate neck skin that allows easy entrance to the jugular vein, have a packed cell volume that is at least 0.40 L/L, have demonstrated a good temperament and be in good physical condition, have no past time history of transfusion or pregnancy, and have got sufficient levels of von Willebrand factor (vWF) [1, 3].

The ideal feline blood donors should be healthy, indoor-only cats with an agreeable temperament for easy handling and restraint. Owned pet cats should be donate maximum once every 2 months [43]. The features of feline donor sould be as follows; weigh more than 4.5 kg, have a packed cell volume that is at least 0.35 L/L, have demonstrated a good temperament, and be in good physical condition [3]. Donor cats can donate between 10 and 12 ml/kg. Adult healthy cats can donate 50 ml every weeks. Donors have to be type A. Type B donors may be demanded depending on breed prevalence and geography. Feline leukemia virus, feline immunodeficiency virus (FIV), feline infectious peritonitis, heartworm disease, and Hemobartonella sp have to be excluded in donor cats [1].

For appropriate care of donors some processes needed. These are current vaccinations, if there is contact with new animals every 6 mo fecal floatation, monitorization of hemogram every year, analysing clinical chemistry, screening for infectious diseases and in the dog preventative heartworm therapy in areas where it is necessary. When blood collection is taken the donor's weight, temperature, and packed cell volume have to be analysed [3, 71]. PCV or Hb are measured by taking a blood sample. Preferentially cats with a PCV of 30–35% are used but cats with low–normal PCVs should not be used [43].

In the cat, blood can be taken by using a 19- to 20 gauge needle or butterfly into a syringe via jugular vein venipuncture. The region over the jugular vein is clipped and prepared aseptically and sedation is administered. It is prefered to use a 1:1 combination of ketamine 100 mg/ml and midazolam 5 mg/ml. It is made up in a small syringe and given intravenously up to a maximum dose of 5 mg/kg ketamine (0.1 ml/kg of combination). Syringe consists of either ACD, CPD, or CPDA- 1 (1 mL/9 mL of blood), or heparin (5 units/mL of blood). Before a preservative solution is used it can be placed in a small blood bag. To access the jugular vein a 19-21G butterfly needle is used. The blood is collected over a total of 10 15 mins. At once a maximum of 10-12 ml/kg blood can be donated. Isotonic crystalloid fluid therapy post-donation at a rate of 60 ml/h for 3 h is given to the cat [3, 43].

5. Administration

Precaution is necessary to prevent damage of the blood product and harm to recipient. Blood typing or crossmatching have to be carried out to provide compatibility before RBC transfusion [41].

Transfusions of red blood cell should be administered through a filter. The filter is arranged to remove clots and particles which are potentially harmful to the patient. Blood infusion sets have in-line filters. These filters trap large cells, cellular debris, and coagulated proteins. The pore size range from 170μm to 260μm. A filter may be used to administer 2-4 units of blood to a patient or for a maximum time limit of 4 hours according to human blood banking standards. High protein concentration at the filter surface and room temperature conditions promote proliferation of any contaminating microorganisms. The rate of flow slowed down by accumulated material. After 5 days or more of refrigerated storage constituted microaggregates composed of degenerating platelets, white blood cells (WBCs), and fibrin strands in blood. They are removed by other blood filters with a pore size of 20-40

Jim. For transfusions of RBCs primarily microaggregate filters are designed. In administering small volumes of blood (<50 mL WB or <25mL pRBCs) to cats and small dogs a pediatric micro-aggregate blood filter (18 um pore size, priming space <lmL) is especially helpful. Because of a progressive decrease in pore size due to increased blood filtered larger volumes of blood administration can result in hemolysis [41].

If plasma is taken from blood preservative solutions can be put in. Blood preservative solutions are dextrose, adenine, mannitol, and the sodium chloride. They are necessary for RBCs to carry on their energy metabolism and viability during storage [3]. Canine pRBCs stored in a RBC preservative can be applied directly. Other pRBC products have to be diluted by putting 10mL of saline feline pRBCs or 100mL of saline to the blood bag so that the viscosity of the donor blood decreased [41].

In the dog, if sedation is needed, butorphanol (0.1 mg/kg BW, IV) is generally used for sedation. But acepromazine should not be used because it may cause platelet function disturbance [72]. In the cat, ketamin may be used 2 to 4 mg/kg BW, IV for sedation. In addition to ketamin is very successful when it is used together with 0.1 to 0.2 mg/kg BW diazepam [3]. Also combinations of ketamine hydrochloride, midazolam and butorphanol tartrate, or mask administration of sevoflurane can be used [73, 74].

Generally, intravenous administration is used for RBC transfusions. In addition intraosseous administration is a perfect alternative. Peripheral veins may be preferred to central veins because of an increased bleeding predisposition [41].

Blood is administered through administration sets containing 0.9% saline intravenously. Contraindications include hypotonic saline, 5% dextrose in water and lactated Ringer's solution. Cardiac arrest may be caused by injection of undiluted citrate containing anticoagulants [1].

Using a syringe driver or by hand the transfusion should begin slowly at 0.25 ml/kg/h. If no adverse affects are encountered after the first 30–60 mins of administration the rate can be increased. Due to the urgency of the requirement for whole blood and any underlying concurrent disease the rate of administration can vary [75].

With a PCV of 20%, dogs and cats with chronic anemia can be cardiovascularly stable [76]. Conversely in patients with an acute onset of anemia and continuing blood loss or hemolysis, transfusion to a higher PCV is necessary for stabilization. Generally administration of 2mL/kg of WB or lmL/ kg of pRBCs will increase the patient's PCV by 1% if there is no continuing hemorrhage or hemolysis [41].

Patient's overall condition determine the rate of blood administration. The maximum rate of transfusion is 10-20mL/ kg/h in normovolemic anemic patients, to avoid circulatory overload [41].

To provide blood volume again fluid therapy with crystalloids or colloids is necessary. If the patient's total blood volume do not decrease under 20% this is usually enough for losses. If losses are more than 20% whole blood or packed red cell transfusion is used. Between 20% and 50% of blood volume losses are treated by crystalloids and packed RBCs [3, 77].

Blood components like cryoprecipitate and platelet-rich plasma are used infrequently. Cryoprecipitate contains vWF, factors VIII, XIII, fibrinogen, and fibronectin. In vWF-deficient patients cryoprecipitate is recommended particularly when surgery is planned or patient affected by blood loss. Bleeding hemophilia A patients, or patients having hypo or dysfibrinogenemia are the other indications for choosing it [3, 78].

Sometimes platelet-rich plasma is used in veterinary practice. In small-sized animals it is more useful because in larger dogs it is difficult to gain enough volume and management of platelet count. An alternative to platelet-rich plasma are frozen platelet concentrates [79].

For expansion of plasma volume, different types of colloids as dextrans and hetastarch are used as alternatives to blood products. Altering hemostasis is one of the problems of dextrans and hetastarch. Oxyglobin is a hemoglobin-based oxygen carrier. It is approved for use in the dog in 1998. In emergency situations it is used instead of blood products when there is limited time for preparing it or performing compatibility testing [3, 80].

In clinical signs of anaemia and as a therapy for carbon monoxide poisoning oxyglobin is used in cats. Because it is a potent colloid (colloid osmotic pressure 43 mmHg), the main risk associated with administration is volume overload. In patients with normovolaemic anaemia conservative administration rates are needed such as as low as 0.2-0.4 ml/kg/h and to a maximum of 1 ml/kg/h. Careful monitorization of patients with paying particular attention to their heart and respiratory rate is recommended [81, 82].

A recent study described the clinical outcome in dogs experiencing massive transfusion. Also this study documented predictable changes in electrolytes and coagulation status. Massive transfusion is different from usual transfusions in terms of volume and rate of blood transfusion and blood components administered. Transfusion of a volume of whole blood or blood components has been described as massive transfusion. The administrated blood is greater than the patient's predicted blood volume within a 24-hour period or arranged as replacement of half the patient's predicted blood volume in 3 hours. In a study, massive transfusion receiving dogs were investigated and in this study the mean volumes of pRBCs was 66.5mL/kg and FFP was 22.2mL/kg. As a result of this mean plasma, RBC ratio was 1:3. After transfusion clinicopathologic changes consists of electrolytes disturbances, dilutional coagulopathy, ionized hypocalcemia and hypomagnesemia and progressive thrombocytopenia and prolongation of prothrombin and activated partial thromboplastin times [41, 83].

6. Preparations used for transfusions and blood transfusions indications

The gold standard approach is that the donor and recipient are cross-matched before administration. Administration is maintained mainly intravascular with the use of peripheral or centrally placed catheter. Also intraosseous catheters can be used to administer all blood products. It is useful in collapsed neonatal patients where vascular access is difficult [43, 75, 84].

In acute hemorrhage, anemia, decreased red cell mass, severe methaemoglobinaemia, paracetamol toxicity, chronic non-regenerative anaemia, coagulation disorders, and thrombocytopenia fresh whole blood is used [1, 45].

The reason of anaemia in cats requiring transfusion are haemorrhage and primary immune-mediated haemolytic anaemia. Hemorrhage is caused as a result of peri- or postoperative bleeding, trauma, gastrointestinal bleeding, abdominal neoplasia, primary immune-mediated thrombocytopenia and coagulopathies [85, 86, 87]. Also in a number of infectious diseases anaemia is reported such as especially feline immuno-deficiency virus (FIV) and feline leukaemia virus (FeLV) infections, and feline infectious peritonitis [88, 89]. Other infectious diseases which cause anemia are Ehrlichia species, Bartonella species, Haemoplasmas (Mycoplasma haemofelis, 'Candidatus Mycoplasma haemominutum' and 'Candidatus Mycoplasma turicensis'), Anaplasma phagocytophilum, Neorickettsia risticii, Cytauxzoon felis and Rickettsia felis have additionally been associated with anaemia [43, 90].

The indication of whole blood is in a patient whom needed several blood components or has acutely lost more than 50% of its total blood volume. When 50% of total blood volume is lost oxygen carrying capacity and oncotic activity should be recovered. In anemia, stored whole blood is used. For anemic animals packed erythrocytes especially those with volume overload are prefered. For tissue reoxygenation the transfusion of packed RBCs are used. They are also useful for normovolemic, anemic patient. Before administration, to dilute any potentially damaging antibodies these erythrocytes can be washed with saline. Refrigerated whole blood should be warmed to room temperature. Before administration it sould be gently agitated to resuspend the red blood cells. Infusion rate is limited by colder blood which has a higher viscosity [3, 41, 91].

The usage of transfusion of fresh-frozen or stored-frozen plasma (FFP) are as follows; lack of coagulation factors associated with hepatic insufficiency, disseminated intravascular coagulation (DIC), vitamin K deficiency, rodenticide toxicosis, liver insufficiency, biliary tract obstruction, sepsis/multiple organ dysfunction syndrome, pancreatitis, hypoalbuminemia, and DIC without associated laboratoryproven coagulopathy, malassimilation syndrome, chronic antibiotic use, a need for plasma volume expansion, or a massive blood loss within a few hours. Other It is also used in congenital or a hereditary deficiency in coagulation factors (i.e hemophilia A, B, or von Willebrand's disease and hypoproteinemia), [1, 3, 39]. Plasma (FP or FFP) is used especially in the emergency conditions like excessive protein loss such as enteropathy, nephropathy, exudative dermatitis or inadequate intake. It is not appropriate for using as long-term source of protein in these patients [3, 92]. In cats, reactions have not been reported following transfusions of FFP [46].

The collection and re-transfusion of the cat's own blood is called autotransfusion. It is a useful technique in an emergency situation. It can be obtained when animals bleed into body cavities. It should not be used if the blood is contaminated with urine, bacteria or bile. Blood is collected from the body cavity in a sterile manner. After that it re-transfused into the patient through an appropriate fitler. To prevent clotting anticoagulant like acid citrate dextrose should be included at a ratio of 1:7 [39, 43].

7. Transfusions reactions

The indication of transfusion reactions can be immunologic or nonimmunologic. They can be immediate or delayed. Antibodies to surface antigens of transfused erythrocytes cause immune-mediated hemolytic reactions. According to surface antigens canine blood is grouped. For six of these antigens typing is available. Except DEA 4, canine universal donor is negative for all dog erythrocyte antigens (DEAs). Universal donors should be examined. If other donors are known to be compatible with the recipient they can be also used. Acute hypersensitivities mediated by IgE antibodies are one of the possible immunologic reaction. The other can be leukocyte or platelet sensitivity caused by recipient antibodies to the donor's white cells or platelets. The mechanisms of nonimmunologic reactions are various. According to the specific reaction the type and severity of clinical signs vary [17] Adverse reaction occurs in 2 types. First one is immediate reaction and following transfusion it occurs within 1 to 2 h. Second is delayed reaction and it may begin within days, months, or years later [17]. Adverse reaction varies from mild (fever) to severe (death). Transfusion reactions can be acute or delayed. In animals receiving incompatible transfusions, acute intravascular hemolysis with hemoglobinemia and hemoglobinuria may be seen. Acute hemolytic reaction is the most serious transfusion reaction that can be prevented. It is an immunological reaction and it happens when circulating natural or acquired antibodies towards donor erythrocytic antigens are given. Hemoglobinuria, vasoconstriction, renal ischemia occur due to intravascular hemolysis. Intravascular hemolysis determine clinical signs. Disseminated intravascular coagulopathy (DIC) can be caused by release of thromboplastic substances. Secondary to the release of vasoactive substances, hypotension and shock can ocur. Also acute renal failure and death can develop. After transfusion a decrease in hematocrit between 2 days and 2 weeks resulted in suspicion of delayed hemolysis. As a result of extravascular hemolysis, hyperbilirubinemia and bilirubinuria may occur. In dogs clinical signs are as follows: fever, tachycardia or bradycardia, hypotension, dyspnea, cyanosis, excessive salivation, tearing, urination, defecation, vomiting, collapse, opisthotonos, cardiac arrest, hemoglobinemia, and hemoglobinuria. When an acute hemolytic reaction occured transfusion sould be interrupted at once and shock should be treated. Also blood product being used sould be checked out and the steps that led to the transfusion sould be examined [1, 3, 17, 93].

To detect transfusion reactions earlier requires careful evaluation of patient's behavior, vital signs, and perfusion before, during, and after a RBC transfusion. Pre- and post-transfusion measurement of PCV and total solids for example instantly and at 24 hours are needed. Also evaluation of the plasma and urine for the presence of Hgb is done [41].

In the dog the acute hemolytic reaction is rare because in this species naturally occurring anti-erythrocytic antibodies prevalence is low [3]. Alloantibodies against the common canine erythrocyte antigens 1.1 and 1.2 do not exist in dogs. As a result of this generally first transfusion can be safely given without regard for donor blood type. Thus the recipient can be sensitized to immunogenic antigens (i.e 1.1, 1.2, 7, and others). On first transfusion it can cause shortened survival times of the transfused cells. Subsequent predisposition to severe transfusion reaction can develop. DEA 1.1 which is the strongest antigen in dogs, leads to the most severe transfusion reaction [1]. In the second transfusion especially when DEA-1 type blood is applied twice to a DEA- 1-negative dog there is more risk [3].

In cats receiving typed or crossmatched transfusions low rates of transfusion reactions have been indicated. Transfusions with whole blood or packed red blood cells transfusion reactions were reported [45]. But transfusions with FFP no reactions have been reported in cats [46].

Initial or subsequent AB-mismatched transfusions in cats can cause acute hemolytic incompatibility reactions. Erythrocytes are destroyed immediately in cats because of alloantibodies. On the contrary in dogs, delayed transfusion reactions are more often occur. A type B transfusion to type A cat causes mild signs. In this situation shortened erythrocyte survival can occur. This causes ineffective therapy. Acute hemolytic transfusion reaction with massive intravascular hemolysis with serious clinical signs occurs in type A transfusion to a type B cat. These symptoms may occur even if it is the first transfusion. Type AB or A blood can be received by type AB cats safely [1, 94].

The transfusion should be stopped immediately if a transfusion reaction is suspected. The recipient sould be monitored continually for follow up. The most severe is acute haemolytic transfusion reactions developing as a result of naturally occurring alloantibodies [32].

Clinical signs are restlessness, vocalisation, tachypnoea, bradycardia, tachycardia, hypotension and hypertension. Pyrexia is seen frequently as a result of reactions to donor leukocytes, platelets and plasma proteins. As a result of binding by citrate, there is potential for hypocalcaemia when administering large volumes of blood products. Thus, if the patient is showing clinical signs of hypocalcaemia calcium should be measured [38, 43].

The next hour after transfusion nonhemolytic fever can ocur as adverse reactions. If contaminated blood products applied by mistake, fever may occur in an acute hemolytic reaction in association with septicemia. Vomiting or diarrhea can be seen after plasma administration. Rarely urticaria may cause trouble to patient. It can be treated with antihistamines, with or without glucocorticosteroids. If whole blood is administered with rapid administration of a large volume of blood component to normovolemic cats or small-sized dogs hypervolemia can be observed. Hypervolemia can result in pulmonary edema. Cough, tachypnea, dyspnea, or cyanosis can occur due to hypervolemia. Treatment can be done by stopping the transfusion, administering diuretics (furosemide) to reduce pulmonary edema, and providing oxygen support [3,72, 93].

The recipient should be carefully examined before the procedure. Its heart rate, respiratory rate, mucous membrane colour, capillary refill time and temperature sould be recorded. Also the PCV and total plasma protein should be recorded [43, 51] .

Delayed adverse transfusion reactions are consist of delayed hemolytic reaction, transmission of infectious disease, and posttransfusion purpura. Posttransfusion purpura has been reported in the dog. It is characterized by the appearance of severe thrombocytopenia in the week following a second transfusion. [3, 95, 96].

Anemia, regardless of underlying cause, is troublesome for clinicians in respect to stabilising and supporting the patient. The survival rate of all reasons for a transfusion is 84% in the first 24 h. It is 75% for blood loss anaemia and 49.6% for ineffective erythropoeisis at 10 days [43, 97].

8. Cross-Matching blood

The incompatibilities between the donor's red blood cells and recipient's plasma are identified by major cross-match. The incompatibilities between the donor's plasma and recipient's red blood cells is identified by a minor cross-match [43].

Cross-Matching usually is identified as either "major" or "minor" cross-matches. A major cross-match include putting patient serum into donor cells and determine the presence of agglutinating and/or hemolytic antibodies in the patient aganist the donor antigens. The principle of this test is hemolytic or agglutinating reaction. In this test the reagent or antibody reacts with the RBCs. Serological discordance between a candidate donor and the patient is identified by the crossmatching. It does not determine the blood group [3]. A positive in vitro reaction is caused by the presence of antibodies. In patients that had no antibodies at the time of transfusion, a mild reaction can be seen in 4 to 14 days after mismatched transfusions. When blood is transfused to a patient in which antibodies are already present, a severe reaction occurs. This antibody can be developed by either naturally occurring or as a result of a previous mismatched transfusion. Furthermore, high concentrations of antibodies can be caused by isosensitization from transplacental immunization. In dogs that have received transfusions before, a crossmatch should always be performed. A minor cross-match include putting donor serum into patient erythrocytes. This step is not necessary for the donor whom previously tested negative for antibodies. Transfusing packed or washed erythrocytes rather than whole blood can prevent administration of antibodies in donor blood against patient erythrocytes [1].

Before transfusion the reason of analysis with these methods are to prevent acute hemolytic reaction due to transfusion, to provide optimal lifetime of the transfused RBCs, to prevent next discordant blood transfusions and to prevent neonatal isoerythrolysis [3].

Because there are blood types that have not been described and it is not possible to type for Mik it is recommended that cross-matching is performed before any transfusion. If the recipient has received a transfusion before more than 4 days cross-matching should be performed [98].

9. Principles of blood transfusion in horses

Horses have eight RBC groups or systems: A, C, D, K, P, Q, U, and T. The first seven systems are recognized by the International Society of Animal Blood Grouping Research.

Blood-typing antiserum is not readily available for horses. Because of this to identify suitable donors equine blood-group testing can be performed by only few diagnostic laboratories. Over 30 different factors have been identified within these seven equine systems. Experimentally many more systems have been identified [99, 100]. Red cell antigens Ca, Aa, and Qa are play an important role in transfusion reactions and neonatal isoerythrolysis. There is no universal equine blood donor. Because of this to prevent inadvertent sensitization of brood mares against the two most common alloantigens (Aa and Qa) involved in neonatal isoerythrolysis, the preferred donor should be negative for factors Aa, Qa, and Ca [100, 101]. Aa and Qa alloantigens are most immunogenic, and most neonatal isoerythrolysis cases are associated with anti-Aa or Qa antibodies. The horse is clinically relevant for blood group incompatibilities. It is the only livestock species for this situation. Blood group antibodies can laed to transfusion reactions or NI and can be found in horses either ''naturally'' or as a result of a blood group incompatible pregnancy [2]. A donkey RBC antigen that has not been found in the horse has been identified, it is unique to the donkey and the mule [1].

In horses, requirement of blood transfusion include correction of anemia arising from acute blood loss secondary to trauma, surgical complications, ruptured uterine artery, guttural pouch mycosis, and neonatal isoerythrolysis [99, 102].

Generally, whole blood transfusions are applied to horses that have acute blood loss caused by trauma, surgery, or some other conditions like splenic rupture or uterine artery hemorrhage. The transfusion recovers blood volume and oxygen-carrying capacity in cases of blood loss. There is no certain indicative variables for the beginning of transfusion so that physical examination and clinicopathologic parameters should be used to make the transfusion decision. In cases of acute hemorrhage one sould remember that the packed cell volume (PCV) may be normal for up to 12 hours because of the time required for fluid redistribution and the effects of splenic contraction. As the horse is rehydrated with intravenous fluids, serial monitoring of PCV and total protein (TP) can estimate the amount of blood loss. The transfusion decision is made by suspection of large volume blood loss, together with tachycardia, tachypnea, pale mucous membranes, lethargy, and decreasing TP. During an acute bleeding episode when the PCV fall under 20%, blood transfusion is probably required. In acute severe cases, transfusion may be required before there is a significant fall in PCV. PVC shows the need for beginning of transfusion in chronic anemia better whereas in acute hemorrhage, with transfusions proposed for horses with demonstration of tissue hypoxia and a PCV less than 10-12% [103, 104].

Blood is collected and stored in glass bottles containing acid–citrate–dextrose (ACD). The method traditionally used for collecting blood from donor horses. Glass bottles containing ACD are easy and suitable for rapid vacuum blood draw. Because of this they are recommended for equine whole-blood collection. For equine whole blood the optimal storage method is commercial citrate–phosphate–dextrose with adenine (CPDA-1) bags [105, 106].

Packed RBCs (pRBCs) are specified for normovolemic anemia (i.e neonatal isoerythrolysis, erythropoietic failure, and chronic blood loss). Markers of tissue oxygenation, for example lactate and oxygen extraction are useful in chronic or hemolytic anemia cases. In horses, disseminated intravascular coagulation, clotting factor deficiency, hypoalbuminemia, decreased colloid oncotic pressure, and failure of transfer of passive immunity (FPT) are treated by plasma [104].

Colloid is usually used in patients with a total protein less than 4.0g/dL or serum albumin concentration less than 2.0g/dL. When there is oncotic pressure less than 14 mmHg, clinical symptoms like ventral edema, and conditions which increase microvascular permeability like sepsis are other indications for colloid usage [104].

According to plasma obtained by plasmapheresis and centrifugation preparations, plasma prepared by gravity sedimentation contains greater numbers of erythrocytes and leucocytes. The risk of a transfusion reaction can be increased by these cells. During storage leukocytes can degranulate and fragment and release pyrogens and proinflammatory substances [107, 108, 112].

Multiple hyperimmune plasma products are avaible with bacterial or viral specific antibodies. For the treatment of equine endotoxemia, the efficacy of E. coli (J5) and Salmonella tiyphiimiriuni hyperimmune plasma has proved to be useful in some reports; in contrast, there are some reports which disapprove the utility of such products. For the protection of R. equi, the use of Rhodococcus equi hyperimmune plasma has also been controversial. For treatment of specific disease additional plasma products like botulism antitoxin, West Nile virus antibody, and Streptococcus equi antibody are usable. In general equine practice plasma is administered to neonates to provide protective immunoglobulins. Protective immunoglobulins are used for treatment of failure of transfer of passive immunity or prophylaxis against Rhodococcus equi. Also, the albumin content of the plasma used as a colloid for circulatory volume support and in the treatment of protein-losing enteropathies. In horses heritable and acquired coagulopathies can occur. Specific coagulation factors are not available for supplementation. Also indications include coagulopathies, protein-losing nephropathy and protein loss through third spacing into a body cavity (occurring with peritonitis or pleuritis) [104, 109-113].

Fresh frozen plasma must be separated and frozen within 8 hours of blood collection. Then it can be colder at -18 °C and stored for up to 1 year. Frozen plasma is considered as plasma separated any time after 8 hours of blood storage [112, 114, 115].

9.1. Blood donor selection

Healthy, young gelding weighing at least 500 kg is the ideal equine blood donor. Donor horses should be performed current vaccinations. To prevent from equine infectious anemia donors should be tested each year. RBC antigens Aa and Qa are the most immunogenic antigens. Because of this in the ideal donor, the Aa and Qa alloantigens should be absent. There are breed-specific blood factor frequencies. Thus a donor of the same breed as the recipient, particularly when blood typing is absent may be preferable. Horses that have taken blood or plasma transfusions and mares that have had foals are not appropriate as donors. Because they have a higher risk of carrying RBC alloantibodies. Donkeys have a RBC antigen known as "donkey factor". Horses do not have this antigen. Thus donkeys or mules should not be used as donors for horses because horses can develop anti-donkey factor antibodies if transfusion takes place [1, 104, 116].

An immediate blood transfusion can be applied for the first time in an emergency situation with a very minor risk of serious transfusion reaction. Horses can develop alloantibodies within 1 week of transfusion. Thus blood typing and crossmatching are recommended before a second transfusion is given. A second blood transfusion may be given confidently without a blood crossmatch within 2-3 days of the first transfusion. Blood typing and alloantibody screening can be used for the transfusion needed patient to find the most suitable donor horse. Blood typing and antibody screening before initial transfusion are more important for horses. Because subsequent blood transfusions are anticipated and if sensitized to other blood group factors broodmares may produce foals with neonatal isoerythrolysis (NI). For detection of equine RBC antigens Ca and Aa, a rapid agglutination method has been developed. It can be more suitable for pretransfusion testing [99, 103, 104].

9.2. Collection techniques

Blood is collected from the jugular vein of the donor horse. For this purpose two way used; direct needle cannulation or catheteri-zation. When a large volume of blood is required, a 10 or 12 gauge catheter is recommended. A 14 gauge catheter is also sufficient. Plastic bags and vacum-collection glass bottles in sizes ranging from 450 mL to 2 L are suitable for blood accumulation. Anticoagulation with 3.2% sodium citrate is enough when blood is received for immediate transfusion. In saline-adenine-glucose-mannitol solution red blood cell concentrates stored and they can be used for transfusion for up to 35 days after blood accumulation. Equine blood storage condition resemble to canine and human blood storage condition. According to both in vitro tests and human parameters after 35 days of storage equine erythrocytes remain appropriate for transfusion. Fresh frozen plasma is obtained by separation of erythrocytes and plasma. Both of them can be used alone. RBC survival evaluation sould be doen in vivo [104, 117].

To allow separation of red blood cells by gravity sedimentation the blood is stored in a refrigerator at 5 °C for 48 hours in an upright position. Then the plasma is decanted into a sterile 3-L bag with sterile plastic connecting tubing using gravity. 3-L bags containes a constant weight of plasma (3.4 kg). The red cell fraction is thrown out. The plasma bags are sealed, labeled with the horse's name and the date of decantation. They are stored at -20 °C until needed for plasma transfusion [112, 118].

9.3. Administration

In acute blood loss cases, PCV is usually impractical for estimation of volume to be transfused because it does not exactly indicate blood loss. Instead of this the volume of blood needed are predicted by estimation of blood loss and evaluation of clinical parameters. Fluid shifts will replace much of the circulating volume so between 25% and 50% of the total blood lost should be replaced by transfusion. Pay attention sould be give to that up to 75% of RBCs lost into a body cavity like hemoperitoneum are within 24-72 hours autotransfused back into circulation. Thus in cases of intracavitary hemorrhage lower percentages of blood volume replacement can be needed. To remove small clots and fibrin blood and plasma products should be given with an in-line filter [104, 119].

9.4. Adverse reactions

Blood should be given at a rate of approximately 0.3mL/ kg over the first 10-20 minutes for monitoring the transfusion reactions. Heart rate, body temperature, and respiratory rate sould be monitored. Additionally horses have to be monitored for signs of muscle fasciculation, piloerection, and urticaria. Urticaria, hemolysis, pruritis, edema, tachycardia, tachypnea, pyrexia, colic, changes in mentation and acute anaphylactic reactions are adverse reactions indicated in horses taking blood transfusions. The rate of adverse reaction to WB transfusion has been reported as 16% which are mild urticarial reactions and worsening hemolysis. Also 1 of 44 horses (2%) exhibit a fatal anaphylactic reaction [103, 113].

Transfusion reactions may vary from mild urticarial reactions to anaphylaxis. They are divided into immunogenic and nonimmunogenic reactions. Immunogenic reactions include anaphylaxis, hemolysis, fever, hives, acute lung injury, posttransfusion purpura, immunosuppression, and neonatal isoerythrolysis. Nonimmunogenic reactions include circulatory overload, bacterial contamination, citrate toxicity, coagulopathy, hyperammonemia, and transmission of disease. In horses that have received fresh frozen plasma serum hepatitis has been observed [52, 93, 112, 120].

In a second plasma or blood transfusion there exists risk for severe adverse reactions in dogs. Also there is a risk of development of neonatal isoerythrolysis in gravid mares. The risk is much more in whole blood transfusions [26, 33, 112].

In horses suffered from normovolemic anemia polymerized ultrapurified bovine hemoglobin (PUBH) improves hemodynamics and oxygen transport parameters. During infusion to be informed about any adverse reactions patients should be monitored closely. Intense pruritus, tachycardia, and tachypnea can be resolved shortly after stopping the infusion [121].

10. Principles of and indications for blood transfusion in ruminants and camelids

Eleven blood groups have been classified in cattle. The greatest clinical relevance is in groups B and J. The B group is extremely complex, thus closely matched transfusions are very difficult. Newborn calves do not have the J antigen. During the first six months of life they generally acquire it. Cows can be sensitized to erythrocyte antigens by vaccinations of blood origin like some anaplasmosis and babesiosis vaccines. As a result of this neonatal isoerythrolysis in subsequent calves occur. [1].

Seven blood groups have been classified in sheep. The B group in these animals is resemble to the B group in cattle, and the R group is resemble to the J group in cattle. For example, antigens are soluble and soluble antigens passively absorbed to erythrocytes. In the goat, five blood groups are identified which resemble to those of sheep [1].

Blood group A–O expression is affected by 16 porcine blood groups and the S gene. Carbohydrate antigens like AO blood group antigens and minor histocompatibility antigens can be important targets for the immune response to transplanted organs or tissues. These antigens remain an unknown and untested variable in many transplant studies using pigs. Depending, on work performed in some Europian country pig blood groups developed and expanded largely. The source of blood typing reagents is especially from isoimmune sera. Most antibodies behave as agglutinins and a few as hemolysins. Internationally sixteen genetic systems are recognized [2, 122-124].

In two domestic South American camelids, Ilama and alpaca, our knowledge is little about group variation. Six blood groups factors were identified (e.g A, B, C, D, E and F) . from iso- and heteroimmune sera constituted for these animals [2].

In ruminants and camelids indications for WB and plasma transfusion are similar to horses. Chronic anemia may be a more common problem in ruminants. Gastrointestinal parasites, particularly Haemonchus contains, and ectoparasites (e.g. Haematopinus spp. and Linognathus spp.) are causes of chronic blood loss anemia, and iron-deficiency anemia. These can affect neonatal calves [104, 121, 125].

Studies with camelids and bovines has showed that the neonatal intestine can only successfully absorb colostral immunoglobulins for 12–24 hours postpartum. Passive transfer (FPT) is failed in 19% to 24% of neonatal camelids. A common indication for plasma transfusion in neonatal calves and crias is failure of transfer of passive immunity. Hyperimmune serum products are existing for subcutaneous and intramuscular dosing in ruminants. These are products with antibodies against E. coli, Pasturella, Aercanobacter pyogenes, Salmonella typhimurium and Clostridium [104, 126-129].

An integral component of neonatal camelid care is IV plasma transfusion. It is used for the purpose of antibody supplementation and fluid resuscitation in critical illness. Neonates are immunocompetent at birth but due to initial postpartum absorption of colostrum for passive acquisition of immunoglobulins (especially IgG) they are severely hypogammaglobulinemic [130, 131].

In cattle, the first blood transfusion should usually be safe, regardless of the donor. J-negative donor is ideal. Because agglutination reactions do not develop, routine crossmatching is not useful in ruminants. First transfusions are usually safe to apply without a blood cross-match but crossmatching is recommended when more than 48-72 hours have passed away since the first blood transfusion. Blood donors should not have disease like bovine leukosis virus, anaplasmosis, and bovine viral diarrhea virus [104].

Total blood volume estimated in cattle is 80 mL/kg. From the donor animal up to 20-25% of total blood volume can be removed. Usually needle cannulation or jugular catheterization used in this situation. Blood can be collected into bottles or bags using citrate anticoagulant (e.g CPDA-1) in equine transfusions [104].

Blood samples can be taken from the jugular vein in sheep. A 500 ml transfer bag system including a needle can use for the storage. These bags include 70 ml of CPDA-1-stabiliser. Then the blood should be put into four 150 ml transfer bags. These bags can be stored on a horizontal shaker. It shows the best preservation of platelet function. Also it can be used for the storage experiment consecutively [132].

Platelet count and aggregability of CPDA-1-stabilised ovine blood is kept most covenient at room temperature. It provides adequate haemostatic function for ex vivo experiments for one working day. In ovine blood functional loss and high percentage of platelets within aggregates can be observed at refrigerator temperature. This should be considered in blood transfusion in sheep [132].

10.1. Administration and adverse reactions

In order to monitor transfusion reactions blood should first be transported slowly. Ruminant blood type discordance result in primarily complement-mediated hemolysis. Volume overload should not be given. Also in neonates and small ruminants volume should carefully be given [104].

Intestinal absorption of antibodies declines sharply within the first 24 hours postpartum. For treatment of crias with failure of passive transfer (FPT) IV or intraperitoneal administration of 20–40 mL/kg of camelid plasma is recommended. In compromised neonates requiring fluid resuscitation IV administration of plasma is generally preferred. It is used for the correction of FPT and colloid support. In foals during extensive plasma volume expansion careful monitoring is needed to prevent cardiopulmonary complications. Following IV plasma administration the cardiovascular and pulmonary effects of plasma volume expansion have not been specifically worked out in camelids. But in several species (i.e sheep and cat) plasma volume overexpansion depending on excessive IV fluid administration has been associated with reduced lung function and pulmonary edema formation in clinical and experimental settings. In addition according to measures in presumed hypovolemic human patients administration of colloids can induce a greater reduction in lung function than crystalloids [130, 133-137].

Measurable plasma volume expansion and a concurrent reduction in pulmonary functional residual capacity (FRC) is caused by IV administration of 30 mL/kg camelid plasma to neonatal crias. In healthy neonatal crias administration of this quantity of plasma seems to be safe. But with underlying cardiopulmonary or systemic disease changes in lung volume associated with plasma administration could create risks for crias (131).

Adverse effects of transfusing blood stored for prolonged periods in lamps is encountered more often in patients with reduced vascular nitric oxide levels because of endothelial dysfunction. These patients can benefit from transfusion of fresh PRBC if available. Also inhaled nitric oxide supplementation can prevent pulmonary hypertension associated with transfusion of stored PRBC [138].

In previously untransfused pigs, hemolytic transfusion reactions do not appear to develop. But there have been two reports about adverse reactions in pigs undergoing liver transplants by the use of A–O incompatible transfusions. Pulmonary hypertension and decreased fibrinogen with an associated increase in fibrin degradation products occured in pigs that received A–O incompatible transfusions [139]. In a study, two pigs that administered A–O incompatible blood transfusions during liver transplants died because of disseminated intravascular coagulation (DIC), bleeding and progressive hypotension [140].

11. Conclusion

Vital part of veterinary emergency and critical care medicine is transfusion medicine. It is also therapy of some disease of patient. Blood and blood products can be obtained through the purchase of blood products or donors. Potentially fatal adverse transfusion reactions risk is higher in cats than in dogs. Also, adverse transfusion reactions are very important for large animals. By using known donors and screening assays that permit detection of incompatibility of blood typing or crossmatching, the risk can be decreased in both species.

Author details

Nuri Mamak
Department of Internal Medicine, Faculty of Veterinary Medicine,
University of Mehmet Akif Ersoy, Turkey

İsmail Aytekin
Department of Internal Medicine, Faculty of Veterinary Medicine,
University of Balikesir, Turkey

12. References

[1] Brown D and Vap L. Principles of Blood Transfusions and Cross-Matching, In: Thrall, M.A., Baker, D.C., Campbell, T.W., DeNicola, D., Fettman, M.J., Lassen, E.D., Rebar, A., and Glade, W. (eds.) Veterinary Hematology and Clinical Chemistry. USA: Blackwell Publishing; 2006. p.197-202.

[2] Andrews GA and Penedo MC. Erythrocyte Antigens and Blood Groups. In: Weiss DJ and Wardrop KJ (eds.) Schalm's Veterinary Hematology (Sixth Edition). USA: Blackwell Publishing Ltd; 2010. p.711-724.

[3] Lanevschi A, Wardrop KJ. Principles of transfusion medicine in small animals. Can Vet J 2001;42 447-454.

[4] Hale AS. Canine blood groups and their importance in veterinary transfusion medicine. Vet Clin North Am (Small Anim Pract) 1995;25 1323-1332.

[5] Symons M, Bell K. Expansion of the canine A blood group system. Anim Genetics 1991;22 227-235.

[6] Arikan, S., Guzel, M., Mamak, N, Ograk, Y.Z.: Frequency of blood types DEA 1.1, 3, 4, 5, and 7 in Kangal dog. Revue De Medecine Veterinaire 2009;160(4) 180-183.

[7] Gracner D, Bedrica L, Labura C, Maticic D, Gracner GG, Samardzija M. Blood groups and hematology in Istrian pointers. Vet Arhiv 2007;77 95-102.

[8] Ferreira RRF, Gopegui RR, Matos AJF. Frequency of dog erythrocyte antigen 1.1 expression in dogs from Portugal. Vet Clin Pathol 2011;40(2) 198–201.

[9] Ejima H, Kurokawa K & Ikemoto S. DEA 1 blood group system of dogs reared in Japan. Jap J Vet Sci 1982;44 815-817.

[10] Andrews GA, Chavey PS, Smith JE. Production, characterization and applications of a murine monoclonal antibody to dog erythrocyte antigen 1.1. J Am Vet Med Assoc 1992;201 1549- 1552.

[11] Corato A, Mazza G, Hale AS, et al. Biochemical characterization of canine blood group antigens; immunoprecipitation of DEA 1.2, 4 and 7 and identification of a dog erythrocyte membrane antigen homologous to human Rhesus. Vet Immunol Immunopathol 1997;59 213-223.

[12] Swisher SL, Young NL. The blood group system of dogs. Physiol. Rev. (Baltimore) 1961;41 495-550.

[13] Novais AA, Fagliari JJ & Santana AE. DEA (dog erythrocyte antigen) prevalence in domestic dogs (Canis familiaris) reared in Brazil. Ars Vet 2004;20 212-218.

[14] Colling DT, Saison R. Canine blood groups. 2. Description of a new allele in the Tr blood group system. Anim Blood Groups Biochem Genet 1980;11 13-2.

[15] Hohenhaus AE. Importance of Blood Groups and Blood Group Antibodies in Companion Animals. Transfusion Medicine Reviews 2004;18(2) 117-126.

[16] Andrews G.A. Red blood cell antigens and blood groups in the dog and cat. In Feldman BF, Zinkl JG and Jain NC (eds.). Schalm's Veterinary Hematology. Philadelphia: Lippincott Williams & Wilkins; 2000. p.767-773.

[17] Harrell K, Kristensen A, Parrow J.: Canine transfusion reactions 1. Causes and consequences. Comp. Cont. Educ. Pract. Vet 1997;19 181-190.

[18] Hashimoto Y, Yamakawa T, Tanabe Y. Further studies on the red cell glycolipids of various breeds of dogs. A possible assumption about the origin of Japanese dogs. J Biochem 1984;96 1777-1782.

[19] Ejima H, Kurokawa K & Ikemoto S. Comparison test of antibodies for dog blood grouping. Jpn J Vet Sci 1980;42 435-441.

[20] Ejima H, Nomura K & Bull RW. Breed differences in the phenotype and gene frequencies in canine D blood system. J Vet Med Sci 1994;56 623-626.

[21] Ikemoto S and Yoshida H. Genetic studies of new blood group C system on red cells of beagles. Jpn J Vet Sci 1981;43 429-431.

[22] Blais MC, Berman L, Oakley DA, et al. Canine Dal blood type: A red cell antigen lacking in some Dalmatians. J Vet Intern Med 2007;21 281-286.

[23] Wardrop KJ. Clinical Blood Typing and Crossmatching. In: Weiss DJ, Wardrop KJ (eds.) Schalm's Veterinary Hematology (Sixth Edition). USA: Blackwell Publishing Ltd, 2010. p.1101-1105.

[24] Weinstein NM, Blais MC, Harris K, Oakley DA, Aronson LR, Giger U. A newly recognized blood group in domestic shorthair cats: the Mik red cell antigen. J Vet Intern Med 2007;21 287–92.

[25] Giger, U. Blood typing and crossmatching to ensure compatible transfusions. In: Kirk's Curr Vet Ther 2000; 13:396–399.

[26] Auer L & Bell, K. The AB blood group system of cats. Animal Blood Groups, Biochemistry and Genetics 1981;12 287-297.

[27] Mylonakis ME, Koitonas AF, Saridomichelakis M, Leontidis M, Papadogiannakis M, Plevraki K. Determination of the prevalence of blood types in the non-pedigree feline population in Greece. Veterinary Record 2001;149 213-214.

[28] Griot-Wenk ME, Callan MB, Casal ML, Chisholm-Chait A, Spitalnik SL, Patterson DF and Giger U. Blood type AB in the feline AB blood group system. American Journal of Veterinary Research 1996;57 1438-1442.

[29] Knottenbelt C.M. The feline AB blood group system and its importance in transfusion medicine. Journal of Feline Medicine and Surgery 2002;4 69-76.

[30] Arikan S, Duru SY, Gurkan M, et al. Blood type A and B frequencies in Turkish Van and Angora cats in Turkey. J Vet Med Ser A 2003;50 303-306.

[31] Arikan S, Gurkan M, . Ozaytekin E, Dodurka T & Giger U. Frequencies of blood type A, B and AB in non-pedigree domestic cats in Turkey. Journal of Small Animal Practice 2006;47 10–13.

[32] Giger, U, Bucheler J. Transfusion of type-A and type-B blood to cats. J Am Vet Med Assoc 1991;198 411–418.

[33] Feldman BF. In-house canine and feline blood typing. J Am Anim Hosp Assoc 1999;35 455-456.

[34] Giger U, Gelens CJ, Callan MB, et al. An acute hemolytic transfusion reaction caused by dog erythrocyte antigen 1.1 compatibility in a previously sensitized dog. J Am Med Assoc 1995;206 1358–1362.

[35] Wilkerson MJ, Wardrop KJ, Meyers KM, et al. Two cat colonies with A and B blood types and a clinical transfusion reaction. Feline Pract 1991;19 22-26.

[36] Giger U, Bucheler J & Patterson DF. Frequency and inheritance of A and B blood types in feline breeds of the United States. J Hered 1991;82 15-20.

[37] Casal ML, Jezyk PF, Giger U. Transfer of colostral antibodies from queens to their kittens. Am J Vet Res 1996;57 1653–1658.

[38] Griot-Wenk ME, Giger U. Feline transfusion medicine. Blood types and their clinical importance. Vet Clin North Am Small Anim Pract 1995;25 1305–1322.

[39] Rozanski E, de Laforcade AM, Transfusion Medicine in Veterinary Emergency and Critical Care Medicine. Clinical Techniques in Small Animal Practice 2004; 19(2) 83-87.

[40] Tocci LJ. Transfusion medicine in small animal practice. Vet Clin North Am Small Anim Pract 2010; 40(3) 485-494.

[41] Callan MB. Red Blood Cell Transfusion in the Dog and Cat. In: Weiss DJ and Wardrop KJ (eds.) Schalm's Veterinary Hematology (Sixth Edition). USA: Blackwell Publishing Ltd; 2010. p.738-743.
[42] Hebert PC, Van der Linden P, Biro G and Hu LQ. Physiologic aspects of anemia. Crit Care Clin 2004;20 187–189.
[43] Barfield D, Adamantos S. Feline Blood Transfusions. A Pinker Shade of Pale. Journal of Feline Medicine and Surgery 2011;13 11-23.
[44] Michael MA, El Masry H, Khan BR, Das MK. Electrocardiographic signs of remote myocardial infarction. Prog Cardiovasc Dis 2007;50 198–208.
[45] Roux FA, Deschamps JY, Blais MC, Welsh DM, Delaforcade- Buress AM, Rozanski EA. Multiple red cell transfusions in 27 cats (2003–2006): indications, complications and outcomes. J Feline Med Surg 2008;10 213–218.
[46] Castellanos I, Couto CG, Gray TL. Clinical use of blood products in cats: a retrospective study (1997–2000). J Vet Intern Med 2004;18 529–32.
[47] Wardrop KJ, Tucker RL, Anderson EP. Use of an in vitro biotinylation technique for determination of posttransfusion viability of stored canine packed red blood cells. Am J Vet Res 1998;59 397-400.
[48] lseron KV, Mueslis DW. Blood warming: current applications and techniques. Transfusion 1991;31 558-569.
[49] Dodd R, Roth KW, Ashford P, Dax EM, Vyas G. Transfusion medicine and safety. Biologicals 2009;37 62-70.
[50] Godinho-Cunha LF, Ferreira RMRF, Silvestre-Ferreira AC. Whole blood transfusion in small animals: indications and effects. An Acad Bras Cienc 2011;83 (2).
[51] Chiaramonte D. Blood-component therapy: selection, administration and monitoring. Clin Tech Small Anim Pract 2004;19 63–67.
[52] Katz LM, Kiss JE. Plasma for transfusion in the era of transfusion-related acute lung injury mitigation. Transfusion 2008;48 393-397.
[53] Brooks MB. Transfusion of Plasma Products. In: Weiss DJ and Wardrop KJ (eds.) Schalm's Veterinary Hematology (Sixth Edition). USA: Blackwell Publishing Ltd; 2010. p.744-745.
[54] Berent AC, Todd J, Sergeeff J, Powell LL. Carbon monoxide toxicity: a case series. J Vet Emerg Crit Care 2005;15 128-135.
[55] Weingart C, Kohn B. Clinical use of haemoglobin-based oxygen carrying solution (Oxyglobin (R)) in cats: 48 cases (2002—2006). J Feline Med Surg 2008;10 431-38.
[56] Logan JC, Callan MB, Drew K, et al. Clinical indications for use of fresh frozen plasma in dogs. J Am Vet Med Assoc 2001;218 1449-1455.
[57] Lucas RL, Lentz KD, Hale AS. Collection and preparation of blood products. Clin Techn Small Anim Pract 2004;19 55-62.
[58] Vigano F, Perissinotto L, Bosco VR. Administration of 5% human serum albumin in critically ill small animal patients with hypoalbuminemia: 418 dogs and 170 cats (1994-2008). J Vet Emerg Crit Care (San Antonio) 2010;20 237-243.
[59] Freireich EJ. Origins of Platelet Transfusion Therapy. Transfusion Medicine Reviews 2011; 25(3) 252-256.

[60] Abrams-Ogg ACG. Plalet and Granulocyte Transfusion. In: Weiss DJ and Wardrop KJ (eds.) Schalm's Veterinary Hematology (Sixth Edition). USA: Blackwell Publishing Ltd; 2010. p.751-756.
[61] Segawa K, Kondo T, Kimura S, Fujimoto A, Kato T, et al. Effects of Prostaglandin E1 on the Preparation of Platelet Concentrates in Dogs. J Vet Intern Med 2012; 26 370–376.
[62] Callan MB, Appleman EH, Shofer FS, et al. Clinical and clinicopathologic effects of plateletpheresis on healthy donor dogs. Transfusion 2008;48 2214-2221.
[63] Hoffmeister KM, Felbinger TW, Falet H, et al. The clearance mechanism of chilled blood platelets. Cell 2003;112 87–97.
[64] Pruss A, Kalus U, Radtke H, et al. Universal leukodepletion of blood components results in a significant reduction of febrile non-hemolytic but not allergic transfusion reactions. Transfusion Apheresis Sci 2004;30 41-16.
[65] Slichter SJ, O'Donnell MR, Weiden PL, et al. Canine platelet alloimmunization: The role of donor selection. Br J Haematol 1986;63 713-727.
[66] Slichter SJ, Fish D, Abrams VK, et al. Evaluation of different methods of leukoreduction of donor platelets to prevent alloimmune platelet refractoriness and induce tolerance in a canine transfusion model. Blood 2005;105 847-854.
[67] Harris DJ The Resurgence of Granulocyte Transfusions. Journal of Infusion Nursing 2009; 32(6) 323-329.
[68] Christensen RD, Bradley PP, Priebat DA, et al. Granulocyte transfusion in septic canine neonates. Pediatr Res 1982;16 57-59.
[69] Head LL, Daniel GB, Becker TJ, et al. Use of computed tomography and radiolabeled leukocytes in a cat with pancreatitis. Vet Radiol Ultrasound 2005;46 263-266.
[70] Bashir S, Stanworth S, Massey E, et al. Neutrophil function is preserved in a pooled granulocyte component prepared from whole blood donations. BrJ Haematol 2008;140 701-711.
[71] Schneider A. Blood components. Collection, processing and storage. In: Kristensen AT, Feldman BF, (eds.). Canine and Feline Transfusion Medicine. Vet Clin North Am Small Anim Pract 1995; 25: 1245-1261.
[72] Hohenhaus AE. Blood banking and transfusion medicine. In: Ettinger SJ and Feldman AC (eds.) Textbook of Veterinary Internal Medicine, (5th ed. vol 1), , Philadelphia: WB Saunders, 2000. p.348-356.
[73] Tzannes S, Govendir M, Zaki S, Miyake Y, Packiarajah P, Malik R. The use of sevoflurane in a 2:1 mixture of nitrous oxide and oxygen for rapid mask induction of anaesthesia in the cat. J Feline Med Surg 2000;2 83–90.
[74] Killos MB, Graham LF, Lee J. Comparison of two anesthetic protocols for feline blood donation. Vet Anaesth Analg 2010;37 230 39.
[75] Knottenbelt C, Mackin A. Blood transfusions in the dog and cat - Part 2. Indications and safe administration. In Pract 1998;20 191-199.
[76] Klaser DA, Reine NJ, Hohenhaus AE. Red blood cell transfusions in cats: 126 cases (1999). J Am Vet Med Assoc 2005;226 920–923.

[77] Kristensen, A.T., Feldman, B.F., General principles of small animal blood component administration. In: Canine and Feline Transfusion Medicine, Kristensen AT, Feldman BF, Vet Clin North Am Small Anim Pract; 1995; 25: 1277-1290.

[78] de Gopegui RR, Feldman BF. Use of blood and blood components in canine and feline patients with hemostatic disorders. In: Canine and Feline Transfusion Medicine, Kristensen AT, Feldman BF, Vet Clin North Am Small Anim Pract., 1995; 25: 1387-1402.

[79] Abrams-Ogg ACG, Kruth SA, Carter RF, Valli VE, Kamel-Reid S, Dube ID. Preparation and transfusion of canine platelet concentrates. Am J Vet Res 1993;54 635-664.

[80] Kirby R and Rudloff, E. Fluid and electrolyte therapy. In: Ettinger SJ and Feldman AC (eds.) Textbook of Veterinary Internal Medicine. (5th ed. vol 1), , Philadelphia: WB Saunders, 2000. p.325-347.

[81] Adamantos S, Boag A, Hughes D. Clinical use of a haemoglobin-based oxygen-carrying solution in dogs and cats. In Pract 2005;27 399-404.

[82] Chan DL, Freeman LM, Rozanski EA, Rush JE. Colloid osmotic pressure of parenteral nutrition components and intravenous fluids. J Vet Emerg Crit Care 2001;11 269-273.

[83] Jutkowitz LA, Rozanski EA, Moreau JA, et al. Massive transfusion in dogs: 15 cases (1997-2001). J Am Vet Med Assoc 2002;220 1664-1669.

[84] Corley EA. Intramedullary transfusion in small animals. J Am Vet Med Assoc 1963;142 1005-1006.

[85] Kohn B, Weingart C, Eckmann V, Ottenjann M, Leibold W. Primary immune-mediated hemolytic anemia in 19 cats: diagnosis, therapy, and outcome (1998–2004). J Vet Intern Med 2006;20 159–66.

[86] Culp WTN, Weisse C, Kellogg ME, et al. Spontaneous hemoperitoneum in cats: 65 cases (1994–2006). J Am Vet Med Assoc 2010;236 978–82.

[87] Wondratschek C, Weingart C and Kohn B. Primary immune-mediated thrombocytopenia in cats. J Am Anim Hosp Assoc 2010;46 12–19.

[88] Shelton GH, Linenberger ML, Persik MT, Abkowitz JL. Prospective hematologic and clinicopathological study of asymptomatic cats with naturally acquired feline immuno - deficiency virus-infection. J Vet Intern Med 1995;9 133–140.

[89] Norris JM, Bosward KL, White JD, Baral RM, Catt MJ, Malik R. Clinicopathological findings associated with feline infectious peritonitis in Sydney, Australia: 42 cases (1990–2002). Aust Vet J 2005;83 666–673.

[90] Reynolds CA, Lappin MR. 'Candidatus Mycoplasma haemominutum' infections in 21 client-owned cats. J Am Anim Hosp Assoc 2007;43 249–257.

[91] Dula DJ, Muller HA & Donovan JW. Flow rate variance of commonly used IV infusion techniques. J Trauma 1981;21 480-82.

[92] Koretz RL. Intravenous albumin and nutrition support: going for the quick fix. J Parenter Enteral Nutr 1995;19 166-171.

[93] Harrell KA, Kristensen AT. Canine transfusion reactions and their management. In: Kristensen AT, Feldman BF (eds.). Canine and Feline Transfusion Medicine. Vet Clin North Am Small Anim Pract 1995;25 1333-1364.

[94] Arikan S, Gurkan M. Kedilerde kan aktarımının klinik uygulama esasları. Ankara Üniv Vet Fak Derg 2009;56 153-157.

[95] Lester SJ, Hume JB, Phipps B. Hemobartonella canis infection following splenectomy and transfusion. Can Vet J 1995;36 444 445.

[96] Wardrop KJ, Lewis D, Marks S, Buss M. Posttransfusion purpura in a dog with hemophilia A. J Vet Intern Med 1997; 1(1) 261-263.

[97] Weingarta C, Gigerb U, Kohn B. Whole blood transfusions in 91 cats: a clinical Evaluation. Journal of Feline Medicine and Surgery 2004;6 139–148.

[98] Tocci LJ, Ewing PJ. Increasing patient safety in veterinary tranfusion medicine: an overview of pretransfusion testing. J VetEmerg Crit Care 2009;19 66-73.

[99] Owens SD, Joy Snipes K, Magdesian G, Christopher MM. Evaluation of a rapid agglutination method for detection of equine red cell surface antigens (Ca and Aa) as part of pretransfusion testing. Vet Clin Pathol 2008;37(1) 49–56.

[100] Mudge MC, Walker NJ, Borjesson DL, Librach F, Johns JL, Owens SD. Post transfusion survival of biotin-labeled allogeneic RBCs in adult horses. Vet Clin Pathol 2012;41(1) 56-62.

[101] Bailey E. Prevalence of anti-red blood cell antibodies in the serum and colostrum of mares and its relationship to neonatal isoerythrolysis. Am J Vet Res 1982;43 1917–1921.

[102] Pusterla N, Fecteau ME, Madigan JE, Wilson WD, Magdesian KG. Acute hemoperitoneum in horses: a review of 19 cases (1992–2003). J Vet Intern Med 2005;19 344–347.

[103] Hurcombe SD, Mudge MC and Hinchcliff KW. Clinical and clinicopathologic variables in adult horses receiving blood transfusions: 31 cases (1999-2005). J Am Vet Med Assoc 2007;231 267-274.

[104] Mudge M.C. Blood Transfusion in Large Animals. In: Weiss DJ and Wardrop KJ (eds.) Schalm's Veterinary Hematology (Sixth Edition), USA: Blackwell Publishing Ltd 2010. p.757-762.

[105] Slovis NM, Murray G: How to approach whole blood transfusions in horses. Proc Am Assoc Equine Practnr 2001;47 266–269.

[106] Mudge M, Macdonald MH, Owens SD, Tablin F. Comparison of 4 Blood Storage Methods in a Protocol for Equine Pre-operative Autologous Donation. Veterinary Surgery 2004;33 475–486.

[107] Sachs UJH. The pathogenesis of transfusion-related lung injury and how to avoid this serious adverse reaction of transfusion. Transfusion Apheresis Sci 2007;37 273–282.

[108] Feige K, Ehrat FB, Kastner SBR, et al. Automated plasmapharesis compared with other plasma collection methods in the horse. J Vet Med 2003;50 185–189.

[109] Durando MM, MacKay RJ, Linda S, et al. Effects of polymyxin B and Salmonella typhimurium antiserum on horses given endotoxin intravenously. Am J Vet Res 1994;55 921-927.

[110] Perkins G A, Yeager A, Erb HN, et al. Survival of foals with experimentally induced Rhodococcus equi infection given either hyperimmune plasma containing R. Equine antibody or normal equine plasma. Vet Ther 2002;3 334-346.

[111] Feige K, Kastner SBR, Dempfle CE, et al. Changes in coagulation and markers of fibrinolysis in horses undergoing colic surgery. J Vet Med 2003;50 30–36.

[112] Wilson EM, Holcombe SJ, Lamar A, Hauptman JG, Brooks MB. Incidence of Transfusion Reactions and Retention of Procoagulant and Anticoagulant Factor Activities in Equine Plasma. J Vet Intern Med 2009;23 323–328

[113] Hardefeldt LY, Keuler N, Peek SF. Incidence of transfusion reactions to commercial equine plasma. Journal of Veterinary Emergency and Critical Care 2010;20(4) 421–425.

[114] O'Neill EM, Rowley J, Hansson-Wicher M, et al. Effect of 24- hour whole-blood storage on plasma clotting factors. Transfusion 1999;39 488–491.

[115] Cardigan R, Lawrie AS, Mackie IJ, et al. The quality of fresh-frozen plasma produced from whole blood stored at 4 1C. Transfusion 2005;45 1342–1348.

[116] McClure JJ, Kock C, Traub-Dargatz J. Characterization of a red blood cell antigen in donkeys and mules associated with neonatal isoerythrolysis. Anim Genet 1994; 25:119-120.

[117] Niinisto K, Raekallio M, Sankari S. Storage of equine red blood cells as a concentrate. The Veterinary Journal 2008;176 227–231.

[118] Eicker SW, Ainsworth DM. Equine plasma banking: Collection by exsanguination. J Am Vet Med Assoc 1984;185 772– 774.

[119] Sellon DC. Disorders of the hematopoietic system. In: Reed SM, Bayly WM. Sellon DC (eds.) Equine Internal Medicine, (2nd ed.). St. Louis: Elsevier 2004. p.728.

[120] Aleman M, Nieto JE, Carr EA, et al. Serum hepatitis associated with commercial plasma transfusion in horses. J Vet Intern Med 2005;19 120–122.

[121] Belgrave RL, Hines MT, Keegan RD, Wardrop KJ, Bayly WM & Sellon DC. Effects of a polymerized ultrapurified bovine hemoglobin blood substitute administered to ponies with normovolemic anemia. J Vet Intern Med. 2002;16(4) 396-403.

[122] Andresen E. Blood groups in pigs. Ann N Y Acad Sci 1962;97 205.

[123] Hojny J, Stratil A. Report on the pig and sheep blood group and polymorphic protein workshops (Libechov, 9 to 11 August 1978). Anim Blood Groups Biochem Genet 1978;9 245.

[124] Smith DM, Newhouse M, Naziruddin B, Kresie L. Blood groups and transfusions in pigs. Xenotransplantation 2006;13 186–194.

[125] Fielding L. A hemoglobin-based oxygen carrier solution for the treatment of parasite-induced anemia in a Barbados sheep. J Vet Emerg Crit Care 2006;16 54-57.

[126] Garmendia AE, Palmer GH, DeMartini JC, et al. Failure of passive immunoglobulin transfer: a major determinant of mortality in newborn alpacas (Lama pacos). Am J Vet Res 1987;48(10) 1472– 1476.

[127] Weaver DM, Tyler JW, Scott MA, et al. Passive transfer of colostral immunoglobulin G in neonatal llamas and alpacas. Am J Vet Res 2000;61(7) 738–741.

[128] Barrington GM, Parish SM. Bovine neonatal immunology. Vet Clin North Am Food Anim Pract 2001;17(3) 463–476.

[129] Calloway CD, Tyler JW, Tessman RK, et al. Comparison of refractometers and test endpoints in the measurement of serum protein concentration to assess passive transfer status in calves. J Am Vet Med Assoc 2002;221 1605-1608.

[130] Wernery U. Camelid immunoglobulins and their importance for the new-born – a review. J Vet Med B Infect Dis Vet Public Health 2001;48(8) 561–568.

[131] Paxson JA, Cunningham SM, Rush JE, Bedenice D. The association of lung function and plasma volume expansionin neonatalalpaca crias following plasma transfusion for failure of passive transfer. Journal of Veterinary Emergency and Critical Care 2008;18(6) 601–607.

[132] Baumgarten A, Wilhelmi M, Ganter M. Rohn K & Mischke R. Changes of platelet function and blood coagulation during short-term storage of CPDA-1-stabilised ovine blood. Research in Veterinary Science 2011;91 150–158

[133] Dellinger RP, Levy MM, Carlet JM, et al. Surviving sepsis campaign: international guidelines for management of severe sepsis and septic shock: 2008. Crit Care Med 2008;36(1) 296–327.

[134] Palmer JE. Fluid therapy in the neonate: not your mother's fluid space. Vet Clin North Am Equine Pract 2004;20(1) 63–75.

[135] Bjorling DE & Rawlings CA. Relationship of intravenous administration of Ringer's lactate solution to pulmonary edema in halothane- anesthetized cats. Am J Vet Res 1983;4(6) 1000–1006.

[136] Wallin CJ, Rundgren M, Hjelmqvist H, et al. Effects of rapid colloid volume expansion on pulmonary microvascular pressure and lung water in the conscious sheep. Respir Physiol 1997;108(3) 225– 231.

[137] Verheij J, van Lingen A, Raijmakers PG, et al. Effect of fluid loading with saline or colloids on pulmonary permeability, oedema and lung injury score after cardiac and major vascular surgery. Br J Anaesth 2006;96(1) 21–30.

[138] Baron DM., Yu B, Lei C, Bagchi A, Beloiartsev A et al. Pulmonary Hypertension in Lambs Transfused with Stored Blood Is Prevented by Breathing Nitric Oxide. Anesthesiology 2012;116 637– 647.

[139] Hunfeld MA, Hoitsma HF, Meijer S, van Haeringen H and Rietveld FW. The role of A–O-incompatible blood transfusions in porcine orthotopic liver transplantations. Eur Surg Res 1984;16 354.

[140] Sheil AG, Halliday JP, Drummond JM, Bookallil MJ, Gaudry PL, Yezerski SD. A modified technique for orthotopic liver transplantation. Arch Surg 1972;104 720.